Anesthesia for
Maternal-Fetal Surgery

Anesthesia for Maternal-Fetal Surgery

Concepts and Clinical Practice

Edited by

Olutoyin A. Olutoye
Texas Children's Hospital Baylor College of Medicine Houston, TX

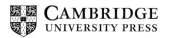

CAMBRIDGE
UNIVERSITY PRESS

University Printing House, Cambridge CB2 8BS, United Kingdom

One Liberty Plaza, 20th Floor, New York, NY 10006, USA

477 Williamstown Road, Port Melbourne, VIC 3207, Australia

314–321, 3rd Floor, Plot 3, Splendor Forum, Jasola District Centre,
New Delhi – 110025, India

103 Penang Road, #05–06/07, Visioncrest Commercial, Singapore 238467

Cambridge University Press is part of the University of Cambridge.

It furthers the University's mission by disseminating knowledge in the pursuit of
education, learning, and research at the highest international levels of excellence.

www.cambridge.org
Information on this title: www.cambridge.org/9781009088909
DOI: 10.1017/9781108297899

First published 2022

Printed in the United Kingdom by TJ Books Limited, Padstow Cornwall

A catalogue record for this publication is available from the British Library.

Library of Congress Cataloging-in-Publication Data
Names: Olutoye, Olutoyin A., editor.
Title: Anesthesia for maternal-fetal surgery : concepts and clinical practice / edited by Olutoyin A. Olutoye.
Description: New York, NY : Cambridge University Press, 2021. | Includes bibliographical references and
index.
Identifiers: LCCN 2021016256 (print) | LCCN 2021016257 (ebook) | ISBN 9781009088909 (paperback) |
ISBN 9781108297899 (ebook)
Subjects: MESH: Fetal Diseases – surgery | Anesthesia – methods | Congenital Abnormalities – surgery |
Fetal Therapies | Fetus – physiology | Pregnancy – physiology
Classification: LCC RG732 (print) | LCC RG732 (ebook) | NLM WQ 211 | DDC 617.9/682–dc23
LC record available at https://lccn.loc.gov/2021016256
LC ebook record available at https://lccn.loc.gov/2021016257

ISBN 978-1-009-08890-9 Paperback

Dedicated to:

– *God Almighty,*

– *My dear late mother, Ebun,*

– *The brave women who give of themselves for the betterment of their fetuses.*

Contents

List of Contributors   viii
List of Abbreviations   x
Preface   xiii
Acknowledgments   xiv

Section 1

1   **Physiology of Pregnancy**   1
    Caitlin Dooley Sutton and David Guye Mann

2   **Fetal Physiology and Fetal Pain**   17
    Olutoyin A. Olutoye, Caitlin Dooley Sutton, and Titilopemi Aina

3   **Ethical Considerations for Maternal-Fetal Surgery**   37
    David Guye Mann

4   **Multidisciplinary Approach to Fetal Surgery**   45
    Lori J. Howell and Susan M. Scully

5   **Intrauterine Transfusion**   64
    Saul Snowise and Ranu Jain

Section 2

6   **Twin-Twin Transfusion Syndrome**   83
    Rupi Mavi Parikh and Jose L. Peiro

7   **Fetal Endoscopic Tracheal Occlusion (FETO)**   95
    Mariatu Verla, Candace C. Style, Olutoyin A. Olutoye, and Oluyinka O. Olutoye

8   **Fetal Cardiac Intervention**   103
    Olutoyin A. Olutoye and Shaine Morris

9   **Antepartum Fetal Monitoring**   119
    Jimmy Espinoza

Section 3

10 **Myelomeningocele Repair**   137
    William Whitehead and Titilopemi Aina

11 **Lung Masses**   152
    Candace C. Style, Mariatu Verla, Olutoyin A. Olutoye, and Oluyinka O. Olutoye

12 **Sacrococcygeal Teratoma**   168
    Kha Tran and Holly Hedrick

13 **Ex-Utero Intrapartum Therapy**   191
    James Fisher, Timothy C. Lee, and Mario Patino

Index   207

Contributors

Titilopemi Aina, MD, MPH, FAAP, FASA
Associate Professor
Department of Anesthesiology
Baylor College of Medicine
Attending Anesthesiologist
Texas Children's Hospital
Houston, TX

Jimmy Espinoza, MD, MSc, FACOG
Professor
Department of Obstetrics and
Gynecology
Baylor College of Medicine
Co-Director, Texas Children's Fetal Center
Texas Children's Hospital
Houston, TX

James Fisher, MD, PhD
Pediatric and Fetal surgeon
Minneapolis Perinatal Physicians
and
The Midwest Fetal Care Center
Minneapolis, MN

Holly Hedrick, MD, FACS
Professor
Department of Surgery
Perelman School of Medicine
The University of Pennsylvania
Louise Schnaufer Endowed Chair in
Pediatric Surgery
Surgical Director, ECMO Program
Children's Hospital of Philadelphia
Philadelphia, PA

Lori J. Howell, DNP, MS, RN
Lynne L. Garbose Endowed Chair in Fetal
Family Care,
Executive Director, The Center for Fetal
Diagnosis and Treatment
Children's Hospital of Philadelphia
Philadelphia, PA

Ranu Jain, MD
Professor
Department of Anesthesiology at
University of Texas
McGovern Medical School
Assistant Division Chief of Pediatric
Anesthesia
Director of Fetal /Maternal Anesthesia
Memorial Hermann Children's Hospital
Houston, TX

Timothy C. Lee, MD, MA
Associate Professor
Department of Surgery, Pediatrics, and
Obstetrics & Gynecology
Baylor College of Medicine
Co-Director, Texas Children's Fetal Center
Texas Children's Hospital
Houston, TX

David Guye Mann, MD, DBe, HEC-C
Associate Professor
Department of Anesthesiology
Baylor College of Medicine
Chief, Clinical Ethics
Chair, Fetal Therapy Board
Texas Children's Hospital
Houston, TX

Shaine Morris, MD, MPH
Associate Professor
Department of Pediatrics
Baylor College of Medicine
Medical Director, Fetal Cardiology
Texas Children's Hospital
Houston, TX

Olutoyin A. Olutoye, MD, MSc, FASA
Professor
Department of Anesthesiology, Pediatrics
and Obstetrics & Gynecology
Baylor College of Medicine

Vice-Chief for Academic Affairs
Division Chief, General Anesthesiology
Texas Children's Hospital
Houston, TX

Oluyinka O. Olutoye, MD, PhD, FACS, FAAP, FWACS
Professor
Department of Surgery, Pediatrics and Obstetrics & Gynecology
The Ohio State University Wexner College of Medicine

Surgeon-in-Chief
E. Thomas Boles, Jr. MD Chair in Pediatric Surgery,
Nationwide Children's Hospital
Columbus, OH

Rupi Mavi Parikh, MD
Associate Professor
Department of Anesthesiology
University of Cincinnati
Director of Fetal Anesthesia
Cincinnati Children's Hospital Medical Center
Cincinnati, Ohio

Mario Patino, MD
Associate Professor
Department of Anesthesiology
University of Cincinnati
Cincinnati Children's Hospital Medical Center
Cincinnati, OH

Jose L. Peiro, MD, PhD, MBA
Professor
University of Cincinnati
Director of Endoscopic Fetal Surgery
Cincinnati Children's Hospital Medical Center Fetal Care Center
Cincinnati, OH

Susan M. Scully, MSN, RN, CNOR
Clinical Nurse Expert
Fetal Surgery Team Lead

Children's Hospital of Philadelphia
Philadelphia, PA

Saul Snowise, MD
Maternal-Fetal Medicine Specialist
Minneapolis Perinatal Physicians
and
The Midwest Fetal Care Center
Minneapolis, MN

Candace C. Style, MD
Postdoctoral Research Fellow
The Abigail Wexner Research Institute
Nationwide Children's Hospital
Columbus, OH

Caitlin Dooley Sutton, MD
Assistant Professor
Department of Anesthesiology
Baylor College of Medicine
Division Chief, Maternal-Fetal Anesthesiology
Texas Children's Hospital
Houston, TX

Kha Tran, MD
Associate Professor
Department of Anesthesiology
Perelman School of Medicine
University of Pennsylvania
Director of Fetal Anesthesia
Children's Hospital of Philadelphia
Philadelphia, PA

Mariatu Verla, MD
Resident
Michael E. DeBakey Department of Surgery
Baylor College of Medicine
Houston, TX

William Whitehead, MD
Professor
Department of Neurosurgery
Baylor College of Medicine
Texas Children's Hospital
Houston, TX

Abbreviations

AA	arterioarterial
AAPSS	American Academy of Pediatrics Surgical Section
ACLS	advanced cardiac life support
AFS	antenatal fetal surveillance
AFV	amniotic fluid volume
AO	ascending aorta
APN	Advanced Practice Nurse
AREDF	absent or reversed end diastolic flow
AV	arteriovenous
BA	bronchial atresia
BC	bronchogenic cyst
BPP	biophysical profile
BPS	bronchopulmonary sequestration
CCA	common carotid artery
CCAM	congenital cystic adenomatoid malformation
CCO	combined cardiac output
CCHD	critical congenital heart disease
CDH	congenital diaphragmatic hernia
CHAOS	congenital high airway obstruction syndrome
CHD	congenital heart disease
CLE	congenital lobar emphysema
CPAM	congenital pulmonary airway malformations
CPR	cerebroplacental ratio
CSF	cerebrospinal fluid
CST	contraction stress test
CT	computed tomography
CVR	CCAM volume ratio
DA	ductus arteriosus
DV	ductus venosus
DVP	deepest vertical pocket
ECG	electrocardiogram
ECMO	extracorporeal membrane oxygenation
EFW	estimated fetal weight
eHLHS	evolving hypoplastic left heart syndrome
ELS	extralobar sequestration
ePPROM	early preterm premature rupture of membranes
EXIT	ex-utero intrapartum therapy
FBS	fetal blood sampling
FETO	fetal endoscopic tracheal occlusion
FEV1	one-second forced expiratory volume
FFP	fresh frozen plasma
FGR	fetal growth retardation
FHR	fetal heart rate
FO	foramen ovale
FOV	foramen ovale valve
FTB	Fetal Therapy Board
FTC	fetal therapy center
FTNC	Fetal Therapy Nurse Coordinator
FVC	forced vital capacity
hCG	human chorionic gonadotropin
HDFN	hemolytic disease of the fetus and newborn

HELLP	hemolysis, elevated platelets, low platelets
HFOV	high-frequency oscillation ventilation
HLHS	hypoplastic left heart syndrome
HPL	human placental lactogen
ILS	intralobar sequestrations
iNO	inhaled nitric oxide
IPT	intraperitoneal transfusion
IUT	intrauterine transfusion
IRB	investigational review board
IUGR	intrauterine growth restriction
IUT	intrauterine transfusion
IVC	inferior vena cava
LA	left atrium
L&D	labor and delivery
LHR	lung-to-head ratio
LHV	left hepatic vein
LUTO	lower urinary tract obstruction
LV	left ventricle
MAC	minimum alveolar concentration
MAC	minimal anesthetic concentration
MAP	mean arterial pressure
MBA	mainstem bronchial atresia
MCA-PSV	middle cerebral artery peak systolic velocity
MCDA	monochorionic and diamniotic
MFM	maternal-fetal medicine
MoM	multiples of the median
MMC	myelomeningocele
MRI	magnetic resonance imaging
NICU	neonatal intensive care unit
NRP	neonatal resuscitation program
NST	nonstress test
NT	nuchal transparency
NTD	neural tube defect
O/E-LHR	observed-to-expected lung-to-head ratio
O/E TFLV	observed-to-expected total fetal lung volume
OFS	open fetal surgery
OOPS	operation on placental support
OR	operating room
PA	pulmonary trunk
PA/IVS	pulmonary stenosis/atresia with intact ventricular septum
PCR	polymerase chain reaction
PI	pulsatility index
PRBC	packed red blood cells
PROM	premature rupture of membrane
RA	right atrium
RBC	red blood cell
RFA	radiofrequency ablation
RP	right portal branch
RV	right ventricle
SCD	sequential compression device
SCT	sacrococcygeal teratoma
S/D ratio	systolic to diastolic ratio
SFLP	selective fetoscopic laser photocoagulation
SIVA	supplemented intravenous anesthesia
SVC	superior vena cava
SVR	systemic vascular resistance

TA	thoracoamniotic
TAPS	twin anemia polycythemia sequence
TEDI	tracheoesophageal displacement index
tPA	tissue plasminogen activator
TR	tricuspid regurgitation
TRAP	twin retrograde arterial perfusion syndrome
TTTS	twin to twin transfusion syndrome
UA	umbilical artery
UV	umbilical vein
VSD	ventriculoseptal defect
VTE	venous thromboembolism
VV	venovenous

Preface

This book provides education about different conditions in pregnancy that constitute a threat to fetal survival or postnatal morbidity and are amenable to repair in-utero. Advances in imaging have allowed for these conditions, and the associated pathophysiology, to be diagnosed early and/or monitored during prenatal care with an accompanying plan for fetal surgical management. This book, contributed to by diverse experts in maternal-fetal care from a variety of fetal programs, provides foundational knowledge to aid anesthetic management for these procedures. Specific nuances for the peri-operative anesthetic care of both the mother and the fetus in this period, and the close multidisciplinary collaboration required, are all discussed in this book. The initial chapters on physiology of pregnancy, fetal physiology and ethics of fetal surgery, are followed by chapters pairing the discussion of a fetal anomaly and its perinatal management with the anesthetic considerations for that particular condition. This material is uniquely crafted for the anesthesia providers, surgeons, obstetricians, pediatricians, nurses and trainees who care for patients who have, or will undergo, fetal surgery.

Acknowledgments

The editor would like to acknowledge the authors and contributors from many institutions and fetal programs who helped make this book a reality. Their willingness to share their research, clinical experience and expertise in various aspects of maternal-fetal surgery is invaluable and greatly appreciated.

Physiology of Pregnancy

Caitlin Dooley Sutton and David Guye Mann

Introduction

Pregnant women undergo significant physiologic changes throughout pregnancy and the peripartum period. These changes impact every organ system, allowing the mother to adapt to the demands of the developing fetus.

Specialists in maternal-fetal anesthesia often care for women with mild pre-existing disease or pregnancy-related pathology, both of which can have significant impact on maternal physiology. While these pathophysiological changes often require alterations in medical management, this chapter focuses on the normal physiologic changes that occur in a healthy woman during pregnancy. A clear understanding of the normal alterations to physiology during pregnancy provides the foundation for managing the full spectrum of patients that can present to the maternal-fetal anesthesia specialist.

Cardiovascular System

Anatomic Changes

During pregnancy, the cardiovascular system must physically adapt to the changes occurring in the body. The heart muscle and vasculature respond to increases in intravascular volume and metabolic demand. As the uterus grows and the diaphragm becomes elevated, the heart's position in the chest changes as well.

Generally, the left ventricle (LV) size increases along with the increased cardiac work of pregnancy, preserving the myocardial oxygen supply–demand relationship. In the setting of increased preload and afterload, this eccentric hypertrophy is thought to be an adaptation to minimize wall stress, and appears similar to the cardiac response to exercise.[1-4] Growth of the left ventricle begins as early as the first trimester, reaching a 15–25% increase in ventricular wall thickness and a 50% increase in overall LV mass at term.[1-3,5,6]

These cardiovascular changes are notable both on physical exam and diagnostic studies, particularly as the pregnancy nears term. Electrocardiogram (ECG) changes include shortening of the PR and QT intervals, QRS axis variability, depressed ST segments, and isoelectric low-voltage T waves in left-sided leads.[7,8] Echocardiography reveals an increase in valve annulus diameters associated with evidence of tricuspid and pulmonic regurgitation in up to 94%, and mitral regurgitation in up to 27% of healthy pregnant women at term.[9]

Hemodynamic Changes

Hemodynamic changes during normal pregnancy are relatively predictable. An overview of these changes is shown in Table 1.1. Generally, cardiac output increases, blood pressure remains relatively stable, and total vascular resistance decreases.[4]

Cardiac Output, Heart Rate, and Stroke Volume

Cardiac output is the quantity of blood pumped by the heart each minute and is the product of heart rate and stroke volume. While the magnitude and time course of changes in heart rate and stroke volume throughout pregnancy are controversial because of variations in measurement, both increase from baseline values during pregnancy. The increase in heart rate begins early in the first trimester and peaks in the third trimester at levels around 15–25% higher than baseline.[1,4,10–12] Stroke volume reaches values of 20–30% above baseline by the second trimester.[4,13–16] Because the left ventricular end-diastolic volume increases but the end-systolic volume remains unchanged, the ejection fraction is increased relative to nonpregnant levels.[13]

As heart rate and stroke volume increase, cardiac output rises, with higher values noted as early as 5 weeks' gestation.[13] By the end of the first trimester, cardiac output reaches up to 30–40% above baseline. Cardiac output continues to increase through the second trimester, reaching up to 50% higher than pre-pregnancy values and remains stable during the third trimester in nonlaboring women.[13,17–19] This rise in cardiac output serves to increase uterine blood flow from 50 mL/min in nonpregnant women to 700–900 mL/min (over 10% of cardiac output) at term.[20,21] Blood flow also increases to the kidneys, skin, and breast tissue.[22–24]

Maintaining cardiac output for adequate uterine perfusion is critical for anesthesiologists when managing hemodynamics during an anesthetic; this is particularly important when neuraxial anesthesia leads to a sympathectomy. Phenylephrine has replaced ephedrine as the preferred first-line vasopressor in pregnant women; it is now commonly used to treat

Table 1.1 Summary of cardiovascular hemodynamic changes during pregnancy

Parameter	Change in pregnancy
Heart rate	⇑
Stroke volume	⇑
Cardiac output	⇑ ⇑
Ejection fraction	⇑
Systemic vascular resistance	⇓
Systolic blood pressure	–
Diastolic blood pressure	⇓
Mean arterial pressure	⇓ –
Central venous pressure	–
Pulmonary vascular resistance	⇓
Pulmonary artery pressure	–

low blood pressure associated with neuraxial anesthesia.[25] Following vasopressor administration, changes in cardiac output correlate with changes in heart rate, making heart rate a surrogate indicator of cardiac output in these patients.[26] That is, when treating decreased systemic vascular resistance, phenylephrine should be dosed with the goal of maintaining heart rate and avoiding reflex bradycardia, which could lead to a decrease in cardiac output.

Systemic Vascular Resistance and Blood Pressure

Systemic vascular resistance (SVR) falls during normal pregnancy, with a resultant increase in arterial compliance. This is an adaptive response to accommodate the significant elevation in intravascular volume that occurs in pregnancy.[4] A nadir of 35% below baseline SVR occurs in the second trimester at around 20 weeks' gestation. Subsequently the SVR begins to rise, returning to approximately 20% less than nonpregnant values at term.[19] The decrease in SVR during pregnancy is thought to be related to hormonally mediated vasodilation, as well as the development of the intervillous space, which serves as a low-resistance vascular bed.[27]

Blood pressure decreases concomitantly with changes in SVR, with a nadir around 28 weeks' gestation. The decrease in diastolic blood pressure is more marked than that of systolic blood pressure, which does not change significantly during pregnancy.[24,28] Mean arterial pressure mirrors the changes in diastolic blood pressure, with a nadir in the second trimester followed by an increase to pre-pregnancy levels by term.[3,29,30]

The gravid uterus can compress the inferior vena cava (IVC) and aorta, with the extent of the compression related to positioning and gestational age. Aortocaval compression may lead to hemodynamic disturbances with resultant uteroplacental hypoperfusion.[31] For this reason, left lateral tilt positioning is often recommended to achieve left uterine displacement, thereby reducing aortocaval compression.[31,32] Recent magnetic resonance imaging studies showed IVC but not aortic compression in term pregnant women; this caval compression was relieved by 30 (but not 15) degree lateral tilt positioning.[33]

Pulmonary Vascular Resistance

Pulmonary vascular resistance decreases during pregnancy.[27] This decrease accommodates the increase in cardiac output without an elevation in pulmonary artery pressure as measured by pulmonary capillary wedge pressure.[24]

Hemodynamic Changes During Labor

Classically, it has been taught that cardiac output increases by as much as 10–25% from pre-labor values in the first stage of labor and by 40% in the second stage of labor.[13,34] However, recent studies using minimally invasive continuous hemodynamic monitoring suggest that the progression of labor does not have a major effect on baseline hemodynamic values between contractions.[35]

During uterine contractions, 300–500 mL of blood is displaced from the intervillous space into the central circulation.[36,37] While studies reporting the absolute changes in cardiac output and stroke volume differ,[27,35] it is agreed that the overall hemodynamic stress is substantially higher during the second stage of labor.[35] Immediately after delivery, cardiac output has been reported to increase up to 75% more than pre-delivery measurements, but more recent studies with different monitoring techniques have questioned this value.[35,37,38] Cardiac output returns to pre-labor values at 24 hours and pre-pregnancy values by 12–24 weeks postpartum.[34,36,37,39]

Respiratory System

Pregnancy impacts both the anatomy and physiology of the respiratory system.

Anatomic Changes

As the rate of general anesthesia for cesarean delivery continues to decrease,[40] anesthesiologists have progressively less experience in managing the airways of pregnant women. The anesthesiologist caring for the patient undergoing fetal intervention, on the other hand, has the unique challenge of facing the obstetric airway on a relatively frequent basis. Thus, maternal-fetal anesthesiologists must be familiar with the changes in the airway during pregnancy to facilitate the often dynamic airway management required in cases ranging from sedation to planned general anesthesia. Anatomic and physiologic factors affecting the obstetric airway are listed in Table 1.2. Upper airway edema occurs in normal pregnancy as a result of capillary engorgement in the laryngeal, nasal, and oropharyngeal mucosa.[41] Pathologic conditions such as pre-eclampsia can exacerbate this edema.[42] Changes in estrogen levels can affect nasal mucosa leading to rhinitis and epistaxis.[43] The thoracic cavity also undergoes mechanical changes related to the hormone relaxin, leading to increases in the circumference of the chest wall of 5–7 cm by term.[44]

The Obstetric Anaesthetists' Association and Difficult Airway Society published joint guidelines for the management of difficult and failed tracheal intubation for obstetrics in 2016.[45] Although it is beyond the scope of this chapter, the algorithm is an excellent resource for the anesthesiologist caring for women undergoing fetal intervention.

Lung Mechanics

During pregnancy, diaphragmatic excursion is the primary contributor to inspiration. This results from the higher resting position combined with increased excursion distance, as well as the limitation of thoracic expansion beyond its already increased resting position.[46]

Most measures of air flow including the one-second forced expiratory volume (FEV1), forced vital capacity (FVC), and their ratio (FEV1/FVC) are largely unchanged throughout pregnancy.[24,47] This contrasts with static lung volumes, which are altered (Table 1.3). These changes are shown in comparison with the volumes in the nonpregnant patient in

Table 1.2 Factors affecting the obstetric airway

Anatomic and physiologic factors affecting the obstetric airway	
Upper airway edema	Decreased functional residual capacity
Breast enlargement	Increased oxygen consumption
Weight gain	Increased risk of aspiration
Cephalad displacement of diaphragm	Cricoid pressure may worsen view

Adapted from, and with permission: Munnur U, Suresh MS. Airway problems in pregnancy. *Crit Care Clin.* 2004;20(4):617–642.

Table 1.3 Lung and chest wall mechanics in pregnancy

Parameter	Change
Diaphragm excursion	↑
Chest wall excursion	↓
Tidal volume	↑
Minute ventilation	↑
VC	↔
FEV1	↔
FEV1/FVC	↔
Closing capacity	↔

VC, vital capacity; FEV1, forced expiratory volume in one second; FVC, forced vital capacity

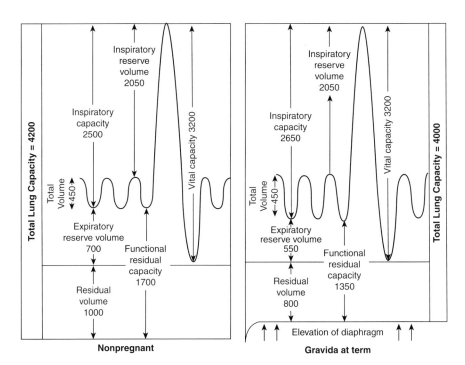

Figure 1.1 Lung volume changes during pregnancy.
With permission from O'Day MP. Cardio-respiratory physiological adaptation of pregnancy. *Semin Perinatol.* 1997;21(4):268–275.

Figure 1.1. The decline in functional residual capacity reaches 80% of the pre-pregnancy value at term, and is worsened in the supine position to just 70% of baseline.[48,49] Adjusting the patient to a 30 degree head up position can increase the supine functional residual capacity (FRC) by 10%.[50]

Table 1.4 Blood gas values during pregnancy

	Nonpregnant adult	First trimester	Second trimester	Third trimester
pH	7.4	7.44	7.44	7.44
pO_2 (mmHg)	90–100	93–107	90–105	92–107
pCO_2 (mmHg)	38–42	30	30	25–33
Bicarbonate (mEq/L)	22–26	21	20	16–22

With permission from Abbassi-Ghanavati M, Greer L, Cunningham F. A reference table for clinicians. *Obstet Gynecol.* 2009;114(6):1326–1331.

Gas Exchange and Arterial Blood Gases

During pregnancy, minute ventilation increases as a result of a 33% increase in tidal volume and an increase in respiratory rate of one to two breaths per minute.[51] These changes, which are related to the direct respiratory stimulant properties of progesterone,[52] occur during the first trimester and do not change significantly throughout the remainder of pregnancy. Up to 75% of women experience symptoms of dyspnea related to awareness of this increased ventilation.[53]

The increase in minute ventilation leads to a slight respiratory alkalosis despite a 30% increase in carbon dioxide production during pregnancy, primarily related to the increased metabolic rate of the fetus. Compared to nonpregnant adults, the $PaCO_2$ decreases, leading to pH increases.[54] The gradient between $PaCO_2$ and end tidal CO_2 that exists in most patients is absent or reversed in many pregnant women, likely because of the increased cardiac output and decreased alveolar dead space that occur during pregnancy.[55] The decline in $PaCO_2$ also leads to a slight increase in PaO_2 initially. As the pregnancy progresses, FRC may be below closing capacity and the PaO_2 can drop below 100 mmHg. Normal blood gas values by trimester are shown in Table 1.4. The anesthesiologist caring for a pregnant patient can use position adjustments such as lateral decubitus to reduce shunting that occurs in the supine position as a result of increased abdominal pressure elevating the diaphragm. This decrease in shunt reduces the alveolar to arterial oxygen gradient, improving oxygen transfer to the fetus.

Neurologic System

Anatomy

Anatomic changes affecting the spine during pregnancy are an important consideration for anesthesiologists caring for patients undergoing fetal intervention. The epidural space, containing both epidural fat and veins, enlarges during pregnancy. Cerebrospinal fluid volume decreases.[56]

Over 50% of pregnant women complain of low back pain, with onset most commonly in the third trimester.[57] In a study of women of childbearing age, MRI revealed a disc bulge or herniation in 53% of pregnant and 54% of nonpregnant women.[58] Lumbar disc bulge or herniation is not a contraindication to neuraxial analgesia or anesthesia.

Central Nervous System

During pregnancy, cerebrovascular resistance decreases, causing an increase in cerebral blood flow from 44 mL/min/100 g in the first trimester to 52 mL/min/100 g in the third trimester.[59] The decreased cerebrovascular resistance, along with increased hydrostatic pressure, also leads to increased permeability of the blood-brain barrier.[60] In normal pregnancies autoregulation is preserved or slightly improved, but in pathophysiologic states such as preeclampsia, autoregulation is abnormal and does not necessarily correlate with blood pressure abnormalities.[61]

As women approach term, elevated levels of endorphins and enkephalins are found in the plasma and CSF. Although a causation mechanism is unclear, the pain threshold increases concurrently with these changes.[62,63] Pregnant women experience more sleep disturbances including insomnia, daytime sleepiness, snoring, and transient restless leg syndrome.[64] These symptoms are caused by mechanical as well as hormonal factors, particularly related to progesterone.[65]

Hematologic System

The anesthesiologist caring for the obstetric patient must be familiar with the myriad of changes in the hematologic system during pregnancy. The increased blood flow to the uterus puts the patient at increased risk of hemorrhage during fetal intervention, and alterations in baseline blood components and coagulation factors in pregnant women have important implications for management should hemorrhage occur.

Blood Volume

Total plasma volume increases throughout pregnancy, starting in the first trimester with a 10–15% increase.[66] By term, pregnant women have a plasma volume of 30–50% above nonpregnant levels.[66–68] Based on plasma renin and atrial natriuretic peptide levels, this increase in plasma volume seems to be in response to systemic vasodilation and increased vascular capacitance rather than a primary blood volume expansion.[69,70]

Red Blood Cells

Red blood cell mass increases in pregnancy, reaching 20–30% above baseline levels at term. The hormonal regulation of this increase is complex: erythropoietin increases from baseline, human placental lactogen augments the action of erythropoietin, estrogen inhibits erythropoietin, and progesterone negates the activity of estrogen on erythropoietin.[71] Despite the increase in red blood cell mass, "dilutional anemia," or physiologic anemia of pregnancy, results from the greater relative increase in plasma volume. Even healthy pregnant women should receive iron supplementation to support this increased erythrocyte production. The nadir of this physiologic anemia occurs between 28 and 36 weeks' gestation.[72] Despite the difficulty of determining when anemia in pregnancy becomes pathologic, the Centers for Disease Control and Prevention has defined anemia as a hemoglobin less than 11 g/dL in the first and third trimesters and less than 10.5 g/dL in the second trimester.[73] The Institute of Medicine has recommended decreasing these thresholds by 0.8 g/dL for African-American adults.[74] Women with hemoglobin levels below these cutoffs should undergo evaluation.

White Blood Cells

An increased level of neutrophils leads to leukocytosis in pregnancy. The rise in white blood cell count begins in the first trimester and plateaus in the second or third trimester between 9,000 and 15,000 cells/μL.[75] During labor, leukocytosis can become more marked, increasing to as high as 29,000 cells/μL.[76,77]

Platelets

Thrombocytopenia in pregnancy is of special concern to the anesthesiologist, especially when considering neuraxial anesthesia or analgesia. Although the exact mechanisms are not completely understood, some etiologies include pregnancy-related pathology such as hypertensive disorders of pregnancy, idiopathic hematologic disorders such as idiopathic thrombocytopenic purpura, or gestational thrombocytopenia. In the setting of thrombocytopenia, both the absolute platelet level and the trend over time contribute to management decisions. Many obstetric anesthesiologists have a "cutoff" for consideration of neuraxial placement at around 70,000 platelets/μL, but this arbitrary cutoff level would be impacted by the risk-benefit ratio for a neuraxial analgesic or anesthetic technique, as well as the trend in the platelet count and overall clotting function demonstrated by thromboelastography.[78]

Coagulation

Circulating levels of multiple coagulation factors change during pregnancy, leading to an overall hypercoagulable state. As a result of hypercoagulability, pregnant women are at increased risk for venous thromboembolism (VTE); VTE has been implicated in 13–15% of maternal deaths in developed countries.[79,80] For this reason, increased emphasis is being placed on decreasing maternal morbidity and mortality related to embolic disease.[81] As guidelines change, it is likely that increasing numbers of pregnant women will receive anticoagulants as prophylaxis against VTE. Although multiple major societies have published guidelines for VTE prophylaxis, recommendations differ, and a task force has formed to define a consensus bundle.[82,83] Given the often unplanned nature of fetal intervention, patients who are receiving ongoing VTE prophylaxis are likely to present for surgery. The implications of anticoagulation on obstetric anesthesia management are significant; therefore, anesthesiologists must carefully consider these medications when electing a neuraxial technique for analgesia or anesthesia.

Table 1.5 shows expected laboratory values in pregnancy.[54] Thromboelastography demonstrates changes associated with hypercoagulability in pregnancy (Figure 1.2). These alterations have implications for management of obstetric hemorrhage. While details on the management of hemorrhage are beyond the scope of this chapter, the anesthesiologist caring for a woman undergoing fetal intervention should be familiar with the differences in the coagulation system, particularly with relation to fibrinogen stores and antifibrinolysis,[84] during pregnancy to facilitate appropriate care in the event of large volume blood loss.

Gastrointestinal System

Gastrointestinal Changes

As the uterus transitions from a pelvic to an abdominal organ, the stomach is displaced upward and leftward, rotating about 45 degrees to the right relative to its normal vertical

Table 1.5 Hematologic laboratory values during pregnancy

	Nonpregnant adult	First trimester	Second trimester	Third trimester
Hemoglobin (g/dL)	12–15.8	11.6–13.9	9.7–14.8	9.5–15
Hematocrit (%)	35.4–44.4	31–41	30–39	28–40
White blood cells (×10³/mm³)	3.5–9.1	5.7–13.6	5.6–14.8	5.9–16.9
Platelets (×10⁹/L)	165–415	174–391	155–409	146–429
Fibrinogen (mg/dL)	233–496	244–510	291–538	373–619
Partial thromboplastin time, activated (sec)	26.3–39.4	24.3–38.9	24.2–38.1	24.7–35
Prothrombin time (sec)	12.7–15.4	9.7–13.5	9.5–13.4	9.6–12.9
INR	0.9–1.04	0.89–1.05	0.85–0.97	0.8–0.94

With permission from Abbassi-Ghanavati M, Greer L, Cunningham F. A reference table for clinicians. *Obstet Gynecol.* 2009;114(6):1326–1331.

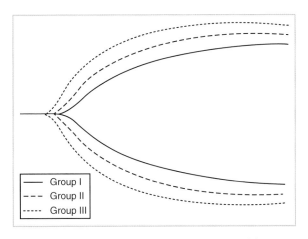

— Group I
--- Group II
----- Group III

Figure 1.2 Comparative thromboelastographs in nonpregnant (Group I), nonlaboring term pregnant (Group II), and laboring (Group III) women.
With permission from Steer PL, Krantz HB. Thromboelastography and Sonoclot analysis in the healthy parturient. *J Clin Anesth.* 1993;5:419–24.

position.[27] This change in position displaces the esophagus upward, with the uppermost intra-abdominal portion moving into the thorax. The tone of the lower esophageal high-pressure zone decreases, leading to higher prevalence of gastric reflux.[85] Between one-third and one-half of pregnant women complain of gastroesophageal reflux disease, with increasing prevalence as the pregnancy progresses.[86]

Studies evaluating gastric acid secretion and gastric pH in pregnancy have conflicting results. However, studies using various methodologies have consistently shown that pregnancy does not alter gastric emptying;[27] and in addition, gastric emptying does not differ between obese and lean patients.[87] On the other hand, esophageal and intestinal transit times are both slowed during pregnancy.[88,89] About 80% of women experience nausea and vomiting in pregnancy, usually starting early in the first trimester and occasionally lasting until 12–16 weeks' gestation.[90] Constipation is also a common complaint of pregnant women.[91]

Liver and Gallbladder Changes

The liver's position in the abdomen changes to be more superior, posterior, and rightward during pregnancy. Liver function tests, including bilirubin, transaminases, and lactate dehydrogenase, remain within the normal nonpregnant limits during pregnancy. Alkaline phosphatase, which is also produced by the placenta, increases twofold.[54]

The risk of gallbladder dysfunction increases during pregnancy, with a 5–12% incidence of gallstones.[92] Cholecystectomy is one of the most common non-obstetric surgeries indicated during pregnancy.

Renal System

Renal blood flow and glomerular filtration rate increase by 50% by the beginning of the second trimester, likely because of vasodilation of both afferent and efferent arterioles.[93] Serum creatinine is thus decreased, with levels greater than 0.8 mg/dL indicating possible renal dysfunction.[94] Hormonal changes also lead to sodium retention in pregnancy, with a consequent increase in total body water by up to 8 L, including that distributed as 1.5 L in plasma volume and 3.5 L in the fetus, placenta, and amniotic fluid.[91] Anesthesiologists caring for pregnant women must consider alterations in renal function and increased volume of distribution when administering medications that are cleared in the urine or that are hydrophilic.

The kidney compensates to maintain the acid–base status during pregnancy. The chronic respiratory alkalosis of pregnancy leads to a compensatory increase in the renal excretion of bicarbonate.[24] This decrease in serum bicarbonate impacts the pregnant patient's buffering capability when faced with an acid load.[27]

Both progesterone and relaxin affect smooth musculature in the urinary system, causing dilation of the collecting system and urinary stasis.[95] The hydronephrosis-related urinary stasis as well as ureterovesical reflux related to decreased ureteral tone and increased rates of glycosuria which encourage bacterial growth, result in pregnant women having a higher likelihood of urinary tract infections.[95,96]

Endocrine System

Many women of childbearing age either have or are at risk of hypothyroidism during pregnancy.[97] One study showed a 15% rate of gestational hypothyroidism in pregnant women, with one-third of these women being symptomatic.[98] Clinical diagnosis is difficult, as many symptoms of hypothyroidism mimic common symptoms of pregnancy, so evaluation of hormone levels is essential for diagnosis during pregnancy.

The changes in estrogen levels during pregnancy cause thyroid-binding globulin to increase, with resultant increases in total triiodothyronine (T_3) and thyroxine (T_4). Normally, the concentrations of free T_3 and T_4 remain unchanged, but the measurement of these levels can be unreliable in pregnancy.[99,97] For this reason, thyroid stimulating hormone (TSH) is the gold standard of thyroid function evaluation during pregnancy. Of note, placental human chorionic gonadotropin (hCG) lowers TSH levels, necessitating pregnancy-specific ranges for evaluation.[97]

Hormonal alterations in pregnancy also result in insulin resistance. Despite a more robust insulin response, blood glucose levels are higher after a carbohydrate load during pregnancy than baseline. Pregnant women are also more prone to ketosis in response to periods of fasting.[100]

Musculoskeletal System

Relaxin, a hormone produced by both the corpus luteum and the placenta, affects collagen remodeling in the pregnant patient.[101] Joint mobility increases via relaxin as well as biomechanical strain from the pregnancy itself.[102] Changes in posture, such as exaggeration of lumbar lordosis, can also lead to nerve injury. Lateral femoral cutaneous nerve stretching can result in meralgia paresthetica; brachial plexus neuropathies can occur from postural alterations as well.[27]

About half of women have back pain during pregnancy, with rates increasing as they approach full term.[57] Anesthesiologists are often asked about back pain in relation to neuraxial anesthesia/analgesia. Patients should be reassured that neuraxial interventions do not increase the likelihood of chronic back pain; multiple prospective reports and randomized controlled trials have failed to show a link between epidural use and long-term back pain.[103–105] Furthermore, while patients with baseline back pain are more likely to have continued or progressive back pain related to pregnancy, surgery, and delivery with the associated limitations on mobility, preexisting low back pain is not a contraindication to neuraxial analgesia or anesthesia.[106,104,103]

Conclusion

As fetal intervention becomes more widely practiced, the field of maternal-fetal anesthesia is rapidly expanding. The maternal-fetal anesthesia specialist has the unique task of caring for two patients, both of whom are undergoing rapid and significant anatomic and physiologic changes. Optimal anesthetic care during a fetal intervention and beyond necessitates a clear understanding of all aspects of the highly dynamic physiology of pregnant women.

References

1. Robson SC, Dunlop W, Moore M, Hunter S. Combined Doppler and echocardiographic measurement of cardiac output: theory and application in pregnancy. *Br J Obstet Gynaecol*. 1987;**94**(11):1014–1027. doi:10.1111/j.1471–0528.1987.tb02285.x.

2. Geva T, Mauer MB, Strikera L, Kirshon B, Pivarnik JM. Effects of physiologic load of pregnancy on left ventricular contractility and remodeling. *Am Heart J*. 1997;**133**(1):53–59. doi:10.1016/S0002–8703(97)70247–3.

3. Simmons LA, Gillin AG, Jeremy RW. Structural and functional changes in left ventricle during normotensive and preeclamptic pregnancy. *Am J Physiol Heart Circ Physiol*. 2002;**283**(4):H1627–1633.

4. Melchiorre K, Sharma R, Thilaganathan B. Cardiac structure and function in normal pregnancy. *Curr Opin Obstet Gynecol*. 2012;**24**(6):413–421. doi:10.1097/GCO.0b013e328359826 f.

5. Vered Z, Mark Poler S, Gibson P, Wlody D, Pérez JE. Noninvasive detection of the morphologic and hemodynamic changes during normal pregnancy. *Clin Cardiol*. 1991;**14**(4):327–334. doi:10.1002/clc.4960140409.

6. Gilson G, Samaan S, Crawford M, Quails C, Curet L. Changes in hemodynamics, ventricular remodeling, and ventricular

contractility during normal pregnancy: A longitudinal study. *Obstet Gynecol.* 1997;**89**(6):957–962. doi:10.1016/S0029–7844(97)85765–1.

7. Carruth JE, Mirvis SB, Brogan DR, Wenger NK. The electrocardiogram in normal pregnancy. *Am Heart J.* 1981;**102**(6):1075–1078. doi:10.1016/0002–8703(81)90497-X.

8. Oram S, Holt M. Innocent depression of the S-T segments and flattening of the T-wave during pregnancy. *J Obstet Gynaecol Br Emp.* 1961;**68**(5):765–770. doi:10.1111/j.1471–0528.1961.tb02807.x.

9. Campos O, Andrade JL, Bocanegra J, et al. Physiologic multivalvular regurgitation during pregnancy: a longitudinal Doppler echocardiographic study. *Int J Cardiol.* 1993;**40**(3):265–272. doi:10.1016/0167–5273(93)90010-E.

10. Duvekot JJ, Cheriex EC, Pieters FAA, Menheere PPCA, Peeters LLH. Early pregnancy changes in hemodynamics and volume homeostasis are consecutive adjustments triggered by a primary fall in systemic vascular tone. *Am J Obstet Gynecol.* 1993;**169**(6):1382–1392. doi:10.1016/0002–9378(93)90405–8.

11. Clapp JF, Capeless E. Cardiovascular function before, during, and after the first and subsequent pregnancies. *Am J Cardiol.* 1997;**80**(11):1469–1473. doi:10.1016/S0002–9149(97)00738–8.

12. Atkins AFJ, Watt JM, Milan P, Davies P, Crawford JS. A longitudinal study of cardiovascular dynamic changes throughout pregnancy. *Eur J Obstet Gynecol Reprod Biol.* 1981;**12**(4):215–224. doi:10.1016/0028–2243(81)90012–5.

13. Robson SC, Hunter S, Boys RJ, Dunlop W. Serial study of factors influencing changes in cardiac output during human pregnancy. *Am J Physiol.* 1989;**256**(4 Pt 2):H1060–1065.

14. Capeless EL, Clapp JF. Cardiovascular changes in early phase of pregnancy. *Am J Obstet Gynecol.* 1989;**161**(6):1449–1453. doi:10.1016/0002–9378(89)90902–2.

15. Rubler S, Damani PM, Pinto ER. Cardiac size and performance during pregnancy estimated with echocardiography. *Am J Cardiol.* 1977;**40**(4):534–540. doi:10.1016/0002–9149(77)90068–6.

16. Pöpping DM, Elia N, Marret E, Wenk M, Tramèr MR. Opioids added to local anesthetics for single-shot intrathecal anesthesia in patients undergoing minor surgery: A meta-analysis of randomized trials. *Pain.* 2012;**153**(4):784–793. doi:10.1016/j.pain.2011.11.028.

17. Laird-Meeter K, van de Ley G, Bom TH, Wladimiroff JW, Roelandt J. Cardiocirculatory adjustments during pregnancy – An echocardiographic study. *Clin Cardiol.* 1979;**2**(5):328–332. doi:10.1002/clc.4960020503.

18. Katz R, Karliner JS, Resnik R. Effects of a natural volume overload state (pregnancy) on left ventricular performance in normal human subjects. *Circulation.* 1978;**58**(3):434–441.

19. Clark SL, Cotton DB, Lee W, et al. Central hemodynamic assessment of normal term pregnancy. *Am J Obstet Gynecol.* 1989;**161**(6):1439–1442. doi:10.1016/0002–9378(89)90900–9.

20. Assali NS, Douglass RA, Baird WW, Nicholson DB, Suyemoto R. Measurement of uterine blood flow and uterine metabolism. *Am J Obstet Gynecol.* 1953;**66**(2):248–253. doi:10.1016/0002–9378(53)90560–2.

21. Thaler I, Manor D, Itskovitz J, et al. Changes in uterine blood flow during human pregnancy. *Am J Obstet Gynecol.* 1990;**162**(1):121–125. doi:10.1016/0002–9378(90)90834-T.

22. Katz M, Sokal MM. Skin perfusion in pregnancy. *Am J Obstet Gynecol.* 1980;**137**(1):30–33. doi:10.1016/0002–9378(80)90381–6.

23. Dunlop W. Serial changes in renal haemodynamics during normal human pregnancy. *Br J Obstet Gynaecol.* 1981;**88**(1):1–9. doi:10.1111/j.1471–0528.1981.tb00929.x.

24. O'Day MP. Cardio-respiratory physiological adaptation of pregnancy. *Semin Perinatol.* 1997;**21**(4):268–275. doi:10.1016/S0146–0005(97)80069–9.

25. Macarthur A, Riley ET. Obstetric anesthesia controversies: vasopressor choice for postspinal hypotension during cesarean delivery. *Int Anesthesiol Clin.* 2007;**45**(1):115–132. doi:10.1097/ AIA.0b013e31802b8d53.

26. Dyer RA, Reed AR, van Dyk D, et al. Hemodynamic effects of ephedrine, phenylephrine, and the coadministration of phenylephrine with oxytocin during spinal anesthesia for elective cesarean delivery. *Anesthesiology.* 2009;**111** (4):753–765. doi:10.1097/ ALN.0b013e3181b437e0.

27. Gaiser R. Physiologic changes of pregnancy. In: Chestnut D, ed. *Chestnut's Obstetric Anesthesia: Principles and Practice.* Fifth ed. Philadelphia: Elsevier Saunders; 2014.

28. Gunderson EP, Chiang V, Lewis CE, et al. Long-term blood pressure changes measured from before to after pregnancy relative to nonparous women. *Obstet Gynecol.* 2008;**112**(6):1294–1302. doi:10.1097/AOG.0b013e31818da09b.

29. Mabie WC, DiSessa TG, Crocker LG, Sibai BM, Arheart KL. A longitudinal study of cardiac output in normal human pregnancy. *Am J Obstet Gynecol.* 1994;**170** (3):849–856. doi:10.1016/S0002–9378(94)70297–7.

30. Report of the National High Blood Pressure Education Program Working Group on High Blood Pressure in Pregnancy. *Am J Obstet Gynecol.* 2000;**183** (1):s1–s22. doi:10.1067/mob.2000.107928.

31. Ansari I, Wallace G, Clemetson CAB, Mallikarjuneswara VR, Clemetson CD. Tilt caesarean section. *J Obstet Gynaecol Br Commonw.* 1970;**77**(8):713–721. doi:10.1111/j.1471–0528.1970.tb03597.x.

32. Kinsella SM. Lateral tilt for pregnant women: why 15 degrees? *Anaesthesia.* 2003;**58**(9):835–836. doi:10.1046/j.1365–2044.2003.03397.x.

33. Abengochea A, Morales-Roselló J, Del Río-Vellosillo M, Argente P, Barberá M. Effect of lateral tilt angle on the volume of the abdominal aorta and inferior vena cava in pregnant and nonpregnant women determined by magnetic resonance imaging. *Anesthesiology.* 2015;**123** (3):733–734. doi:10.1097/ ALN.0000000000000791.

34. Kjeldsen J. Hemodynamic investigations during labour and delivery. *Acta Obstet Gynecol Scand.* 1979;**58**(89):218–249.

35. Kuhn JC, Falk RS, Langesæter E. Haemodynamic changes during labour: continuous minimally invasive monitoring in 20 healthy parturients. *Int J Obstet Anesth.* 2017;**31**:74–83. doi:10.1016/ j.ijoa.2017.03.003.

36. Hendricks CH. The hemodynamics of a uterine contraction. *Am J Obstet Gynecol.* 1958;**76**(5):969–982. doi:10.1016/0002–9378(58)90181–9.

37. Adams J, Alexander A. Alterations in cardiovascular physiology during labor. *Obstet Gynecol.* 1958;**12**(5):542–548.

38. Filippatos G, Baltopoulos G, Lazaris D, et al. Cardiac output monitoring during vaginal delivery. *J Obstet Gynaecol.* 2009;**17** (3):270–272.

39. Robson SC, Dunlop W, Boys RJ, Hunter S. Cardiac output during labour. *Br Med J.* 1987;**295**(6607).

40. Palanisamy A, Mitani AA, Tsen LC. General anesthesia for cesarean delivery at a tertiary care hospital from 2000 to 2005: a retrospective analysis and 10-year update. *Int J Obstet Anesth.* 2011;**20**(1):10–16. doi:10.1016/j.ijoa.2010.07.002.

41. Leontic E. Respiratory disease in pregnancy. *Med Clin North Am.* 1977;**61**:111–128.

42. Munnur U, Suresh MS. Airway problems in pregnancy. *Crit Care Clin.* 2004;**20** (4):617–642. doi:10.1016/j.ccc.2004.05.011.

43. Wise RA, Polito AJ, Krishnan V. Respiratory physiologic changes in pregnancy. *Immunol Allergy Clin North Am.* 2006;**26**(1):1–12. doi:10.1016/ j.iac.2005.10.004.

44. Contreras G, Gutiérrez M, Beroíza T, et al. Ventilatory drive and respiratory muscle function in pregnancy. *Am Rev Respir Dis.* 1991;**144**(4):837–841. doi:10.1164/ajrccm/ 144.4.837.

45. Mushambi MC, Kinsella SM, Popat M, et al. Obstetric Anaesthetists' Association and Difficult Airway Society guidelines for the management of difficult and failed tracheal intubation in obstetrics. *Anaesthesia*. 2015;**70** (11):1286–1306. doi:10.1111/anae.13260.

46. Grenville-Mathers R, Trenchard HJ. The diaphragm in the puerperium. *J Obstet Gynaecol Br Emp*. 1953;**60**(6):825–833.

47. Russell IF, Chambers WA. Closing volume in normal pregnancy. *Br J Anaesth*. 1981;**53** (10):1043–1047.

48. Alaily AB, Carrol KB. Pulmonary ventilation in pregnancy. *Br J Obstet Gynaecol*. 1978;**85**(7):518–524.

49. Gee JB, Packer BS, Millen JE, Robin ED. Pulmonary mechanics during pregnancy. *J Clin Invest*. 1967;**46**(6):945–952. doi:10.1172/JCI105600.

50. Hignett R, Fernando R, McGlennan A, et al. A randomized crossover study to determine the effect of a 30° head-up versus a supine position on the functional residual capacity of term parturients. *Anesth Analg*. 2011;**113**(5):1098–1102. doi:10.1213/ANE.0b013e31822bf1d2.

51. Bobrowski RA. Pulmonary physiology in pregnancy. *Clin Obstet Gynecol*. 2010;**53** (2):285–300. doi:10.1097/GRF.0b013e3181e04776.

52. Zwillich CW, Natalino MR, Sutton FD, Weil JV. Effects of progesterone on chemosensitivity in normal men. *J Lab Clin Med*. 1978;**92**(2):262–269.

53. Jensen D, Duffin J, Lam Y-M, et al. Physiological mechanisms of hyperventilation during human pregnancy. *Respir Physiol Neurobiol*. 2008;**161** (1):76–86. doi:10.1016/j.resp.2008.01.001.

54. Abbassi-Ghanavati M, Greer L, Cunningham F. A reference table for clinicians. *Obstet Gynecol*. 2009;**114** (6):1326–1331.

55. Shankar KB, Moseley H, Vemula V, Ramasamy M, Kumar Y. Arterial to end-tidal carbon dioxide tension difference during anaesthesia in early pregnancy. *Can J Anaesth*. 1989;**36**(2):124–127. doi:10.1007/BF03011432.

56. Hirabayashi Y, Shimizu R, Fukuda H, Saitoh K, Igarashi T. Soft tissue anatomy within the vertebral canal in pregnant women. *Br J Anaesth*. 1996;**77**(2):153–156.

57. Ansari NN, Hasson S, Naghdi S, Keyhani S, Jalaie S. Low back pain during pregnancy in Iranian women: Prevalence and risk factors. *Physiother Theory Pract*. 2010;**26** (1):40–48. doi:10.3109/09593980802664968.

58. Weinreb JC, Wolbarsht LB, Cohen JM, Brown CE, Maravilla KR. Prevalence of lumbosacral intervertebral disk abnormalities on MR images in pregnant and asymptomatic nonpregnant women. *Radiology*. 1989;**170**(1):125–128. doi:10.1148/radiology.170.1.2521192.

59. Nevo O, Soustiel JF, Thaler I. Maternal cerebral blood flow during normal pregnancy: a cross-sectional study. *Am J Obstet Gynecol*. 2010;**203**(5):475.e1–6. doi:10.1016/j.ajog.2010.05.031.

60. Johnson AC, Cipolla MJ. The cerebral circulation during pregnancy: adapting to preserve normalcy. *Physiology*. 2015;**30** (2):139–147. doi:10.1152/physiol.00048.2014.

61. van Veen TR, Panerai RB, Haeri S, Griffioen AC, Zeeman GG, Belfort MA. Cerebral autoregulation in normal pregnancy and preeclampsia. *Obstet Gynecol*. 2013;**122**(5):1064–1069. doi:10.1097/AOG.0b013e3182a93fb5.

62. Cogan R, Spinnato JA. Pain and discomfort thresholds in late pregnancy. *Pain*. 1986;**27** (1):63–68.

63. Abboud TK, Sarkis F, Hung TT, et al. Effects of epidural anesthesia during labor on maternal plasma beta-endorphin levels. *Anesthesiology*. 1983;**59**(1):1–5.

64. Manconi M, Govoni V, De Vito A, et al. Restless legs syndrome and pregnancy. *Neurology*. 2004;**63**(6):1065–1069.

65. Pien GW, Schwab RJ. Sleep disorders during pregnancy. *Sleep*. 2004;**27** (7):1405–1417.

66. Bernstein IM, Ziegler W, Badger GJ. Plasma volume expansion in early pregnancy. *Obstet Gynecol*. 2001; **97** (5 Pt 1): 669–672.

67. Lund CJ, Donovan JC. Blood volume during pregnancy. Significance of plasma and red cell volumes. *Am J Obstet Gynecol.* 1967;**98**(3):394–403.

68. Pritchard JA. Changes in the blood volume during pregnancy and delivery. *Anesthesiology.* 1965;**26**:393–399.

69. Schrier RW, Fassett RG. Pathogenesis of sodium and water retention in cardiac failure. *Ren Fail.* 1998;**20**(6):773–781.

70. Nadel AS, Ballermann BJ, Anderson S, Brenner BM. Interrelationships among atrial peptides, renin, and blood volume in pregnant rats. *Am J Physiol.* 1988; **254** (5 Pt 2): R793–800.

71. Peck TM, Arias F. Hematology changes associated with pregnancy. *Clin Obstet Gynecol.* 1979;**22**(4):785–798.

72. Whittaker PG, Macphail S, Lind T. Serial hematologic changes and pregnancy outcome. *Obstet Gynecol.* 1996;**88**(1):33–39. doi:10.1016/0029-7844(96)00095-6.

73. Centers for Disease Control (CDC). CDC criteria for anemia in children and childbearing-aged women. *MMWR Morb Mortal Wkly Rep.* 1989;**38**(22):400–404.

74. Earl R, Woteki C. Iron deficiency anemia: recommended guidelines for the prevention, detection, and management among U.S. children and women of childbearing age. In: *Institute of Medicine (US) Committee on the Prevention, Detection, and Management of Iron Deficiency Anemia Among U.S. Children and Women of Childbearing Age.* Washington, D.C.: National Academies Press; 1993. doi:10.17226/2251.

75. Kuvin SF, Brecher G. Differential neutrophil counts in pregnancy. *N Engl J Med.* 1962;**266**(17):877–878. doi:10.1056/NEJM196204262661708.

76. Molberg P, Johnson C, Brown TS. Leukocytosis in labor: what are its implications? *Fam Pract Res J.* 1994;**14** (3):229–236.

77. Acker DB, Johnson MP, Sachs BP, Friedman EA. The leukocyte count in labor. *Am J Obstet Gynecol.* 1985;**153** (7):737–739.

78. Camann W. Obstetric neuraxial anesthesia contraindicated? Really? Time to rethink old dogma. *Anesth Analg.* 2015;**121** (4):846–848. doi:10.1213/ANE.0000000000000925.

79. Khan KS, Wojdyla D, Say L, Gulmezoglu AM, Van Look PF. WHO analysis of causes of maternal death: a systematic review. *Lancet.* 2006;**367** (9516):1066–1074. doi:10.1016/S0140-6736(06)68397-9.

80. Say L, Chou D, Gemmill A, et al. Global causes of maternal death: a WHO systematic analysis. *Lancet Glob Heal.* 2014;**2**(6):e323–e333. doi:10.1016/S2214-109X(14)70227-X.

81. D'Alton ME, Friedman AM, Smiley RM, et al. National Partnership for Maternal Safety: Consensus Bundle on Venous Thromboembolism. *J Midwifery Womens Health.* 2016;**61**(5):649–657. doi:10.1111/jmwh.12544.

82. Palmerola K, D'Alton M, Brock C, Friedman A. A comparison of recommendations for pharmacologic thromboembolism prophylaxis after caesarean delivery from three major guidelines. *BJOG.* 2016;**123** (13):2157–2162. doi:10.1111/1471-0528.13706.

83. D'Alton ME, Friedman AM, Smiley RM, et al. National Partnership for Maternal Safety Consensus Bundle on Venous Thromboembolism. *Obstet Gynecol.* 2016;**128**(4):688–698. doi:10.1097/AOG.0000000000001579.

84. Shakur H, Roberts I, Fawole B, et al. Effect of early tranexamic acid administration on mortality, hysterectomy, and other morbidities in women with post-partum haemorrhage (WOMAN): an international, randomised, double-blind, placebo-controlled trial. *Lancet.* 2017;**389** (10084):2105–2116. doi:10.1016/S0140-6736(17)30638-4.

85. Van Thiel DH, Gavaler JS, Stremple J. Lower esophageal sphincter pressure in women using sequential oral contraceptives. *Gastroenterology.* 1976;**71** (0016–5085;2):232–234.

86. Richter JE. Review article: The management of heartburn in pregnancy. *Aliment Pharmacol Ther.* 2005;**22**(9):749–757. doi:10.1111/j.1365–2036.2005.02654.x.

87. Wong CA, McCarthy RJ, Fitzgerald PC, Raikoff K, Avram MJ. Gastric emptying of water in obese pregnant women at term. *Anesth Analg.* 2007;**105**(3):751–755. doi:10.1213/01.ane.0000278136.98611.d6.

88. Chiloiro M, Darconza G, Piccioli E, De Carne M, Clemente C, Riezzo G. Gastric emptying and orocecal transit time in pregnancy. *J Gastroenterol.* 2001;**36** (8):538–543. doi:10.1007/s005350170056.

89. Derbyshire EJ, Davies J, Detmar P. Changes in bowel function: Pregnancy and the puerperium. *Dig Dis Sci.* 2007;**52**(2):324–328. doi:10.1007/s10620–006–9538-x.

90. Gill SK, Maltepe C, Koren G. The effect of heartburn and acid reflux on the severity of nausea and vomiting of pregnancy. *Can J Gastroenterol.* 2009;**23**(4):270–272.

91. Costantine MM. Physiologic and pharmacokinetic changes in pregnancy. *Front Pharmacol.* 2014;**5**:65. doi:10.3389/fphar.2014.00065.

92. Mendez-Sanchez N, Chavez-Tapia NC, Uribe M. Pregnancy and gallbladder disease. *Ann Hepatol.* 2006;**5**(3):227–230. doi:457963 [pii].

93. Davison JM, Dunlop W. Renal hemodynamics and tubular function in normal human pregnancy. *Kidney Int.* 1980;**18**:152–161.

94. Mattison DR. *Clinical Pharmacology During Pregnancy.* Elsevier; 2013. doi:10.1016/C2010–0-67194-X.

95. Rasmussen PE, Nielsen FR. Hydronephrosis during pregnancy: a literature survey. *Eur J Obstet Gynecol Reprod Biol.* 1988;**27**(3):249–259. doi:10.1016/0028–2243(88)90130-X.

96. Delzell JE, Lefevre ML. Urinary tract infections during pregnancy. *Am Fam Physician.* 2000;**61**(3):713–720.

97. Dichtel LE, Alexander EK. Preventing and treating maternal hypothyroidism during pregnancy. *Curr Opin Endocrinol Diabetes Obes.* 2011;**18**(6):389–394. doi:10.1097/MED.0b013e32834cd3d7.

98. Blatt AJ, Nakamoto JM, Kaufman HW. National status of testing for hypothyroidism during pregnancy and postpartum. *J Clin Endocrinol Metab.* 2012;**97**(3):777–784. doi:10.1210/jc.2011–2038.

99. Harada A, Hershman JM, Reed AW, et al. Comparison of thyroid stimulators and thyroid hormone concentrations in the sera of pregnant women. *J Clin Endocrinol Metab.* 1979;**48**(5):793–797. doi:10.1210/jcem-48-5-793.

100. Fisher PM, Sutherland HW, Bewsher PD. The insulin response to glucose infusion in gestational diabetes. *Diabetologia.* 1980;**19**(1):10–14.

101. Kristiansson P, Nilsson-Wikmar L, Von Schoultz B, Svardsudd K, Wramsby H. Back pain in in-vitro fertilized and spontaneous pregnancies. *Hum Reprod.* 1998;**13**(11):3233–3238.

102. Berg G, Hammar M, Möller-Nielsen J, Lindén U, Thorblad J. Low back pain during pregnancy. *Obstet Gynecol.* 1988;**71**(1):71–75. doi:10.1097/01.AOG.0000129403.54061.0e.

103. Loughnan BA, Carli F, Romney M, Doré CJ, Gordon H. Epidural analgesia and backache: A randomized controlled comparison with intramuscular meperidine for analgesia during labour. *Br J Anaesth.* 2002;**89**(3):466–472. doi:10.1093/bja/aef215.

104. Russell R, Dundas R, Reynolds F. Long term backache after childbirth: prospective search for causative factors. *BMJ* 1996;**312**(7043):1384–1388. doi:10.1136/bmj.312.7043.1384a10.1136/bmj.312.7043.1384.

105. Breen TW, Ransil BJ, Groves PA, Oriol NE. Factors associated with back pain after childbirth. *Anesthesiology.* 1994;**81**(1):29–34. doi:10.1097/00000542–199407000–00006.

106. Howell CJ, Kidd C, Roberts W, et al. A randomised controlled trial of epidural compared with non-epidural analgesia in labour. *Br J Obstet Gynaecol.* 2001;**108** (1):27–33. doi:10.1016/S0306–5456(00)00012–7.

Fetal Physiology and Fetal Pain

Olutoyin A. Olutoye, Caitlin Dooley Sutton, and Titilopemi Aina

Introduction

Fetal physiology is markedly distinct from that of the neonate in both structure and function. The transition from fetal to neonatal physiology is triggered by increased oxygen concentration induced by inspiration at delivery. The maternal-fetal anesthesia specialist should be conversant with the unique fetal physiology and the changes that occur following delivery. This may be of importance in the management of an infant undergoing surgery immediately after delivery; a scenario which occasionally occurs if a baby requires additional surgery after an Ex Utero Intrapartum Therapy (EXIT) procedure.

Fetal Environment

The uterus provides a stable thermal environment for the fetus. The mother's body supplies an appropriate amount of heat to the amnion via the placental surface and the umbilical circulation. A lot of information regarding fetal temperature has been obtained from animal experiments including studies of the fetal lamb, which is commonly utilized to study maternal fetal interactions.[1] The temperature of the fetus is typically 3–5 degrees Celsius higher than that of the mother; this is as a result of the fetal metabolic rate being higher than oxygen consumption, and the transfer of heat to the fetus via the placenta and the uterus.[2] Fetal temperature is therefore maternally dependent. This must be kept in mind during fetal procedures as maternal hypothermia may result in fetal bradycardia if not effectively managed.[3] The fetus and neonate are not capable of nonshivering thermogenesis in-utero, and this further contributes to fetal hypothermia if the mother becomes cold during a procedure.

The Placenta

The placenta is the specialized maternal-fetal unit that supports the development and growth of the fetus during pregnancy. It serves different functions:

(i) *Exchange of nutrients and waste products between the maternal and fetal circulatory systems.* Oxygen and nutrients are provided to the fetus and carbon dioxide and waste products are removed from the fetus via the placenta. Several metabolic substances are also metabolized in the placenta and some metabolic products are released into the maternal and/or fetal circulation.[4]

(ii) *Protection of the fetus* by reducing the transfer of potentially toxic substances such as xenobiotic molecules, infections, and maternal diseases to the fetus.[5,6]

(iii) *Secretion of hormones* such as progesterone, estrogen, human placental lactogen (HPL), and human chorionic gonadotropin (hCG).[7,8] The secretion of hCG supports the corpus luteum, which continues to produce progesterone in the first few weeks of pregnancy. It also supports differentiation of the placenta. After approximately nine weeks' gestation, the placenta takes over progesterone production which serves to inhibit uterine contractions. Estrogen is secreted by the placenta as a special growth hormone to support the mother's reproductive organs.

The placenta comprises two main parts. A portion of this unit contains fetal tissue derived from the chorionic sac. This develops into the chorionic plate or chorion frondosum, housing the chorionic blood vessels which are branching radials from the umbilical vessels. The maternal aspect of the placenta, derived from the endometrium, is called the basal plate or decidua basalis and this section contains the maternal blood supply (Figure 2.1). The intervillous space lies between the chorionic and basal plates and contains the main functioning unit of the placenta, namely the tightly packed and extensively branched villous structures which contain fetal blood vessels. It is at the tip of these chorionic villi that maternal-fetal exchange of nutrients and gas occurs.[5,9] Maternal blood fills the intervillous space and bathes the villi, allowing exchange of nutrients, gases, and waste. The maternal and fetal blood circulations are thus in proximity allowing for exchange of important elements for growth, but no actual exchange of fluid.

Fertilization of the sperm and ovum results in eventual formation of a morula which enters the uterus as a blastocyst on day five following fertilization. The blastocyst then divides into the trophoblast and embryoblast. On day six to seven following fertilization, the blastocyst implants into the uterine decidua. This implantation stimulates differentiation of trophoblasts along villous and extra villous pathways: cytotrophoblasts fuse and develop

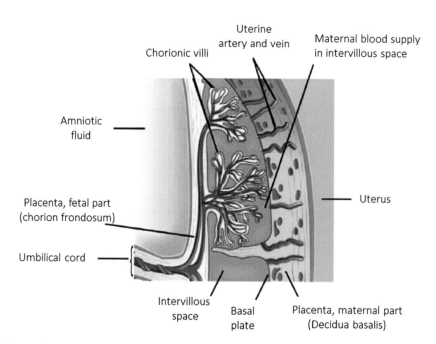

Figure 2.1 Schematic diagram of the anatomy of the placenta showing the maternal and fetal compartments. With permission from Wassenaar TM, Panigrahi P. Is a foetus developing in a sterile environment? *Lett Appl Microbiol.* 2014;59:572–579.

into multinucleated nonmigratory syncytiotrophoblasts, which line the outer surface of the villi and form the fetal components of the placenta. Extra villous trophoblasts migrate into the uterine decidua and remodel the uterine arteries.

Remodeling of the uterine arteries occurs as the placenta adapts to the increasing metabolic demands of the fetus, and converts the arteries from high-resistance, low-capacity vessels to low-resistance, high-capacity vessels. The change in capacity of the vessels increases uterine blood flow with advancing gestation and promotes placental and fetal growth.[10] Impaired remodeling of the uterine arteries is believed to play an integral part in the etiology and pathophysiology of placental-mediated disorders such as early-onset preeclampsia.[11–13]

At delivery, the placenta separates cleanly from the myometrium. However, in conditions of abnormal placental adherence, such as placenta accreta, inadequate separation may lead to significant postpartum hemorrhage. Placenta accreta spectrum, as it is now commonly referred to, encompasses varying degrees of placental infiltration into the myometrium. In placenta accreta, the placenta invades the endometrium. Placenta increta, characterized by a firm adherence and infiltration into the myometrium, and placenta percreta characterized by growth of the placenta into and through the uterine wall to attach to surrounding organs, are more severe types of placenta accreta spectrum (Figure 2.2).

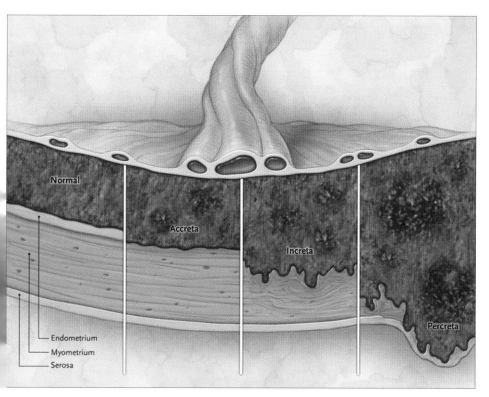

Figure 2.2 Placenta accreta spectrum includes placenta accreta (invasion of placenta to the myometrium), placenta increta (invasion of the placenta into the myometrium), and placenta percreta (invasion of placenta through the myometrium, serosa and into the surrounding structures).
With permission from Silver RM, Branch DW. Placenta accreta spectrum. *N Engl J Med*. 2018;378:1529–1536.

Patients are at risk for placenta accreta if they have a previous history of placenta previa or have undergone invasive uterine procedures such as hysteroscopic surgery, uterine curettage, endometrial ablation, myomectomy, uterine artery embolization as well as a previous history of cesarean section or open fetal surgery.[14,15] These predisposing conditions for placenta accreta may not be contraindications for fetal surgery but should increase scrutiny on the examination of the placenta during ultrasound assessment. Placenta accreta is typically diagnosed by ultrasound in the late second or third trimester with a sensitivity and specificity of 80% and 90%, respectively.[16,17] Ultrasound is complemented by magnetic resonance imaging (MRI) for diagnosis, in instances where ultrasound assessment is inconclusive.[18]

The incidence of placenta accreta has increased exponentially with the increase in cesarean deliveries over the years,[19] and this condition has become the leading cause of postpartum hemorrhage.[15,20] In-utero fetal surgery is usually performed during mid-gestation and does not involve separation of the placenta. Therefore, the complications of abnormal placental implantation are not a major concern for mid-gestation fetal surgery. If placenta accreta spectrum is present, there is a risk of profuse bleeding at the time of delivery or during ex-utero intrapartum therapy, which occurs near term. Such patients are best cared for in facilities prepared to handle severe maternal blood loss, which have ready access to the advanced surgical management required to manage accreta cases. Definitive treatment of the abnormally implanted placenta is surgical hysterectomy after delivery of the fetus.

Uteroplacental Blood Flow

Invasion of the trophoblasts into the endometrium, myometrium, and selectively into the uterine vessels is key to the modification or remodeling of the uterine spiral arteries.[21,22] This modification results in the arteries becoming high-capacity, low-resistance arteries, which allow for the increased maternal blood volume and blood flow to the placenta observed in term pregnancies. At term, a pregnant mother's total blood volume has increased by 40% compared to the nonpregnant state. The cardiac output also increases by 30–35% and the uteroplacental blood flow increases to 25% of cardiac output to accommodate the increased blood volume in the pregnant mother.[23-25] Studies using transvaginal duplex Doppler ultrasound have shown that there is a 3.5-fold increase in blood flow in the gravid uterus compared to the non-gravid uterus. Blood flow to the placenta gradually increases starting from the 12th week of gestation. While little is known about regulation of uteroplacental blood flow in normal pregnancy, several factors have been found to alter uteroplacental flow ex vivo. Utero placental flow can be affected by systemic or local factors:

(i) Change in resistance of the vascular bed: the uteroplacental circulation is maximally dilated so any changes in arterial pressure can easily affect placental flow. A decrease in systemic vascular resistance for example, caused by antihypertensives, will result in a decrease in uteroplacental flow.

(ii) Circulating vasoactive substances such as angiotensin II.

(iii) Locally produced hormones such as prostacyclin and nitric oxide.

(iv) Vasoactive intestinal polypeptide, substance P, and magnesium, which can dilate the isolated uterine artery,[26,27] and endothelin 1 and endothelin 3 which both cause vasoconstriction of the uterine arteries; an action that can be reversed by calcium channel blockers such as nifedipine and diltiazem.[28,29]

While there is no standard definition for placental insufficiency, it is commonly agreed that it is characterized by a reduction in transfer of nutrients and oxygen to the fetus resulting in decompensated fetal hypoxia and acidosis.[30,31] This leads to downregulation of metabolic demands by the fetus and intrauterine growth restriction ensues. Placental insufficiency not only results in intrauterine growth restriction but may also result in preterm labor, preeclampsia, and stillbirth. As the fetus matures during gestation, Doppler ultrasound has become a valuable tool in detecting the many circulatory changes that can occur during this period. Four Doppler techniques are fundamental in providing information about fetal-maternal circulation. These include assessments of the uterine artery, umbilical artery, middle cerebral artery, and the ductus venosus.[32] Use of Doppler ultrasound examination of the umbilical artery decreases the risk of prenatal death as well as the rate of obstetric interventions.[33] For example, absent or reversed end diastolic flow (AREDF) in the umbilical artery is associated with increased perinatal mortality in fetuses with intrauterine growth restriction. These assessments of uteroplacental sufficiency are incorporated into the management and surveillance of the fetal patient and play a role in the treatment algorithms for different conditions. Fetuses undergoing anesthesia for myelomeningocele repair were found to commonly have umbilical artery abnormalities which varied with anesthetic agent; however, all abnormalities were reversed by postoperative day one.[34] Analysis of the umbilical artery waveform has also been determined to be helpful for monitoring the progression of fetuses with sacrococcygeal teratoma. Abnormal umbilical artery waveforms have heralded reversed diastolic umbilical arterial blood flow and subsequent fetal demise in fetuses with large sacrococcygeal teratoma.[35] Interrogation of the middle cerebral artery is useful in the diagnosis and monitoring of fetal anemia. Fetal anemia may occur as a result of alloimmunization to anti-D, and less commonly, anti-Kell and other antibodies. Serial Doppler examination of the peak systolic velocity in the middle cerebral artery has become the standard method to determine fetal anemia and the need for intrauterine transfusion.[36,37] The presence and/or persistence of ductus venosus abnormalities in the recipient twin, before and after laser photocoagulation for twin-twin transfusion syndrome, is associated with poor outcomes.[38]

Fetal Drug Administration and Pharmacology

Drugs may exert effects on the fetus directly or indirectly. Drugs that decrease the uteroplacental blood flow and subsequently decrease fetal perfusion invariably affect the fetus as they reduce the rate of uteroplacental transfer.

Drugs such as angiotensin-converting enzyme inhibitors directly affect the fetus. They block the fetal renin-angiotensin system and may cause acute renal failure, oligohydramnios, and secondary pulmonary hypoplasia in the fetus through pre- and postglomerular effects. Beta-blockers also affect the fetus directly causing fetal hypoglycemia.[39]

Most of the available information about the effects of anesthetic drugs on the fetus has been obtained from animal studies,[40,41] isolated human placenta models,[42–45] and human in vivo peripartum studies.[46–48].

The extent of placental transfer of a drug depends on its physicochemical properties including the molecular weight, lipid solubility, partition coefficient, degree of ionization, and spatial configuration.[47] Many anesthetic drugs are lipophilic and can cross the placenta to have some effect on the fetus. Fetal acidosis which occurs because of fetal stress, can lead to an accumulation of drugs such as local anesthetics in the fetal circulation. The concern about transplacental passage of drugs is of importance when the baby will be delivered as many of the anesthetic agents can cause depression of the respiratory system, cardiovascular system, or both. One benefit of in-utero fetal surgery with regards to drug transfer, is that surgical procedures are commonly performed during mid-gestation and the focus is fetal treatment without interruption of pregnancy. Thus, respiratory suppression is less of a concern, but cardiac suppression remains hazardous.

Cardiac depression that occurs during fetal surgery, because of maternal anesthesia, eventually resolves once the anesthetic is discontinued. Procedures performed at term, or near term, such as the EXIT procedure, will require direct administration of additional medications to the fetus in addition to those received from the mother via transplacental passage. Additional medications typically administered to the fetus during fetal surgery include an analgesic, muscle relaxant, and an anticholinergic agent (latter medication helps decrease a vagal response). This cocktail is necessary to provide anesthesia and analgesia for airway interventions during the EXIT procedure, surgical resection of fetal head/neck and lung masses, or cannulation in preparation for extracorporeal membrane oxygenation (ECMO). Additional discussion on the basis for direct analgesia and anesthesia for the fetus during fetal surgery occurs later in this chapter.

Fetal Physiology by System

Cardiovascular System

The development of the cardiovascular system begins as early as 20 days' gestation, and by 44 days it has transitioned into a four-chambered structure.[49] A heartbeat can be detected by ultrasound at around seven weeks' gestation.[50]

Cardiac Development and Performance

The myocardium grows by hyperplasia (cell division) until birth, after which growth can be attributed to hypertrophy (cell enlargement).[51] The fetal heart is generally described as noncompliant or "stiff" for several reasons. The number of cardiac myofibrils and the type of cardiac troponins (fetal versus adult) can alter contractility of the heart.[49] In-utero, the pericardium, lungs, and chest wall have low compliance, restricting the fetal myocardium.[52] Additionally, the contractile apparatus of fetal troponin is more sensitive to calcium than adult troponin.[49] The fetal heart does appear to respond to changes in intravascular volume in a manner consistent with the Frank-Starling curve.[53,54] It has been suggested that the limited capacity to increase stroke volume in vivo may result from the fetal heart functioning near the peak of the Frank-Starling curve.[52] This leaves heart rate as the primary determinant of cardiac output.[55,56]

Changes in heart rate, therefore, have significant impact on fetal cardiac output. While a slower heart rate does theoretically allow for extended diastolic filling time as in adults, the noncompliant ventricles have limited ability to distend. Thus, fetal bradycardia leads to a significant decrease in cardiac output.

The fetal circulation comprises two circuits in parallel (Figure 2.3). For this reason, cardiac output is expressed as combined cardiac output (CCO). The right ventricle accounts

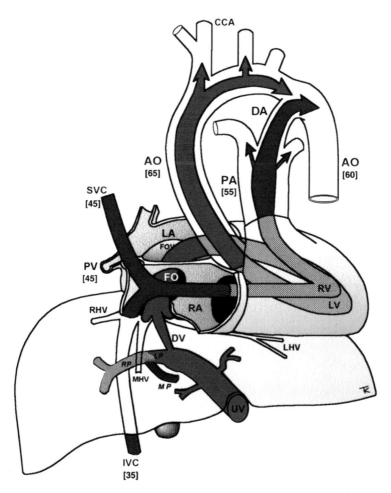

Figure 2.3 Pathways of the fetal heart and representative oxygen saturation values (in brackets). The via sinistra (red) directs well-oxygenated blood from the umbilical vein (UV) through the ductus venosus (DV) or (left half of the liver) across the inferior vena cava (IVC), through the foramen ovale (FO), left atrium (LA) and ventricle (LV), and up the ascending aorta (AO) to reach the descending AO through the isthmus aortae. De-oxygenated blood from the superior vena cava (SVC) and IVC forms the via dextra (blue) through the right atrium (RA) and ventricle (RV), pulmonary trunk (PA) and ductus arteriosus (DA). CCA, common carotid arteries; FOV, foramen ovale valve; LHV, left hepatic vein; RP, right portal branch.
Copied and modified with permission from Kiserud T. Physiology of the fetal circulation. *Semin Fetal Neonatal Med.* 2005;10:493–503.

for slightly more of the CCO than does the left ventricle.[51] During fetal life, the CCO increases from 210 mL/min at mid-gestation to 1,900 mL/min at 38 weeks' gestation.[55,57]

The fetal cardiac output is regulated by the neurologic and endocrine systems. The primary sensors for neural regulation are baroreceptors and chemoreceptors, which are primarily found in the aortic arch and common carotid arteries.[49] The autonomic nervous system also plays a critical role in cardiovascular hemodynamic regulation. The parasympathetic nervous system appears earlier than the sympathetic nervous system (8 versus 9–10 weeks).[58,59] As gestation progresses, the parasympathetic system continues to become more dominant and is more functionally complete than the sympathetic nervous system at birth. This is demonstrated by the earlier response of the fetus to atropine when compared to a beta-adrenergic receptor antagonist.[58] Endocrine regulation occurs through vasoactive hormones such as vasopressin, renin, angiotensin, and aldosterone.

Circulation

The fetal circulation differs greatly from postnatal circulation (Figure 2.3). Three anatomic connections are present in the normal fetal cardiovascular system, and they shunt the blood such that the right and left ventricle work in parallel rather than in series. These anatomic connections are the ductus venosus, the foramen ovale, and the ductus arteriosus. The ductus venosus connects the umbilical vein to the inferior vena cava, allowing oxygenated blood from the placenta to bypass the liver and portal circulation. This oxygenated blood enters the right atrium and flows preferentially through the foramen ovale, a connection between the right and left atria, and then proceeds through the left ventricle and out the aorta. This flow pattern allows for delivery of oxygen-rich blood from the placenta to the heart and brain.

Deoxygenated blood from the head and upper extremities flows from the superior vena cava into the right atrium and is directed into the right ventricle and pulmonary artery. Most of this blood flows from the pulmonary artery across the ductus arteriosus into the descending aorta, bypassing the lungs because of high pulmonary vascular resistance. Only a small portion travels through the lungs to the left heart and the ascending aorta. Oxygen-poor blood returns through the umbilical arteries to the placenta, where they undergo gas and nutrient exchange.[49]

Blood Volume and Pressure

Fetal blood volume comprises approximately 10–12% of the total body weight (90–115 mL/ kg fetal body weight), in contrast to approximately 7–8% (70 mL/kg) for adults.[60-62] This difference is because of the large blood volume within the placenta, with an estimated 80 mL/kg within the fetal body itself.[60,62] Because of high diffusion rates, the fetus is able to adapt to changes in intravascular volume more quickly than adults.[62]

Studies evaluating fetal blood pressure have used values obtained from cordocentesis as well as intrauterine recording of intraventricular pressure. Around 16 weeks the systolic pressure is approximately 15–20 mmHg and increases to around 30–40 mmHg at 28 weeks.[63] When fetal arterial pressure drops, fetal plasma renin increases, leading to increases of angiotensin I and II and resultant intravascular volume expansion.[49]

Pulmonary System

The fetal lung begins to develop as early as three weeks' gestation. It begins as a ventral evagination from the endoderm called the respiratory diverticulum or lung bud (Figure 2.4), which is covered in a layer of the mesoderm. This mesodermal layer will later give rise to the pulmonary vasculature and connective tissue. By around four weeks' gestation, the lung bud splits into two primary bronchial buds, which will become the left and right lungs. These bronchial buds continue to divide further into the future lobes of the lungs and continue dividing throughout most of the development in-utero. By the 28th week, the divisions have led to branching into terminal bronchioles, which will then divide into respiratory bronchioles. By week 36, capillaries are associated with the bronchioles, which are now primitive alveoli.[64] The alveoli mature as the gestation continues to term. As

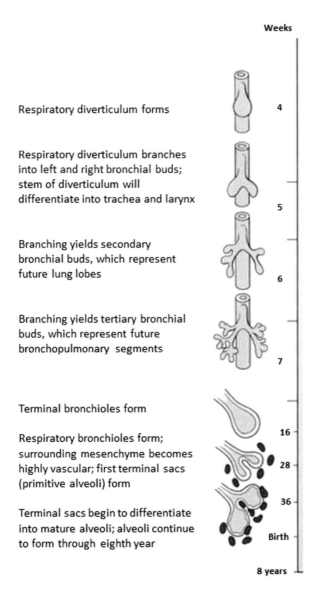

Weeks

Respiratory diverticulum forms — 4

Respiratory diverticulum branches into left and right bronchial buds; stem of diverticulum will differentiate into trachea and larynx — 5

Branching yields secondary bronchial buds, which represent future lung lobes — 6

Branching yields tertiary bronchial buds, which represent future bronchopulmonary segments — 7

Terminal bronchioles form — 16

Respiratory bronchioles form; surrounding mesenchyme becomes highly vascular; first terminal sacs (primitive alveoli) form — 28

— 36

Terminal sacs begin to differentiate into mature alveoli; alveoli continue to form through eighth year — Birth

8 years

Figure 2.4 Timeline. Development of the lungs, respiratory tree, and body cavities.
Adapted from Schoenwolf GC, Bleyl SB, Brauer PR, Francis-West PH, eds. *Larsen's human embryology*. Fifth ed. Philadelphia, PA: Elsevier.

only 5–20% of the total alveoli develop before birth, more alveoli will continue to develop throughout early childhood.[65]

As the fetus approaches term, many rapid changes occur in the lungs in preparation for postnatal life. During fetal life, the alveoli are filled with fluid. This fluid is the basis for the fetal endoscopic tracheal occlusion (FETO) procedure. Tracheal occlusion prevents the egress of lung fluid, which in turn, results in stretching of the lung and encourages lung development in fetuses with congenital diaphragmatic hernia.[66] At birth, this fluid is absorbed, and the alveoli fill with air, greatly increasing the surface area available for alveolar gas exchange. If a fetus is born preterm, the stage of lung development has a large impact on the postnatal outcome. Infants born before 24 weeks have a poorer chance at survival relative to infants born between 24 weeks and term. Advances in neonatal intensive care continue to improve survival rates in preterm infants, but pulmonary complications associated with preterm birth can lead to long-term respiratory problems.[64]

In the weeks before birth, alveolar cells begin to secrete a mixture of phospholipids and proteins called surfactant, which reduces the surface tension in the alveoli. This decreased surface tension facilitates inflation of the alveoli during inspiration after birth. In its absence, the alveoli tend to collapse, greatly increasing the work of breathing.[64] Administration of antenatal steroids to the mother, which increases the production of surfactant, is the most effective prenatal strategy to decrease the morbidity of preterm birth.[67] A 2017 *Cochrane Review* concluded that a single course of antenatal steroids should be considered routine for women at risk for preterm delivery.[68] As women undergoing fetal intervention are at increased risk of preterm birth, antenatal administration of steroids is commonplace in this patient population. For the anesthesiologist caring for the mother undergoing fetal intervention, it is important to note the multiple case reports of pulmonary edema in women receiving antenatal corticosteroids and tocolytics.[69]

Renal System

The fetal urinary system develops from the intermediate mesoderm. After several transformations (from pronephros to mesonephros to metanephros) it ultimately develops into two components, the excretory and collecting portions, which form the definitive kidneys. By the time the fetus is born, nephrogenesis is complete. However, neonatal kidneys do not concentrate or filter urine as well as adults do, and renal function does not reach adult levels until after 12 months of age.[70]

Amniotic Fluid

By the 10th week of gestation, plasma is filtered through the renal corpuscle creating a glomerular filtrate, which is concentrated into urine. The urine that passes through the collecting system into the bladder then contributes to the amniotic fluid. However, the function of the kidneys during fetal life is not to clear waste from the blood as that is primarily done by the placenta.[64]

As the fetus nears term, the kidneys produce 600–700 mL of urine per day. The lungs produce approximately 250 mL of fluid per day. To counterbalance this fluid production, the fetus swallows approximately 500 mL of fluid per day and about 350–450 mL of fluid is absorbed across the placenta. These fluid dynamics contribute to homeostasis of amniotic fluid volume.[71]

Oligohydramnios, or a low volume of amniotic fluid, can suggest a renal problem such as obstruction.[64] This may be seen in patients undergoing fetal intervention such as vesico-amniotic shunt placement for lower urinary tract obstruction (LUTO). Polyhydramnios, or a high volume of amniotic fluid, can be caused by the inability to swallow.[64] This can be a presenting symptom for a fetus with an airway anomaly such as a large neck mass. Mothers undergoing ex-utero intrapartum therapy (EXIT) for such anomalies have often undergone multiple amnioreductions prior to presenting for the EXIT procedure because of polyhydramnios.

Fetal Pain

The ability of a fetus to experience pain has been heavily argued over the years partly because it is ethically challenging to study the concept of pain in human fetuses. Information regarding fetal pain and its consequences is based on, and inferred from, animal studies,[72,73] in-utero studies,[74–77] and studies in the preterm neonate.[78–80]

Basic components of reactions to noxious stimuli have been described and they include: a spinal reflex, cortical perception of pain, and a hormonal response to noxious stimuli that is ablated with the administration of analgesics.[81]

The spinal reflex involves the physical activation of nociceptive pathways which do not involve the emotional response or experience of pain. This occurs when there is a reflex withdrawal from a noxious stimulus without the perception of pain. This process involves peripheral receptors (which start developing at the 7th week of gestation and are fully established by the 20th week of gestation) whose afferent fibers synapse within the spinal cord on interneurons, which in turn synapse on motor neurons that also reside in the spinal cord (Figure 2.5A). This pathway develops much earlier than the pathways necessary for the cortical perception of pain.

The cortical perception or conscious recognition of pain requires cortical connections to be present and functional to establish the capacity for pain perception. The axons from the spinal cord neurons above, project to the thalamus starting from the 14th week of gestation until the 20th week of gestation. This period is followed by the development of afferent fibers from the thalamus to the cerebral cortex (Figure 2.5B), a process that starts from the 17th week of gestation and is completed between 26 and 30 weeks' gestation.[82–85] An indirect connection between the thalamus and the cortex has been proposed by some to occur via the synapse of thalamic afferents on the subplate neurons, which then synapse on cortical neurons.[86] However, the subplate is a transient fetal structure which has not been proven to exist in humans.[81] Despite the establishment of thalamocortical connections, the exact period of functionality, where these connections are involved in the transmission and perception of pain, is gauged roughly by an amalgamation of supporting evidence. This evidence includes the presence of synchronous interhemispheric electroencephalography initially around 34 weeks and then consistently at term, and an EEG pattern suggestive of wakefulness at 30 weeks' postconceptual age (a time when consciousness is believed to be first possible).[87,88]

The evidence stated thus far delineates the development of physical structures necessary for the transmission of pain impulses as well as the perception of pain. Studies performed during fetal procedures such as transabdominal intrauterine fetal blood transfusion, have allowed for some understanding of the effect of noxious stimuli, such as needling, on the fetal hormonal response and the impact of analgesia.[89] Hormones secreted by the hypothalamic-pituitary axis have been used as a surrogate marker for pain, specifically the physiological response to painful stimuli. Fisk and colleagues demonstrated that the administration of fentanyl 10 mcg/kg mitigated the release of β endorphins and cortisol and also decreased the shunting of cerebral blood flow to the brain.[89] Shunting of blood flow to protect vital organs such as the brain and heart has been demonstrated to occur in periods of stress such as hypoxemia, intrauterine growth retardation, and intrauterine fetal needling.[76,89,90] Indeed, at as early as 16 weeks, increased fetal cerebral blood flow has been observed following needling of the intrahepatic vein during intrauterine transfusion, in contrast to needling of the noninnervated umbilical cord during the same procedure. In

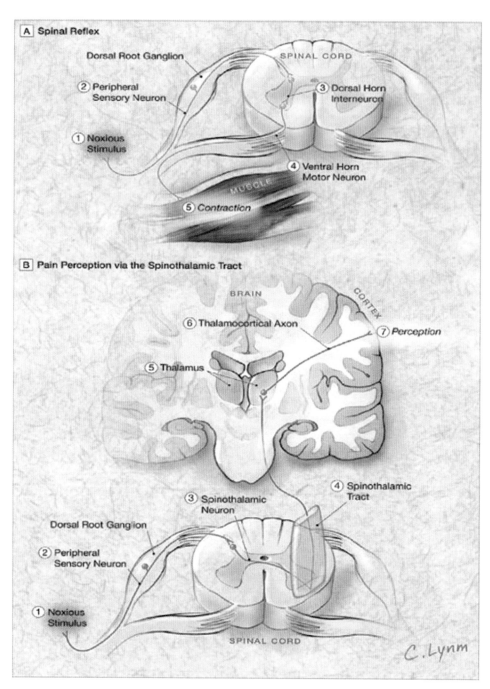

Figure 2.5 Spinal reflex and pain perception pathway. (A) Reflex responses to noxious stimuli occur early in development, before thalamocortical circuits are functional, noxious stimuli trigger reflex movement without cortical involvement. Activated by a noxious stimulus (1), a peripheral sensory neuron (2) synapses on a dorsal horn interneuron (3) that in turn synapses on a ventral horn motor neuron (4), leading to reflex muscle contraction and limb withdrawal (5). (B) Later in development, noxious stimuli (1) activate peripheral sensory neurons (2) that synapse on spinothalamic tract neurons (3), the axons of which extend up the spinal cord as the spinothalamic tract (4) to synapse on neurons of the thalamus (5). From here, thalamocortical axons (6) synapse on subplate and cortical neurons, resulting in the conscious perception of pain (7).

With permission from Lee SJ, Ralston HJ, Drey EA, et al. Fetal pain: a systematic multidisciplinary review of the evidence. *JAMA*. 2005;294:947–54.

addition, elevated levels of cortisol, β endorphins, and adrenaline have occurred with needling of the innervated intrahepatic vein and not with the noninnervated umbilical cord.[89] These increased levels of hormones do not translate directly to the evidence of pain, as there is no conscious cortical processing of hormonal release from the hypothalamic-pituitary axis. Studies in laboratory animals and adult humans have shown a decrease in stress hormones released because of surgical injury, in response to either regional anesthesia of the affected area or opioid analgesic suppression of the cerebral cortex and hormonal release from the hypothalamic-pituitary axis. Both result in an absence of pain following surgery. It follows, therefore, that pain is an important factor that accompanies the release of stress hormones.[78,91]

Plasticity of the developing brain is believed to lead to an alteration of the pain response center, which may place infants, subjected to noxious stimuli at an early age, at risk for stress disorders and anxiety-mediated adult behavior.[92,93] Considering the developmental timeline of the nervous system, the hormonal response to noxious stimuli and the timing at which fetal procedures can occur (as early as 16 weeks' gestation for intrauterine transfusion), medications are routinely administered to provide analgesia and anesthesia to the fetus during fetal surgery, even for procedures that may not directly involve the fetus. These medications serve one or all of the following purposes: (i) prevention of hormonal stress responses which have been associated with poor neonatal surgical outcomes,[78,94] (ii) prevention of possible adverse effects on long-term neurodevelopment and behavioral responses to pain,[72,73] and (iii) minimization of fetal movement during procedures.[95] The opioids, fentanyl and or remifentanil, with or without muscle relaxants are typically administered during fetal surgery for the above reasons.

For percutaneous procedures in which the fetus is not the main target of operation, such as in selective laser photocoagulation of abnormal placental anastomoses for twin-twin transfusion, opioids are administered for maternal comfort and in this case, transplacental passage of remifentanil offers the additional benefit of decreasing fetal movement.[95]

When the fetus undergoes a therapeutic intervention such as fetal endotracheal balloon occlusion or intracardiac intervention, direct administration of a fetal medication cocktail containing an opioid such as fentanyl, a muscle relaxant (vecuronium or rocuronium), with or without an anticholinergic, is frequently employed. Procedures requiring maternal general anesthesia, for example, in-utero fetal myelomeningocele repair and in-utero fetal mass resection also incorporate the direct administration of this medicine cocktail to the fetus.

The Achilles' heel of fetal surgery remains preterm labor which occurs regardless of the nature of fetal anomaly, timing of surgery, and other variables.[96,97] Prostaglandins and hormones released via activation of corticotropin releasing hormone play a significant role in the development of preterm labor.[98,99] Under normal circumstances the chorionic membrane forms a barrier between these hormones and the myometrium, but fetal surgery causes a disruption to this barrier. While the surgical wound created for fetal surgical access is closed after surgery, the disruption to the protective barrier may result in passage of fetal corticotropins into the myometrium and contribute to preterm labor. If this hypothesis holds true, it becomes necessary to mitigate possible elevation of fetal hormones because of noxious stimuli.

In the past several years, the effect of anesthetics including some analgesics on the developing human brain has come under question. This concern is based on findings in which neonatal animals exposed to anesthesia subsequently developed challenges in learning and reflex deficits; these findings have been corroborated in small and large animal models, respectively.[100,101] Such impairments result from anesthesia-induced neuroapoptosis, which is an exaggeration of the normal developmental apoptotic processes.[102,103] The effects of anesthesia on the animal fetal brain vary with dosing and frequency.[101,104] When the administration of anesthesia was combined with surgery on the ovine fetus, normal developmental apoptosis was found to be decreased,[105] the consequences of which (if any) are yet to be determined. Large cohort studies in children have shown that brief exposure to anesthetics in the perinatal period[106] or early childhood[107] does not adversely affect long-term neurodevelopmental outcomes.[107,108] Nevertheless, in December 2016, the Food and Drug Administration released a drug safety communication that "repeated or lengthy use of general **anesthetic** and sedation drugs during surgeries or procedures in children younger than 3 years or in **pregnant women** during their third trimester may affect the development of children's brains."[109] While the long-term effects of anesthesia on the fetal brain are yet to be fully elucidated, anesthesia should not be withheld when procedures are truly indicated.[110] Efforts should be made to minimize the duration and concentration of anesthetic agents and to consider alternative agents that are not implicated in the FDA warning.[111]

References

1. Asakura H. Fetal and neonatal thermoregulation. *J Nippon Med Sch.* 2004;71(6):360–370.

2. Power GG. Biology of temperature: The mammalian fetus. *J Dev Physiol.* 1989;12 (6):295–304.

3. Mann DG, Nassr AA, Whitehead WE, Espinoza J, Belfort MA, Shamshirsaz AA. Fetal bradycardia associated with maternal hypothermia after fetoscopic repair of neural tube defect. *Ultrasound Obstet Gynecol.* 2018;51(3):411–412. doi: 10.1002/ uog.17501 [doi].

4. Wassenaar TM, Panigrahi P. Is a foetus developing in a sterile environment? *Lett Appl Microbiol.* 2014;59(6):572–579.

5. Gude NM, Roberts CT, Kalionis B, King RG. Growth and function of the normal human placenta. *Thromb Res.* 2004;114(5–6): 397–407. doi: S0049-3848(04)00342-1 [pii].

6. Robbins JR, Bakardjiev AI. Pathogens and the placental fortress. *Curr Opin Microbiol.* 2012;15(1):36–43. doi: 10.1016/j. mib.2011.11.006 [doi].

7. Cross JC. Placental function in development and disease. *Reprod Fertil Dev.* 2006;18(1–2): 71–76. doi: RD05121 [pii].

8. Theofanakis C, Drakakis P, Besharat A, Loutradis D. Human chorionic gonadotropin: The pregnancy hormone and more. *Int J Mol Sci.* 2017;18 (5):10.3390/ijms18051059. doi: E1059 [pii].

9. Benirschke K, Kaufmann P. Anatomy and pathology of the umbilical cord and major fetal vessels. In: *Pathology of the human placenta.* Springer; 2000:335–398.

10. Albrecht ED, Pepe GJ. Regulation of uterine spiral artery remodeling: A review. *Reprod Sci.* 2020;27(10):1932–1942. doi: 10.1007/s43032-020-00212-8 [doi].

11. Pijnenborg R, Vercruysse L, Hanssens M. The uterine spiral arteries in human pregnancy: Facts and controversies. *Placenta.* 2006;27(9–10):939–958. doi: S0143-4004(05)00320-6 [pii].

12. Lyall F, Robson SC, Bulmer JN. Spiral artery remodeling and trophoblast invasion in preeclampsia and fetal growth restriction: Relationship to clinical outcome. *Hypertension.* 2013;62 (6):1046–1054. doi: 10.1161/ HYPERTENSIONAHA.113.01892 [doi].

13. Brosens I, Puttemans P, Benagiano G. Placental bed research: I. the placental bed: From spiral arteries remodeling to the great obstetrical syndromes. *Am J Obstet*

Gynecol. 2019;**221**(5):437–456. doi: S0002-9378(19)30746-X [pii].

14. Miller DA, Chollet JA, Goodwin TM. Clinical risk factors for placenta previa-placenta accreta. *Am J Obstet Gynecol.* 1997;**177**(1):210–214. doi: S0002-9378(97)70463-0 [pii].

15. Silver RM, Branch DW. Placenta accreta spectrum. *N Engl J Med.* 2018;**378**(16):1529–1536. doi: 10.1056/NEJMcp1709324 [doi].

16. Berkley EM. Prenatal diagnosis of placenta accreta: Is sonography all we need? *J Ultrasound Med.* 2013;**32**(8):1345–1350. doi: 10.7863/ultra.32.8.1345 [doi].

17. Comstock CH, Bronsteen RA. The antenatal diagnosis of placenta accreta. *BJOG.* 2014;**121**(2):171–81;discussion 181–2. doi: 10.1111/1471-0528.12557 [doi].

18. Warshak CR, Eskander R, Hull AD, et al. Accuracy of ultrasonography and magnetic resonance imaging in the diagnosis of placenta accreta. *Obstet Gynecol.* 2006; **108**(3 Pt 1): 573–581. doi: 108/3/573 [pii].

19. Goh WA, Zalud I. Placenta accreta: Diagnosis, management and the molecular biology of the morbidly adherent placenta. *J Matern Fetal Neonatal Med.* 2016;**29**(11):1795–1800. doi: 10.3109/14767058.2015.1064103 [doi].

20. Publications Committee, Society for Maternal-Fetal Medicine, Belfort MA. Placenta accreta. *Am J Obstet Gynecol.* 2010;**203**(5):430–439. doi: 10.1016/j.ajog.2010.09.013 [doi].

21. Kliman HJ. Uteroplacental blood flow. The story of decidualization, menstruation, and trophoblast invasion. *Am J Pathol.* 2000;**157**(6):1759–1768.

22. Soares MJ, Chakraborty D, Kubota K, Renaud SJ, Rumi MK. Adaptive mechanisms controlling uterine spiral artery remodeling during the establishment of pregnancy. *Int J Dev Biol.* 2014;**58**:247. Accessed 10/23/2020 4:46:27 PM.

23. Metcalfe J, Ueland K. Maternal cardiovascular adjustments to pregnancy. *Prog Cardiovasc Dis.* 1974;**16**(4):363–374. doi: 0033-0620(74)90028-0 [pii].

24. Ueland K, Metcalfe J. Circulatory changes in pregnancy. *Clin Obstet Gynecol.* 1975;**18**(3):41–50. doi: 10.1097/00003081-197509000-00007 [doi].

25. Ueland K. Maternal cardiovascular dynamics. VII. intrapartum blood volume changes. *Am J Obstet Gynecol.* 1976;**126**(6):671–677. doi: 0002-9378(76)90517-2 [pii].

26. Hansen V, Maigaard S, Allen J, Forman A. Effects of vasoactive intestinal polypeptide and substance P on human intramyometrial arteries and stem villous arteries in term pregnancy. *Placenta.* 1988;**9**(5):501–506. doi: 0143-4004(88)90022-7 [pii].

27. Skajaa K, Forman A, Andersson KE. Effects of magnesium on isolated human fetal and maternal uteroplacental vessels. *Acta Physiol Scand.* 1990;**139**(4):551–559. doi: 10.1111/j.1748-1716.1990.tb08958.x [doi].

28. Wolff K, Nisell H, Modin A, Lundberg JM, Lunell NO, Lindblom B. Contractile effects of endothelin 1 and endothelin 3 on myometrium and small intramyometrial arteries of pregnant women at term. *Gynecol Obstet Invest.* 1993;**36**(3):166–171. doi: 10.1159/000292619 [doi].

29. Fred G, Liu YA. Effect of endothelin, calcium blockade and EDRF inhibition on the contractility of human placental arteries. *Acta Physiol Scand.* 1994(151):477–484.

30. Gagnon R. Placental insufficiency and its consequences. *Eur J Obstet Gynecol Reprod Biol.* 2003;**110** Suppl 1: S99–107. doi: S0301211503001799 [pii].

31. Mazarico E, Molinet-Coll C, Martinez-Portilla RJ, Figueras F. Heparin therapy in placental insufficiency: Systematic review and meta-analysis. *Acta Obstet Gynecol Scand.* 2020;**99**(2):167–174. doi: 10.1111/aogs.13730 [doi].

32. Harman CR, Baschat AA. Comprehensive assessment of fetal wellbeing: Which doppler tests should be performed? *Curr Opin Obstet Gynecol.* 2003;**15**(2):147–157.

doi: 10.1097/00001703-200304000-00010 [doi].

33. Alfirevic Z, Stampalija T, Dowswell T. Fetal and umbilical doppler ultrasound in high-risk pregnancies. *Cochrane Database Syst Rev.* 2017;**6**:CD007529. doi: 10.1002/14651858.CD007529.pub4 [doi].

34. Sinskey JL, Rollins MD, Whitlock E, et al. Incidence and management of umbilical artery flow abnormalities during open fetal surgery. *Fetal Diagn Ther.* 2018;**43**(4):274–283. doi: 10.1159/000477963 [doi].

35. Olutoye OO, Johnson MP, Coleman BG, Crombleholme TM, Adzick NS, Flake AW. Abnormal umbilical cord doppler sonograms may predict impending demise in fetuses with sacrococcygeal teratoma. A report of two cases. *Fetal Diagn Ther.* 2004;**19**(1):35–39. doi: 10.1159/000074257 [doi].

36. Mari G, Deter RL, Carpenter RL, et al. Noninvasive diagnosis by doppler ultrasonography of fetal anemia due to maternal red-cell alloimmunization. collaborative group for doppler assessment of the blood velocity in anemic fetuses. *N Engl J Med.* 2000;**342**(1):9–14. doi: 10.1056/NEJM200001063420102 [doi].

37. Moise KJ, Jr., Argoti PS. Management and prevention of red cell alloimmunization in pregnancy: A systematic review. *Obstet Gynecol.* 2012;**120**(5):1132–1139. doi: http://10.1097/AOG.0b013e31826d7dc1 [doi].

38. Gil Guevara E, Pazos A, Gonzalez O, Carretero P, Molina FS. Doppler assessment of patients with twin-to-twin transfusion syndrome and survival following fetoscopic laser surgery. *Int J Gynaecol Obstet.* 2017;**137**(3):241–245. doi: 10.1002/ijgo.12143 [doi].

39. Lumbers ER. Effects of drugs on uteroplacental blood flow and the health of the foetus. *Clin Exp Pharmacol Physiol.* 1997;**24**(11):864–868. doi: 10.1111/j.1440-1681.1997.tb02706.x [doi].

40. Musk GC, Netto JD, Maker GL, Trengove RD. Transplacental transfer of medetomidine and ketamine in pregnant ewes. *Lab Anim.* 2012;**46**(1):46–50. doi: 10.1258/la.2011.010179 [doi].

41. Ngamprasertwong P, Dong M, Niu J, Venkatasubramanian R, Vinks A, Shamdasimvam S. Propofol pharmacokinetics and estimation of fetal propofol exposure during mid-gestational fetal surgery: A maternal-fetal sheep model. *PLOS One.* 2016;**11**(1):e0146563.

42. He YL, Tsujimoto S, Tanimoto M, Okutani R, Murakawa K, Tashiro C. Effects of protein binding on the placental transfer of propofol in the human dually perfused cotyledon in vitro. *Br J Anaesth.* 2000;**85**(2):281–286. doi: S0007-0912(17)37318-X [pii].

43. He YL, Seno H, Tsujimoto S, Tashiro C. The effects of uterine and umbilical blood flows on the transfer of propofol across the human placenta during in vitro perfusion. *Anesth Analg.* 2001;**93**(1):151–156. doi: 10.1097/00000539-200107000-00030 [doi].

44. Ueki R, Tatara T, Kariya N, Shimode N, Hirose M, Tashiro C. Effect of decreased fetal perfusion on placental clearance of volatile anesthetics in a dual perfused human placental cotyledon model. *J Anesth.* 2014;**28**(4):635–638. doi: 10.1007/s00540-013-1777-3 [doi].

45. Koren G, Ornoy A. The role of the placenta in drug transport and fetal drug exposure. *Expert Rev Clin Pharmacol.* 2018;**11**(4):373–385. doi: 10.1080/17512433.2018.1425615 [doi].

46. Gregory MA, Davidson DG. Plasma etomidate levels in mother and fetus. *Anaesthesia.* 1991;**46**(9):716–718. doi: 10.1111/j.1365-2044.1991.tb09762.x [doi].

47. Satoh D, Iwatsuki N, Naito M, Sato M, Hashimoto Y. Comparison of the placental transfer of halothane, enflurane, sevoflurane, and isoflurane during cesarean section. *J Anesth.* 1995;**9**(3):220–223. doi: 10.1007/BF02479867 [doi].

48. de Barros Duarte L, Moisés ECD, Cavalli RC, Lanchote VL, Duarte G, Da Cunha SP. Distribution of fentanyl in the placental intervillous space and in the different maternal and fetal compartments in term pregnant women. *Eur J Clin Pharmacol.* 2009;**65**(8):803–808.

49. Soens M, Tsen L. Fetal physiology. In: Chestnut D, Wong C, Tsen L, et al, eds. *Chestnut's Obstetric Anesthesia: Principles and Practice*. Fifth ed. USA: Saunders; 2014:75–91.

50. Cadkin AV, McAlpin J. Detection of fetal cardiac activity between 41 and 43 days of gestation. *J Ultrasound Med*. 1984;**3** (11):499–503. doi: 10.7863/ jum.1984.3.11.499 [doi].

51. Kiserud T. Physiology of the fetal circulation. *Semin Fetal Neonatal Med*. 2005;**10**(6):493–503. doi: S1744-165X(05) 00068-5 [pii].

52. Grant DA, Fauchere JC, Eede KJ, Tyberg JV, Walker AM. Left ventricular stroke volume in the fetal sheep is limited by extracardiac constraint and arterial pressure. *J Physiol*. 2001;**535**(Pt1): 231–239. doi: PHY_12256 [pii].

53. Kirkpatrick SE, Pitlick PT, Naliboff J, Friedman WF. Frank-Starling relationship as an important determinant of fetal cardiac output. *Am J Physiol*. 1976;**231** (2):495–500. doi: 10.1152/ ajplegacy.1976.231.2.495 [doi].

54. Weil SR, Russo PA, Heckman JL, Balsara RK, Pasiecki V, Dunn JM. Pressure-volume relationship of the fetal lamb heart. *Ann Thorac Surg*. 1993;**55** (2):470–475. doi: 0003-4975(93)91021-E [pii].

55. Gilbert RD. Control of fetal cardiac output during changes in blood volume. *Am J Physiol*. 1980;**238**(1):H80–86. doi: 10.1152/ajpheart.1980.238.1.H80 [doi].

56. Thornburg KL, Morton MJ. Filling and arterial pressures as determinants of RV stroke volume in the sheep fetus. *Am J Physiol*. 1983;**244**(5):H656–663. doi: 10.1152/ajpheart.1983.244.5.H656 [doi].

57. Rudolph AM, Heymann MA. Circulatory changes during growth in the fetal lamb. *Circ Res*. 1970;**26**(3):289–299. doi: 10.1161/ 01.res.26.3.289 [doi].

58. Papp JG. Autonomic responses and neurohumoral control in the human early antenatal heart. *Basic Res Cardiol*. 1988;**83** (1):2–9. doi: 10.1007/BF01907099 [doi].

59. Hildreth V, Anderson RH, Henderson DJ. Autonomic innervation of the developing heart: Origins and function. *Clin Anat*. 2009;**22**(1):36–46. doi: 10.1002/ ca.20695 [doi].

60. Brace RA. Fetal blood volume responses to intravenous saline solution and dextran. *Am J Obstet Gynecol*. 1983;**147**(7):777–781. doi: 0002-9378(83)90036-4 [pii].

61. Nicolaides KH, Clewell WH, Rodeck CH. Measurement of human fetoplacental blood volume in erythroblastosis fetalis. *Am J Obstet Gynecol* 1987;**151**(1):50–53.

62. Brace R. Regulation of blood volume in utero. In: Hanson M, Spencer J, Rodeck C, eds. *The circulation, fetus and neonate*. UK: Cambridge University Press; 1993:75–99.

63. Johnson P, Maxwell DJ, Tynan MJ, Allan LD. Intracardiac pressures in the human fetus. *Heart*. 2000;**84**(1):59–63.

64. Schoenwolf GC, Bleyl SB, Brauer PR, Francis-West PH, eds. *Larsen's Human Embryology*. Fifth ed. Philadelphia, PA: Elsevier; 2015.

65. Burri P. Postnatal lung development and modulation of lung growth. In: *Physiology of the Fetal and Neonatal Lung*. Springer; 1987:39–59.

66. Deprest J, Jani J, Cannie M, et al. Prenatal intervention for isolated congenital diaphragmatic hernia. *Curr Opin Obstet Gynecol*. 2006;**18**(3):355–367. doi: 10.1097/ 01.gco.0000193000.12416.80.

67. Merrill JD, Ballard RA. Antenatal hormone therapy for fetal lung maturation. *Clin Perinatol*. 1998;**25**(4):983–997.

68. Roberts D, Brown J, Medley N, Dalziel SR. Antenatal corticosteroids for accelerating fetal lung maturation for women at risk of preterm birth. *Cochrane Database Syst Rev*. 2017;**3**:CD004454. doi: 10.1002/14651858. CD004454.pub3 [doi].

69. Stubblefield PG. Pulmonary edema occurring after therapy with dexamethasone and terbutaline for premature labor: A case report. *Am J Obstet Gynecol*. 1978;**132**(3):341–342. doi: 0002-9378(78)90907-9 [pii].

70. Arant BS, Jr. Postnatal development of renal function during the first year of life. *Pediatr Nephrol.* 1987;**1**(3):308–313. doi: 10.1007/BF00849229 [doi].

71. Modena AB, Fieni S. Amniotic fluid dynamics. *Acta Biomed.* 2004;**75** Suppl 1:11–13.

72. Anand KJ, Coskun V, Hrivikraman KV, Nemeroff CB, Plotsky PM. Long-term behavioral effects of repetitive pain in neonatal rat pups. *Physiol Behav.* 1999;**66** (4):627–637.

73. Bhutta AT, Rovnaghi C, Simpson PM, Gossett JM, Scalzo FM, Anand KJ. Interactions of inflammatory pain and morphine in infant rats: Long-term behavioral effects. *Physiol Behav.* 2001;**73** (1–2):51–58.

74. Radunovic N, Lockwood CJ, Ghidini A, Alvarez M, Berkowitz RL. Is fetal blood sampling associated with increased beta-endorphin release into the fetal circulation? *Am J Perinatol.* 1993;**10** (2):112–114. doi: 10.1055/s-2007-994640.

75. Giannakoulopoulos X, Teixeira J, Fisk N, Glover V. Human fetal and maternal noradrenaline responses to invasive procedures. *Pediatr Res.* 1999; **45** (4 Pt 1): 494–499.

76. Teixeira JM, Glover V, Fisk NM. Acute cerebral redistribution in response to invasive procedures in the human fetus. *Obstet Gynecol.* 1999;**181**(4):1018–1025.

77. Carrasco GA, Van de Kar LD. Neuroendocrine pharmacology of stress. *Eur J Pharmacol.* 2003;**463**(1–3):235–272. doi: S0014299903012858 [pii].

78. Anand K. Sippell WG, and Aynsley-Green A. Randomised trial of fentanyl anaesthesia in preterm babies undergoing surgery: effects on the stress response. *Lancet.* 1987;**1**:62–66.

79. Anand K. Neonatal analgesia and anesthesia. Introduction. *Semin Perinatol.* 1998;**22**(5):347.

80. Anand KJ, Maze M. Fetuses, fentanyl, and the stress response: Signals from the beginnings of pain? *Anesthesiology.*

81. Lee SJ, Ralston HJP, Drey EA, Partridge JC, Rosen MA. Fetal pain: A systematic multidisciplinary review of the evidence. *JAMA.* 2005;**294**(8):947–954.

82. Mrzljak L, Uylings HB, Van Eden GG, Judáš M. Neuronal development in human prefrontal cortex in prenatal and postnatal stages. *Prog Brain Res.* 1991;**85**:185–222.

83. Krmpotić-Nemanić J, Kostović I, Kelović Z, Nemanić Đ, Mrzljak L. Development of the human fetal auditory cortex: Growth of afferent fibres. *Acta Anat (Basel).* 1983;**116**(1):69–73.

84. Kostovic I, Rakic P. Development of prestriate visual projections in the monkey and human fetal cerebrum revealed by transient cholinesterase staining. *J Neurosci.* 1984;**4**(1):25–42.

85. Van de Velde M, De Buck F. Fetal and maternal analgesia/anesthesia for fetal procedures. *Fetal Diagn Ther.* 2012;**31** (4):201–209.

86. Kostovic I, Judas M. Correlation between the sequential ingrowth of afferents and transient patterns of cortical lamination in preterm infants. *Anat Rec.* 2002;**267** (1):1–6. doi: 10.1002/ar.10069 [doi].

87. Clancy RR, Bergqvist AGC, Dlugos DJ. Neonatal electroencephalography. In: Ebersole JS, Pedley TA, eds. *Current Practice of Clinical Electroencephalography.* 3rd ed. Philadelphia, PA: Lippincott Williams & Wilkins; 2003:160–234.

88. Torres F, Anderson C. The normal EEG of the human newborn. *J Clin Neurophysiol.* 1985;**2**(2):89–103. doi: 10.1097/00004691-198504000-00001 [doi].

89. Fisk NM, Gitau R, Teixeira JM, Giannakoulopoulos X, Cameron AD, Glover VA. Effect of direct fetal opioid analgesia on fetal hormonal and hemodynamic stress response to intrauterine needling. *Anesthesiology.* 2001;**95**(4):828–835.

90. Schenone MH, Mari G. The MCA doppler and its role in the evaluation of fetal anemia and fetal growth restriction. *Clin Perinatol.*

2011;**38**(1):83–102, vi. doi: 10.1016/j.clp.2010.12.003 [doi].

91. Kehlet H, Brandt MR, Hansen AP, Alberti KG. Effect of epidural analgesia on metabolic profiles during and after surgery. *Br J Surg*. 1979;**66**(8):543–546. doi: 10.1002/bjs.1800660807 [doi].

92. Johnston CC, Stevens BJ. Experience in a neonatal intensive care unit affects pain response. *Pediatrics*. 1996;**98**(5):925–930.

93. Lowery CL, Hardman MP, Manning N, Hall RW, Anand KJ, Clancy B. Neurodevelopmental changes of fetal pain. *Semin Perinatol*. 2007;**31**(5):275–282. doi: S0146-0005(07)00068-7 [pii].

94. Robinson S, Gregory GA. Fentanyl-air-oxygen anesthesia for ligation of patent ductus arteriosus in preterm infants. *Anesth Analg*. 1981;**60**(5):331–334.

95. Van de Velde M, Van Schoubroeck D, Lewi LE, et al. Remifentanil for fetal immobilization and maternal sedation during fetoscopic surgery: A randomized, double-blind comparison with diazepam. *Anesth Analg*. 2005;**101**(1):251–8. doi: 10.1213/01.ANE.0000156566.62182.AB.

96. Danzer E, Sydorak RM, Harrison MR, Albanese CT. Minimal access fetal surgery. *Eur J Obstet Gynecol Reprod Biol*. 2003;**108**(1):3–13. doi: S0301211502004219 [pii].

97. Golombeck K, Ball RH, Lee H, et al. Maternal morbidity after maternal-fetal surgery. *Obstet Gynecol*. 2006;**194**(3):834–839.

98. Pomini F, Noia G, Mancuso S. Hypothetical role of prostaglandins in the onset of preterm labor after fetal surgery. *Fetal Diagn Ther*. 2007;**22**(2):94–99. doi: 97104 [pii].

99. Ruiz RJ, Dwivedi AK, Mallawaarachichi I, et al. Psychological, cultural and neuroendocrine profiles of risk for preterm birth. *BMC Pregnancy Childbirth*. 2015;**15**:204–015–0640-y. doi: 10.1186/s12884-015-0640-y [doi].

100. Jevtovic-Todorovic V, Hartman RE, Izumi Y, et al. Early exposure to common anesthetic agents causes widespread neurodegeneration in the developing rat brain and persistent learning deficits. *J Neurosci*. 2003;**23**(3):876–882. doi: 23/3/876 [pii].

101. Coleman K, Robertson ND, Dissen GA, et al. Isoflurane anesthesia has long-term consequences on motor and behavioral development in infant rhesus macaques. *Anesthesiology*. 2017;**126**(1):74–84. doi: 10.1097/ALN.0000000000001383 [doi].

102. Rizzi S, Carter LB, Ori C, Jevtovic-Todorovic V. Clinical anesthesia causes permanent damage to the fetal guinea pig brain. *Brain Pathol*. 2008;**18**(2):198–210. doi: 10.1111/j.1750-3639.2007.00116.x.

103. Loepke AW, Soriano SG. An assessment of the effects of general anesthetics on developing brain structure and neurocognitive function. *Anesth Analg*. 2008;**106**(6):1681–1707. doi: 10.1213/ane.0b013e318167ad77 [doi].

104. Olutoye OA, Sheikh F, Zamora IJ, et al. Repeated isoflurane exposure and neuroapoptosis in the midgestation fetal sheep brain. *Am J Obstet Gynecol*. 2016;**214**(4):542.e1–542.e8. doi: 10.1016/j.ajog.2015.10.927 [doi].

105. Olutoye OA, Cruz SM, Akinkuotu AC, et al. Fetal surgery decreases anesthesia-induced neuroapoptosis in the mid-gestational fetal ovine brain. *Fetal Diagn Ther*. 2019;**46**(2):111–118. doi: 10.1159/000491925 [doi].

106. Sprung J, Flick RP, Wilder RT, et al. Anesthesia for cesarean delivery and learning disabilities in a population-based birth cohort. *Anesthesiology*. 2009;**111**(2):302–310. doi: 10.1097/ALN.0b013e3181adf481 [doi].

107. Davidson AJ, Disma N, de Graaff JC, et al. Neurodevelopmental outcome at 2 years of age after general anaesthesia and awake-regional anaesthesia in infancy (GAS): An international multicentre, randomised controlled trial. *Lancet*. 2016;**387**(10015):239–250. doi: 10.1016/S0140-6736(15)00608-X [doi].

108. McCann ME, de Graaff JC, Dorris L, et al. Neurodevelopmental outcome at 5 years

of age after general anaesthesia or awake-regional anaesthesia in infancy (GAS): An international, multicentre, randomised, controlled equivalence trial. *Lancet*. 2019;**393**(10172):664–677. doi: S0140-6736(18)32485-1 [pii].

109. United States Food and Drug Administration. FDA drug safety communication: FDA review results in new warnings about using general anesthetics and sedation drugs in young children and pregnant women. Updated 2017. Accessed 07/06/2017.

110. Andropoulos DB. Effect of anesthesia on the developing brain: Infant and fetus. *Fetal Diagn Ther*. 2018;**43**(1):1–11. doi: 10.1159/000475928 [doi].

111. Olutoye OA, Baker BW, Belfort MA, Olutoye OO. Food and drug administration warning on anesthesia and brain development: Implications for obstetric and fetal surgery. *Am J Obstet Gynecol*. 2018;**218**(1):98–102. doi: S0002-9378(17)31094-3 [pii].

Ethical Considerations for Maternal-Fetal Surgery

David Guye Mann

Introduction

The founders of fetal interventions collectively understood the necessity of a formal ethics review for the novel therapies that they ultimately intended to offer. Providers from 13 fetal treatment centers in five countries convened in 1982 from July 19–23, at the "Unborn: Management of the fetus with a correctable congenital defect" conference to intensively review the experimental and clinical experience with fetal treatments. Those attending this conference highlighted and reported a number of relevant ethical issues.

Their stated purpose was to assess the potential benefits and liabilities of the various interventions, the appropriate directions to be pursued, and the problems to be avoided. They recognized "the most difficult problem in prenatal management [would be] how to select only the fetuses that might benefit from treatment." They further recognized that an ethically appropriate way to manage this and other uncertainties would be to establish criteria to be universally applied for identifying appropriate potential candidates for these novel interventions. The general criteria put forward included: a singleton fetus with no concomitant anomalies; the family would be fully counseled on the risks and benefits, and would agree to treatment including long-term follow-up to determine treatment efficacy; a multidisciplinary team, including a perinatal obstetrician experienced in fetal diagnosis and intrauterine transfusion, an ultrasonographer experienced in the diagnosis of fetal anomalies, and both the pediatric surgeon and neonatologist managing the infant after birth should concur on the plan for innovative treatment, there would be access to a high-risk obstetrical unit and intensive-care nursery, and there would be access to bioethical and psychosocial consultation.[1]

Bioethical Consultation

Fetal Therapy Board

Why It Is Necessary

Maternal-fetal medicine specialists predominately manage pregnancies that constitute a higher risk for the pregnant woman, although some interventions are directed toward mitigating fetal risk. The relationship that exists between a pregnant woman and her fetus is unique in law, medicine, and ethics. Contained in one body there is a person and a potential person with similar and separate interests, as well as developing fetal rights. This circumstance makes the maternal-fetal patient biologically, psychologically, morally, and legally unique. While the maternal-fetal relationship gives certain moral rights to the fetus and moral obligations to the woman, these are not legal rights and obligations; hence, there is little guidance on how to manage these moral duties or responsibilities.[2]

The pioneering maternal-fetal providers, recognizing the lack of guidance for managing maternal-fetal moral duties, saw the need for formal ethics consults to address these responsibilities. The concept of a Fetal Therapy Board (FTB) resulted from this vision. Each fetal center was to assemble a group of interested individuals to review and address the separate, and possibly conflicting, interests for a potential maternal-fetal patient who might be eligible to undergo a novel fetal intervention.

Composition

Although no strict criteria have been established to determine the composition of this group of interested individuals, there are some logical candidates. Ideally, someone with formal training in ethics, and/or philosophy, with a specific interest in the unique issues presented by the maternal-fetal patient, should lead the group. Some specific clinicians that might logically be desirable within this group include a maternal-fetal medicine (MFM) specialist, an anesthesiologist comfortable with managing both pregnant women and critically ill neonates, a clinical geneticist, a pediatric cardiologist comfortable with interpreting fetal echocardiography, a neonatologist, a pediatric surgeon, and a pediatric critical care specialist. The intent for each of these specialists would be to identify risks or burdens to the pregnant woman, the fetus, the maternal-fetal patient, or the neonate and ultimate child. An MFM would be able to identify risks or burdens to the pregnant woman and her fetus during the procedure as well as during the period between the procedure and delivery. The anesthesiologist would be able to assess risks related to the anesthetic for both the pregnant woman and her fetus. Both the clinical geneticist and pediatric cardiologist would be able to assess and interpret any genetic anomaly (geneticist) and/or structural cardiovascular anomaly (cardiologist) that may preclude an ethical justification for offering a novel intervention to a specific maternal-fetal patient. The benefits to the born child following a technically successful novel fetal intervention would be assessed by a neonatologist, a pediatric surgeon, and a pediatric critical care specialist. Collectively this group would assess the risks and/or burdens of performing the novel intervention, any potentially confounding factors related to either the pregnant woman or her fetus, and the benefits early in life to the born child.

The last component, benefits to the born child following a successful novel fetal intervention, is particularly important. For example, a child that is dependent on extracorporeal membrane oxygenation (ECMO) until death, suffers from supra-systemic pulmonary hypertension, or requires a solid organ transplant early in life might not be the outcome goal that the parent(s) were seeking through a novel fetal intervention. Such specific specialists who may provide insight into these conditions, should be included among the FTB group on an as-needed basis. For example, a pediatric nephrologist and/or urologist could contribute significantly, along with the pediatric anesthesiologist, neonatologist, pediatric surgeon, and pediatric critical care specialist, to the ethical analysis of a novel maternal-fetal intervention where "success" results in a neonate that is hemodialysis-dependent until a solid organ transplant can be performed.

Other potential candidates to participate in the ethical analysis by a FTB might include a community representative, a member of the clergy, and/or a social worker. These individuals would tend to view the pregnant woman and her fetus in a more holistic way, instead of identifying them solely by a pathology or lesion. All participants on the FTB should represent a spectrum of ethnicities, cultures, and religious backgrounds. This may be much more significant for some potential maternal-fetal patients. For example, including an Imam during the ethical analysis for a pregnant woman who is a practicing Muslim may be obligatory to address any specific issue related to Islamic bioethics.

Maternal-Fetal Ethics

Consent

Any pregnant woman with decision-making capacity can provide informed consent to medical treatment related to her pregnancy. This would include fetal interventions that are considered standard of care treatments based on published Levels 1 and 2 evidence of benefit. Currently these conditions[3] include:
  (i)   twin to twin transfusion syndrome (TTTS)
 (ii)   myelomeningocele (MMC)
(iii)   lower urinary tract obstruction (LUTO)
 (iv)   congenital diaphragmatic hernia (CDH)
  (v)   intrauterine transfusion (IUT) for fetal alloimmune anemia and parvovirus B19 infection
 (vi)   medical therapy for fetal tachycardia.

Even an adolescent, a woman who has not reached the legal age of majority, would be able to consent to these fetal medical treatments. However, she would not necessarily be able to consent to participate in an experimental fetal intervention. All states enable pregnant adolescents to utilize decision-making capacity to provide consent for pregnancy-related treatments. However, only some states confer complete emancipation to an adolescent female based on her pregnancy status.

State laws variably give adolescents the legal authority to provide informed consent for medical treatment under three general categories as: (1) an emancipated minor, (2) a mature minor, and (3) a public health measure. State laws vary with regard to emancipated minor status. Some require a court ruling, which sometimes requires parental permission: others grant a de facto court ruling of emancipated minor status when certain conditions are met, such as pregnancy.[4]

The adolescent's surrogate decision-maker, in the majority of cases, her parent(s), would need to provide informed consent for any experimental fetal intervention offered in states where pregnancy does not confer complete emancipation. This would be analogous to parental permission for an adolescent to participate in any investigational review board (IRB) approved research trial. With parental (surrogate) informed consent, the adolescent would be able to enroll as a study participant, if she chooses. However, if for any reason the adolescent does not want to enroll, she cannot be coerced or forced by parental informed consent to do so.

Fetal Status

Considering the ethical justification for a fetal intervention is to some extent linked to the moral status afforded to the fetus. Most people would agree that in today's medical world, the fetus has become a patient. The idea that the fetus is a patient has been delineated by McCullough and Chervenak.[5,6] Given the deep-seated metaphysical disagreement about the moral status of the fetus; is the fetus a person with moral standing or not; the authors focus on the concept of patient-hood, not personhood. Even a previable fetus can be a patient when (1) the pregnant woman presents her fetus to the physician as a patient, and (2) a clinical intervention exists to benefit the fetus (patient). This affords the fetus a "dependent moral status" because it is conferred only by the pregnant woman's choice to present her fetus as a patient. Hence the physician has beneficence-based obligations to protect and promote the best interest of the fetus only if the pregnant woman presents her fetus as a patient.[7] This paradigm has been criticized as risking treating the pregnant woman and the fetal patient separately.

There are other paradigms for treating the fetus. Lyerly et al.[8] argue for a single patient, the pregnant woman; whereas, others argue for recognizing the fetus as a person, not because we view it as a person but because we treat it as a person.[9] However, the fetal "patient" concept proposed by McCullough and Chervenak works well provided the recognition that fetal patient-hood does not necessarily imply that the pregnant woman and her fetus are separate patients.

The Ethics Work-Up

Demonstrating an ethical justification for a fetal intervention is predicated upon a number of ethical appeals. The primary appeal is to consequences, both positive and negative. The desired positive consequence is that the intervention actually accomplishes the goal of ameliorating the detrimental fetal effects resulting from the identified lesion. The negative consequences are those identified literally or theoretically involving an elevated maternal-fetal burden compared to a postnatal treatment. Clearly the positive consequence must be greater than any small elevation in the potential negative consequence with the novel intervention. After demonstrating fetal benefit significant enough to outweigh the mater-nal-fetal burdens under the novel intervention, the goal becomes reducing (hopefully to zero) the small increase in negative maternal consequences.

An ethical justification for a maternal-fetal surgical intervention requires balancing the pregnant woman's autonomy and beneficence/nonmaleficence with fetal beneficence/non-maleficence. The fetal benefit (principle of beneficence) must be demonstrated using animal models unless there are human data available. Human data or experience may be available for ethical reviews involving a compassionate care exception to an IRB protocol as opposed to a proposed but, "untried in humans," novel procedure that if successful will be submitted for IRB approval as an experimental protocol. The fetal burdens (principle of nonmalefi-cence), such as preterm delivery, must be anticipated and minimized; a preterm delivery that is less preterm than experienced under an earlier novel intervention would qualify as anticipated and minimized. However, a less preterm delivery is not sufficient for ethical justification. The life experienced by the neonate must also be considered; hence, input from the MFM, neonatologist, pediatric surgeon, and pediatric critical care physician becomes key when determining the ultimate balance between fetal benefits/burdens.

Beneficence to the pregnant woman for most fetal interventions is the indirect benefit of a better outcome for her fetus. Nonmaleficence to the pregnant woman involves minimizing burdens/risks to her during the process of providing the indirect benefit to her and the direct benefit to her fetus. Certain maternal burdens are ethically unacceptable; the novel interven-tion must not cause mortality or significant morbidity to the woman, nor can it be expected to remove her future fertility. Significant morbidity does not necessarily include a commitment to a surgical (cesarean) delivery for any future pregnancies. Also excluded from significant morbidity is the potential for an abnormal placentation resulting from a novel intervention that commits the woman to a surgical delivery for the pregnancy under intervention. Some possible benefits that would give a positive beneficence/nonmaleficence balance for the pregnant woman would include: a theoretically longer gestation by a decreased rate of preterm delivery for obstetric indications, a less invasive technique for entering the uterus, and a novel technique that affords a standard vaginal delivery for this and/or subsequent pregnancies. Further, the principle of beneficence/nonmaleficence for the pregnant woman would mandate pursuing techniques that afford the possibility of decreased postoperative pain, decreased opioid use, decreased time to full functional and opioid-free recovery, and a decreased risk of abnormal placentation with future pregnancies.

The pregnant woman's autonomy must be respected and her decisional rights upheld through a valid informed consent process. Of note, for research subjects enrolled into a study in the US, a paternal informed consent would also be necessary in accordance with the "Common Rule" in 45CFR46 Subpart A[10]

45 CFR 46.204(e) states, "If the research holds out the prospect of direct benefit solely to the fetus then the consent of the pregnant woman *and the father* (italics added) is obtained in accord with the informed consent provisions of subpart A of this part, except that the father's consent need not be obtained if he is unable to consent because of unavailability, incompetence, temporary incapacity or in situations where the pregnancy resulted from rape or incest."

If the pregnant woman, after considering the possible risks and burdens to herself during and after the procedure as well as the expected indirect benefits to herself and the direct benefits to her fetus, provides informed consent to undergo the novel intervention, the principle of autonomy would be positively balanced. If the pregnant woman provides informed refusal to the intervention, no amount of benefit to herself or her fetus would provide a positive balance for the procedure.

Twin Ethics

Maternal-fetal-fetal conflicting obligations (an autonomy-based obligation to the mother, a beneficence-based obligation to co-twin x, and a nonmaleficence obligation to co-twin y), arguably represent one of the most morally challenging dilemmas an ethicist can address. In the case of TTTS, both the donor and recipient co-twin are at risk of demise; therefore, the beneficence and nonmaleficence-based obligations are equivalent for each co-twin; they both stand to benefit and both experience some risk during the procedure.

When the beneficence and nonmaleficence-based obligations between the co-twins are discordant, determining the morally "right" thing to do gets complicated. To a large degree, tradeoffs among the well-being of two fetuses are a values decision (rather than a clinical one) and so would be within the purview of the pregnant woman. In other words, this decision could fall under parental authority because it turns on how the pregnant woman wants to balance the obligations of beneficence and nonmaleficence for her fetuses' well-being during an innovative procedure despite risk to the twins.

Examples of Possible FTB case reviews

FTB Review Question #1

The hypothetical question: Would it be ethically justified to place a vesico-amniotic shunt in a fetus diagnosed with lower urinary tract obstruction (LUTO) and Trisomy 21?

A number of assumptions need to be made:

1. The patient presents to a Fetal Center experienced in this intervention; the procedural risks to the pregnant woman and fetus are <u>minimal</u>.
2. The Fetal Center only offers this intervention under an approved research protocol.
3. This fetus meets the protocol's clinical inclusion criteria.
4. A congenital anomaly (either chromosomal or a physical deformity with physiologic significance) is an absolute exclusion criterion from the protocol.
5. Imaging, ultrasonography or magnetic resonance imaging (MRI), at this gestational age is diagnostic for cardiac anomalies.

Under these assumptions, a fetus without congenital anomalies, diagnosed with LUTO and otherwise meeting inclusion criteria should be offered a shunt under the protocol at the Center. However, the fetus in question carries the diagnosis of Trisomy 21 without cardiac anomalies. Hence, it is absolutely excluded from the protocol. Exclusion is based on the chromosomal anomaly, even without a physical deformity of physiologic significance.

An ethical justification for offering the vesico-amniotic shunt under an exception to the protocol will necessarily address separately, two spectra of the exclusion criteria: (1) the chromosome anomaly and its expected sequela, and (2) the physical deformity with physiologic significance. The chromosomal anomaly (Trisomy 21) involves some expected degree of intellectual deficit (known as mentally impaired). The physical deformity with physiologic significance would include some cardiac lesions; however, it would not include a web-neck (or isolated extranumerary digits, for example). The benefits (preserved or promoted renal function) to a fetus without associated congenital anomalies overwhelmingly outweigh the burdens/risks that shunt placement may pose to the pregnant woman and her fetus.

The first question becomes: how does an expected intellectual deficit alter this benefits/burdens ratio? The benefits/burden (B/B) ratio would be unchanged by minimal intellectual deficit, where the individual can enjoy the social benefits of appropriate education, employment, and relationships. Hence, it would be difficult to ethically justify treating this fetus differently from one that is not expected to have an intellectual deficit and shunt placement will be offered. For a fetus with expected significant intellectual deficit, it can be argued that the balance actually shifts toward benefits by offering the shunt – therefore shunt placement should be offered. Renal dysfunction requiring hemodialysis three times per week could potentially be more traumatic to a person with limited intellect because they do not or cannot understand what is happening or why. This trauma would be expected to extend over years unless a matched designated donor is identified for transplant.

The second question about physiologic significance becomes: how would a small isolated ventriculoseptal defect (VSD) alter the benefits/burdens ratio? To isolate the ethical issues, a small VSD means a hemodynamically insignificant (fetal and postnatal) lesion that will likely resolve spontaneously. Again the hemodynamic insignificance argues toward treating such a fetus in a manner equivalent to a fetus without a small VSD and shunt placement would be recommended in this instance. The more troubling dilemma would involve the B/B ratio shift as the VSD enlarges hypothetically, ultimately becoming a complete AV canal. At some point a postnatal surgical cardiac intervention would become necessary. A further question would be estimating how preservation of renal function by shunt placement might (or might not) impact such a patient's candidacy for cardiac surgery.

In conclusion, intellectual impairment at worst does not change the B/B ratio – so shunt placement will be recommended. The physiological significance of a non-existent cardiac lesion at worst does not change the B/B ratio – and shunt placement will be recommended. Therefore, for this hypothetical case (not a hypothetically more severe expected manifestation of Trisomy 21) – shunt placement will be offered. If successful, it will maximize the child's quality of life. If unsuccessful, the burdens/risks assumed by the mother and fetus by placing the shunt are no different from those for a fetus without a congenital anomaly; however, the quality of life for the child on hemodialysis would be equivalent to not offering the shunt.

FTB Review Question #2

The hypothetical question: Is it ethically justifiable to attempt a laser ablation targeting a donor umbilical artery that "dives" into the placental parenchyma, and is therefore difficult to visualize, but is presumed to be the feeding residual placental anastomoses?

Given that the TTTS has recurred following a prior attempt at separation by ablation, the therapeutic options include:

a. expectant management, most likely associated with worsening TTTS leading to demise for one or both twins as well as premature delivery from recurrent polyhydramnios

b. serial amnioreductions, possibly offering some survival benefit to both twins, but also may result in possible premature delivery

c. fetoscopic laser ablation of the "presumed feeding" (and diving) artery within the placental parenchyma

d. selective fetocide of the donor twin hoping to improve survival of the recipient twin

e. a trial of fetoscopic laser ablation, and if unsuccessful, proceed with selective fetocide.

The ethical considerations may lead to opposing conclusions:

Conclusion 1 – The benefit to the recipient twin of selective fetocide is recognized; however, if the innovative intervention fails and is followed by selective reduction of the donor twin, it is unclear how much additional risk would be assumed by the recipient during the attempt at the innovative intervention. It is also recognized that if the donor twin survives the procedure, and the anhydramnios reverses, then there would be a slight, but (at some centers) real, possibility of "donor" viability. This makes the pregnant woman's desire to attempt an innovative intervention aimed at saving both twins, without ruling out a selective reduction, significant. Hence, a fully counseled pregnant woman who understands the risks and benefits may be allowed to proceed with an innovative procedure despite the risk to the twins.

Conclusion 2 – These fetuses have been presented to the physician as patients, and so the physician has obligations of beneficence and nonmaleficence to both of them. It would therefore violate the obligation of nonmaleficence, to the twin likely to survive with selective reduction, to place that twin at substantial risk through intervention. It is for this reason that we are generally reluctant to intervene (medically or surgically) to save one twin when doing so threatens the co-twin. The duty of beneficence to the less-well-off twin does not override the duty of nonmaleficence to the better-off twin. Therefore the question becomes, how much risk should the better-off twin assume to benefit the co-twin? Only if the available literature suggests that this risk is insignificant would this innovative procedure be ethically justifiable.

Conclusion

As fetal interventions are viewed with the intent to become the standard of care, the FTB necessarily becomes more obligatory because the moral status of a fetus and the choices available to a pregnant woman are socially, culturally, and politically evolving. Novel fetal interventions, research protocols involving a fetus, as well as deviations from the standard of care involving fetuses present sometimes subtle but significant moral dilemmas; as such, performance of these interventions requires deliberate thought and frequently a formal review to determine an ethical justification to proceed.

References

1. Harrison MR, Filly RA, Golbus MS, et al. Fetal treatment 1982. *N Engl J Med.* 1982;**307**(26): 1651–1652.

2. Post LF. Bioethical consideration of maternal-fetal issues. *Fordham Urban Law J.* 1996;**24**(4):757–776.

3. Moaddab A, Nassr AA, Belfort MA, Shamshirsaz AA. Ethical issues in fetal therapy. *Best Pract Res Clin Obstet Gynaecol.* 2017;**43**:58–67.

4. English A, Bass L, Boyle AD, Eshrage F. *State Minor Consent Laws: A Summary.* 3rd ed. Center for Adolescent Health & the Law;2010.

5. Chervenak FA, McCullough LB. Ethics of maternal-fetal surgery. *Semin Fetal Neonatal Med.* 2007;**12**(6):426–431.

6. Chervenak FA, McCullough LB. An ethically justified framework for clinical investigation to benefit pregnant and fetal patients. *Am J Bioethics.* 2011;**11**(5):39–49.

7. Chervenak FA, McCullough LB. Ethical issues in recommending and offering fetal therapy. *Western J Med.* 1993;**159**:396–399.

8. Lyerly AD, Little MO, Faden RR. A critique of the "fetus as patient." *Am J Bioethics.* 2008;**8**(7):42–44.

9. Antiel RM. Ethical challenges in the new world of maternal-fetal surgery. *Semin Perinatol.* 2016;**40**:227–233.

10. Department of Health and Human Services, National Institutes of Health, and Office for Human Research Protections. The Common Rule, Title 45 (Public Welfare), Code of Federal Regulations, Part 46 (Protection of Human Subjects). [Online] 13 May 2018. Available: https://www.hhs.gov/ohrp/regulations-and-policy/regulations/45-cfr-46/index.html

Multidisciplinary Approach to Fetal Surgery

Lori J. Howell and Susan M. Scully

Introduction

The number of fetal therapy centers (FTCs) has grown worldwide as a result of pioneering and ongoing work which established the fetus as a patient.[1] The mission of specific FTCs varies from those providing prenatal diagnosis and testing to centers that offer a full range of fetal interventions.[2] Previous publications have described the requirements of a FTC in which fetal surgery is performed.[3-6] Recently, Moon-Grady et al., representing the International Fetal Medical and Surgical Society (IFMSS) and the North American Fetal Therapy Network (NAFTNet) described the evolution of Fetal Therapy Centers over nearly three decades.[7] However, the initial and basic tenets of offering fetal therapy, including identification of life-threatning or severely debilitating anomalies, reporting of all outcomes, definition of the natural history of the disease, performance of basic and translational research to discover the appropriate mechanisms to intervene, and establishment of maternal safety,[1] continue to be appropriate principles for those FTCs wishing to perform fetal interventions. This chapter will explore the requirements and the role of the multidisciplinary team for a FTC offering prenatal diagnosis and the full range of fetal interventions including open fetal surgery, fetoscopic fetal surgery, shunt placement, and EXIT procedures. Specific anesthesia and operative techniques are detailed elsewhere in the text.

Fetal Therapy Center

A number of opinion statements exist from various specialty organizations regarding this rather young field, seeking to update basic tenets, standardize selection criteria and/or seek collaboration to address the growth of FTCs from three in 1995 to over 45 in 2018.[3,7,8] Creating a vision and mission for a FTC, which should not be entered into lightly, is the first step. A FTC offering fetal surgery should provide comprehensive care to both mother and fetus, neonate and family across the life span. Those seeking to develop a FTC should explore, investigate, and prepare a plan to assess the necessity and feasibility of services, personnel, and facility requirements. In addition, robust administrative support is critical, and philanthropic support is very helpful. Important questions to consider as plans for the FTC are being contemplated include: Will the proposed FTC offer fetal imaging and prenatal diagnosis, minimally invasive fetoscopic procedures, open fetal surgery, all or part of the above? Will a research infrastructure be put into place or will the FTC collaborate with other centers through an organization such as NAFTNet to pool outcome data?,[8,9] and rely on other centers that perform basic and translational research? Are the appropriate, expert team members available and/or attainable? Once the type of FTC is confirmed and

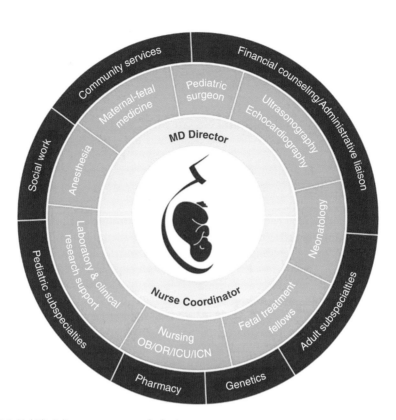

Figure 4.1 Multidisciplinary components of a fetal treatment center.

interventions to be offered are decided upon, the clinical team can be identified, and appropriate infrastructure and facilities can be designed, developed, and built.

An expert multidisciplinary team focused on fetal disease is the key to the ultimate success of any FTC. Although there are many members of the team (Figure 4.1), the following clinical team members will be described in detail as they pertain to fetal interventions: fetal/pediatric surgery, maternal-fetal medicine (MFM), anesthesiology, radiology, genetics, cardiology, nursing, and psychosocial services. The FTC should have a high referral volume to support the multidisciplinary team, to ensure appropriate and necessary services can be offered.

Clinical Team

The ability to perform fetal interventions is a specialized surgical subset. Adherence to guidelines established by the American College of Obstetrics and Gynecology (ACOG) and the American Association of Pediatrics (AAP) for perinatal care is the entry level when establishing a FTC within the United States.[10] The team required for fetal interventions requires substantially more resources and must possess a focus on fetal disease. Each participant in the multidisciplinary team involved in fetal interventions represents their respective clinical specialty. Specialists from anesthesiology, pediatric surgery, maternal-fetal medicine, fetal cardiology, ultrasonography, and nursing undergo additional focused training to safely care for the maternal-fetal dyad. Members of each respective specialty should receive ample time and training to observe the entire team during a procedure and work in tandem with an experienced team member to learn their respective responsibilities. As these procedures are high risk and relatively low volume, there is no "time limit" set to any of the training, as it is impossible to predict the volume and timing of fetal procedures. In addition, because of the variability of these procedures, senior members of the team should develop a competency checklist for an inexperienced provider as it relates to their specialty. Once the new team member has gained necessary experience and comfort with each procedure they become a primary member delivering care, but always with an experienced resource available as needed. The objective of additional subspecialized training is to gain enough experience to maintain that skill set.

Fetal/Pediatric Surgery

Pediatric surgeons routinely operate on children from newborns to adolescents. These surgeons have completed a five year general surgery residency with an additional two years in a surgical laboratory. Those wishing to perform fetal surgery often choose to work in a lab where a FTC performing fetal surgery exists. These general surgeons go on to complete a two year Pediatric Surgical Fellowship and are credentialed both in General and Pediatric Surgery. Those wishing to perform fetal surgery should obtain additional training at a FTC either before or after their fellowship. Pediatric surgeons have specialized knowledge in the surgical repair of birth defects in premature and term neonates. Furthermore, in the prenatal period, pediatric surgeons provide counseling to prospective parents about the birth defect and corrective surgery.[11] A prenatal fetal anomaly diagnosis rarely results in fetal surgery. Typically, fetal surgeons will pursue further research into fetal disease using basic, translational, and clinical research methodologies. Unique and key within a FTC is the pediatric/fetal surgeon role as a general surgeon in which they are able to care for both adults and children.

Fetal Imaging

The fetal radiologist will have completed one year in medicine and an additional three years of residency training in all radiology modalities. Those pursuing prenatal diagnosis will have completed an additional fellowship in pediatric radiology and developed expertise in ultrasound, fetal magnetic resonance imaging (MRI), and fetal computed tomography (CT). Various models exist within FTCs. One should consider that the fetal radiologist's sole clinical responsibility is to obtain the best imaging to confirm the prenatal diagnosis acting independently of a potential proposed procedure. In addition, fetal radiologists are continuing to improve imaging technology from the type of transducer to the machine itself.[12,13]

Some FTCs may have MFMs in the sonography role. The best model incorporates those physicians, sonographers, and radiologic technicians (MRI/CT) who can solely focus on diagnosing fetal disease and confirm the diagnosis particularly under complex conditions (body habitus, fetal position), and have the requisite clinical time to do so. A several hour scan by an MFM is not feasible when seeing many patients per day. One should not embark on providing fetal surgical interventions unless and until expert diagnostics are available and a subspecialty team for counseling can be provided.

Maternal/Fetal Medicine

Maternal-fetal medicine (MFM) specialists undergo a four year obstetric residency and training in high-risk obstetrics and fetal disease as well as research during their four year MFM fellowship. At a FTC, the MFM may be more focused on fetal therapy than a pregnancy complicated by diabetes, hypertension, and other maternal high-risk problems. This expertise, however, is crucial in advising whether a woman is a candidate for a fetal intervention. MFM training is focused on maternal safety, performing minimally invasive procedures such as amniocentesis, vesicoamniotic and throacoamniotic shunt procedures, as well as fetoscopic procedures. MFMs have many additional roles within a FTC from counseling and managing high-risk pregnancies to performing procedures and deliveries. Dependent upon the FTC, during open fetal surgery and EXIT procedures, MFMs can be responsible for ascertaining placental position and assessing uterine tone, can serve as mediators for balancing risks and benefits of fetal therapy for the maternal-fetal dyad and determining delivery and therapy plans based on these risk/benefit calculations. In addition, MFMs play an essential role in postoperative care including the use of tocolytics to prevent preterm labor, management of chorioamniotic separation, and prevention of/or attending to, any obstetric emergency.

Genetics

The field of genetics is rapidly evolving. Fetal therapy for genetic disease will soon be commonplace. It is essential to include a reproductive/clinical geneticist and a genetic counselor on the multidisciplinary team. Their role in analysis of invasive and noninvasive testing and whether or not fetal surgery should be offered, is critical to avoid performing an unwarranted fetal intervention. In addition, obtaining the family pedigree during the evaluation may be key in understanding all the components of the fetal disease, for example, is the condition syndromic or not? Finally, the genetics team has a role to play in reproductive risk counseling for future pregnancies.

Obstetrics

Obstetricians on the FTC team, in addition to their four year residency caring for the general obstetric patient, must know the details of the disease processes of the fetus and be able to translate this knowledge to adapt obstetric care to decisions about inductions, cesarean section, and classical cesarean section deliveries. Careful delivery of fetuses with bone issues, potential liver rupture with giant omphalocele or sac rupture in myelomeningocele (MMC), require this adaptation skill. Further, performing a hysterotomy after a fetal surgery for MMC requires additional skills such as taking down the omental flap, inspection of the fetal surgery hysterotomy site and potential repair to avoid future conception and subsequent delivery issues.

Anesthesia

The anesthesia team that cares for fetal surgical patients should have specialized training in either obstetric anesthesia and/or pediatric anesthesia with a special interest in obstetric anesthesia. The models for staffing fetal surgical procedures can vary between two broad models. One model involves dedicating one anesthesia team to the mother, and a separate anesthesia team to the fetus. The second model utilizes one anesthesia care team for both the mother and fetus. These models are more clearly illustrated in a case of a fetus with a large microcystic lung lesion causing hydrops in mid-gestation. The indicated procedure would be open fetal surgery with hysterotomy to perform a fetal thoracotomy and pulmonary lobectomy.

Using the first staffing model, an anesthesiologist would be dedicated to maternal perioperative care, placing the epidural and intravenous access, and inducing and maintaining general anesthesia. A second anesthesia team would be scrubbed into the sterile field, and this team is responsible for care of the fetus. The pediatric/fetal team would obtain fetal intravenous access, manage fluid and blood administration, and administer fetal medications as needed to alleviate the stress response, mitigate movement, fetal bradycardia, or cardiac depression. Both of these anesthesia teams would be in communication with the pediatric surgeon, MFM, and cardiologists throughout the case. With this first model, the anesthesia subspecialties will collaborate for optimal care of both the mother and fetus. One advantage of this model is the optimal maintenance of skill sets of the two teams. A disadvantage is the communication challenge when more members are involved in decision-making and care of the mother and fetus.

If the second staffing model is used, one anesthesia team cares for both the mother and the fetus simultaneously. The team may be an experienced obstetric anesthesia team that has familiarity with fetal surgical cases and a willingness to participate in the care of the fetus or an experienced pediatric anesthesia team that is willing and able to participate in the care of a pregnant patient. One advantage of the second model is that with an appropriately experienced team, the communication and decision-making will occur much more rapidly. Technical aspects of fetal care such as securing fetal intravenous access will depend on the institution. The surgical team may insert a fetal intravenous catheter or umbilical venous access and/or intubate a fetus during an EXIT procedure (particularly that of a fetus with a difficult airway requiring specialized surgical equipment), while on the sterile field.

The minimally invasive fetal procedures are not as procedurally demanding as open fetal surgery, and these cases can often be cared for by one anesthesia team. In the case of an EXIT procedure, even if the second model is used (one team for mother and fetus together), a second anesthesia and nursing team must be ready to provide care for the fetus in a second operating room (OR) if the fetus requires additional surgery following the EXIT or if the fetus does not tolerate the EXIT procedure. A second anesthesia team may also be necessary if the mother is going to have a cesarean delivery and immediate intervention is planned for the neonate, such as intubation, bronchoscopy, pulmonary lobectomy, cardiac catheterization, or debulking of a sacrococcygeal teratoma. Regardless of the model, the anesthesia team(s) must all have a thorough understanding of the fetal procedure to be performed, the fetal pathophysiology, maternal and fetal physiology, and an excellent working relationship with the operative teams.

Cardiology

The fetal cardiologist is first trained as a pediatrician with subspecialty training in pediatric cardiology. Those pursuing fetal cardiology undergo additional training. The fetal cardiology team interfaces with the members of the FTC in several capacities. They serve as primary decision makers for managing the fetus with prenatally diagnosed cardiac disease. The cardiologists may be able to directly treat the cardiac lesion of the fetus, and with their MFM colleagues, may prescribe medications for the mother to help the fetus. They can also help optimize delivery planning and ensure the appropriate team is ready to resuscitate the newborn with prenatally diagnosed cardiac disease.

As consultants, the cardiologist's interpretation of the fetal echocardiogram will certainly inform the outpatient management of fetuses at risk for hydrops fetalis from any of a number of processes, including but certainly not limited to twin-twin transfusion syndrome, large pulmonary lesions, congenital high airway obstruction (CHAOS), and sacrococcygeal teratoma. The frequency of follow-up fetal echocardiograms will be dictated by the aggressiveness of the disease process. The cardiologists are also important consultants in the OR during surgery, as real-time fetal echocardiography is critical during open fetal surgery and in some EXIT procedures.[14,15] The echocardiographic determination of fetal cardiac function is useful to the anesthesia team as they manage the maternal and fetal administration of medications, fluids, and blood. The echocardiographic data are also used by the surgical and MFM team in positioning the fetus together with communication with the anesthesia team. Echocardiography is also extremely helpful in the diagnosis and management of impending fetal bradycardia or cardiac arrest.

Neonatology

The neonatologist's training includes a three year pediatric residency followed by three years of training in neonatal intensive care. The neonatology role within the FTC is to provide prenatal counseling[16] typically as it relates to prematurity, but they also serve as the experts in neonatal resuscitation and management at delivery and in the neonatal intensive care unit (NICU). For any fetal intervention occurring in a viable fetus, a neonatologist is present during the procedure in the event of a precipitous delivery.

Nursing
Fetal Therapy Nurse Coordinator

Prior to a patient evaluation at a FTC, a prospective patient will speak with the Fetal Therapy Nurse Coordinator (FTNC). In the authors' experience, the majority of questions relate to the fetal condition. A FTNC, preferentially with a master's degree and specialty knowledge in neonatal and pediatric surgery is ideal.[17] This nurse is integral to assuring an expeditious evaluation is scheduled with the appropriate testing and subspecialist consultation. Many factors are taken into consideration. For example, if the fetus is hydropic, surgery may need to be scheduled urgently, leaving little time for parental reflection. Informing the pregnant patient during the referral call, that at times things move quickly, and that the rapidity of events is not an unusual occurrence, may provide some comfort during this stressful time especially if events occur at a rapid pace. Conversely, in a fetus with a nonlife-threatening abnormality such as a myelomeningocele, there is ample time to adhere to the standards established by the Management of Myelomeningocele Study (MOMS) trial.[18] A karyotype can be performed as well as imaging and the procedure can be electively scheduled after appropriate counseling.

In addition to discussing with the family, the FTNC obtains and reviews prenatal records to determine the urgency of the fetal condition prior to the patient appointments and sees to it that the evaluation is tailored to the particular diagnosis and family needs. Assistance and advice is also provided for travel and/or lodging concerns. It is helpful for the FTNC to be about knowledgeable about fetal disease as well.

Perinatal Advance Practice Nurse

This specialty nurse has completed undergraduate nursing education and obtained graduate education training and certification in perinatal, women's health, or midwifery. These graduate programs are typically two years in length and require previous experience in obstetric nursing. Their role can be key in providing prenatal care, normalizing an abnormal pregnancy, performing nonstress tests or biophysical profiles, providing ongoing education and support and in the case of a nurse midwife, assisting at a vaginal delivery or first assisting in a cesarean section delivery. The Advance Practice Nurses will meet all the requirements of an obstetric nurse as listed below.

Obstetric Nurse

The FTC obstetric nurse should be an experienced Labor and Delivery nurse with certification in advanced cardiac life support (ACLS), neonatal resuscitation program (NRP) and Phase I recovery. Generally, obstetric nursing results in the immediate gratification at the delivery of healthy baby and ensuing happiness. This normal birthing process may be experienced later in life for a baby that has undergone a mid-gestation procedure as the gratification in this instance will occur when a baby leaves the NICU following an in-utero procedure. The FTC obstetric nurse is caring for the most difficult end of the fetal/neonatal disease spectrum, and requires acute skills in providing complex antepartum, intrapartum, and postpartum care using a family-centered approach. Further, the obstetric nurse must provide exemplary care to the mother pre- and post-operatively following fetal surgical interventions. These nurses are not trained in neonatal or pediatric surgical interventions.

Fetal Operating Room Nurse

The Fetal Operating Room (OR) RN has education and training in perioperative nursing and should be certified by the American Association of Operating Room Nurses. Further, they possess extremely specialized skills and knowledge in neonatal and pediatric perioperative care. Fetal Surgery nurses should have ample experience in neonatal and pediatric general surgery to be expert both in circulating and scrubbing for the procedures performed on the fetus or neonate during fetal surgery. Special orientation to the team including observation and educational sessions focusing on the history, theory, potential risks, instrumentation, and procedural steps is imperative to ensure competency.

As fetal centers develop, a FTC OR RN team lead role should be created. Responsibilities include overseeing orientation for new nurses, rotation of team members to appropriate cases to maintaining competency, organizing call schedules as necessary, maintaining instrumentation sets, ordering appropriate supplies, and coordinating education of new procedures as applicable. Operating Room nurses that have been at a facility with at least two years of solid foundational neonatal/pediatric surgical experience may be considered for the Fetal Surgery Team.

Neonatal Surgical Advance Practice Nurse

This specialty Advanced Practice Nurse (APN) has completed a baccalaureate and master's program, typically as a Neonatal or Acute Care Nurse Practitioner and has specialty certification. They possess NRP certification, attend deliveries, and are skilled at neonatal resuscitation. The Neonatal Surgical APN will have additional education in neonatal surgery and provide primary neonatal surgical care with the attending neonatologist and pediatric surgeon while the baby is in the NICU. Further, they are integral to the education of neonatal surgical nurses. There may be a large number of surgical neonates in a FTC, and provision of 24/7 care with a surgical APN is a methodology for expert, continuous care.

Neonatal ICU Nurse

Ideally, the Neonatal ICU RN will have a baccalaureate or higher education and experience in caring for neonates. Additionally, they should possess education and training in the care of surgical neonates. They must be NRP-certified and skilled at resuscitation and attending deliveries. Finally, they will provide the requisite care during the neonatal time in the NICU and prepare the family for discharge to home or perinatal palliative care or bereavement expertise as the situation demands.

Psychosocial Services

Psychosocial services are needed to provide emotional and social support for mothers and families during a particularly stressful time in their lives. These services are also necessary to assess the suitability of mothers and families for fetal interventions. As FTCs commonly serve a wide geographic area, families often travel great distances to reach the center for appropriate diagnosis and treatment. Traveling long distances can impose challenging situations on family structure, in terms of care of other dependents left at home, lodging, and employment. These logistical factors add to the stress of learning about and processing the news of the fetal diagnosis. The psychosocial team can help the mother and family cope with uncertainty, fears, and stressors about the fetal diagnosis.[19] Concerns about invasive procedures for the mother, the fetus itself, invasive procedures for the neonate after delivery, communication issues and differences in coping by various family members all require support. Hospital stays can be long and may be even longer for the neonate. Some fetuses may die in the course of treatment or recovery, so palliative care and bereavement services should also be readily available.[20]

Serious fetal diagnoses requiring open fetal surgery can take a heavy emotional and physical toll on the mother and family as a result of the period of prolonged bed rest/ restricted movement that usually follows surgical intervention. Careful and thorough assessment of the mother and her social support system will help identify patients who may not be best served by undertaking open fetal surgery. Ideally, the FTC psychosocial team consisting of a psychologist as manager as well as a psychiatrist, child life specialist, chaplain, and social worker can adequately assess the patient, the patient's support system and the feasibility of the patient undergoing fetal intervention.

Phases of Fetal Intervention

Before a patient undergoes any fetal surgery procedure, the basic tenets of fetal surgery should be upheld. These include awareness of the natural history of the disease, and an appropriate intervention without which the fetus will die or have a significant compromise in quality of life. The planned intervention must be safe for the mother, and both basic and translational research work must have been performed to ensure the appropriate approach and all results must have been reported.[1] Similarly, long-term follow-up programs should be established so that prenatal counseling not only addresses the procedure, but also the risk and benefits to the pregnant woman and her fetus across the life span. With the rapid advancement of fetal imaging, confirmation of the radiological findings as these relate to a particular diagnosis is critical. For example, confirming the bone and skin level of a MMC is crucial to avoid an unnecessary intervention, for example, a lesion below the second sacral vertebrae would exclude a fetus from fetal MMC repair. The fetal MRI must also confirm hindbrain herniation.[18] To offer open fetal surgery, expert diagnostics must be present. However, future interventions as determined through research may change the current accepted criteria.

Prenatal Assessment for Fetal Intervention

The fetal imaging team is critical to ensuring an accurate fetal diagnosis prior to any fetal intervention so essential counseling can be provided. Prenatal imaging can also determine the viability of the options presented during counseling such as whether a short cervix is present or if advanced fetal hydrops exist, both of which will make the woman and her fetus ineligible for fetal surgery. Conversely, fetal imaging is essential to the operative plan such as the determination of placental location and margins for the uterine incision, side of lesion such as in congenital diaphragmatic hernia, and/or the presence of a pedicle in the case of a sacrococcygeal teratoma. At a FTC that offers fetal interventions, every prospective fetal surgery patient should undergo detailed fetal imaging including high resolution ultrasound, fetal echocardiography, and in many instances, an ultrafast MRI. Imaging diagnostics are best performed by experts in fetal imaging, typically a fetal radiologist for ultrasound and MRI and a fetal cardiologist for a fetal echocardiogram. In addition, while a radiologist or a fetal cardiologist performing the diagnostic exams is focused on imaging for fetal disease, they should remain impartial in their recommendations on fetal intervention.

Upon arrival at the FTC, the patient undergoing an evaluation for a fetal intervention will have had her prenatal records reviewed by an MFM specialist looking for any medical contraindications to surgery. An MFM prepared in reproductive genetics will work with the genetic counselor to ensure a complete karyotype, microarray, and/or other laboratory testing such as acetylcholinesterase or amniotic fluid alpha-feto protein have been performed. The genetic counselor, as a member of the team, performs a complete pedigree, ensures genetic results are available and provides genetic counseling on the day of the evaluation. Depending on the setup of the center, the MFM will review all prenatal imaging and testing, and discuss these results with the pediatric surgeon, or they each review the images and consult with the family separately. The prospective parents then meet with MFM, pediatric surgery, and the fetal treatment center nurse coordinator, to discuss the results of the evaluation, confirm the diagnosis and outline options for the pregnancy which include letting nature take its course, fetal intervention, or interruption of the pregnancy.[4–6]

Preoperative Preparation

If fetal intervention is the option chosen, the woman and her support person will meet with a maternal-fetal anesthesiologist to assess for any increased risks the patient may have for the procedure as well as postoperative care. Additional members of the team including social work and psychology also meet with the family to determine coping mechanisms, support structure, and any mental health history. These members of the team may detect warning signs and alert a psychosocial issue and a risk for the fetal surgery outcome to the pediatric surgeon and MFM.

The patient undergoes a thorough history and physical by both anesthesia and MFM specialists to ensure she is an appropriate surgical candidate. Coexisting conditions such as asthma or cardiac disease require further evaluation from an adult subspecialist. Blood work, chest X-ray, and ECG are performed as for any standard surgery. If all evaluation and testing as discussed above indicate the patient is an appropriate fetal surgery candidate, arrangements will proceed for surgery with the multidisciplinary team, the OR, Labor and Delivery (L&D) staff, and as appropriate, the neonatology team. A team meeting is arranged and is typically attended by the FTNC, fetal surgeon, maternal-fetal medicine specialist, maternal and fetal anesthesiologist, genetic counselor, social worker, psychologist, OR and L&D nurses who all meet together and discuss the case, prior to meeting with the family. This pre-meeting provides a critical opportunity for any team member to voice any concerns about the proposed intervention. The family is then subsequently brought into the room to meet the multidisciplinary team. They are prepared in advance that they will be meeting with a large team, but it is also explained that the purpose of the team is to answer any and all questions they may have and that everyone is there for the patients' well-being. The fetal surgeon reviews the procedure again in detail with the family and the team present, discussing all prior outcomes, good and bad, and provides additional opportunity for questions. The preoperative preparation is discussed further including NPO status, pre-operative bath, arrival time, and advance directives by the Perinatal APN and consents are obtained for surgery and anesthesia as applicable.

Day of Fetal Surgical Intervention

The patient arrives on the L&D unit and is escorted to her room by the obstetric nurse. Standardized, preoperative orders, approved by the multidisciplinary physician and nursing teams are activated in the electronic medical record. To ensure privacy, postoperative pain control, and the least amount of OR time, an epidural is placed by the anesthesiologist in the patient room. Once placed, the patient is then transported to the OR. An appropriate handoff is performed and documented between the L&D nurse and the circulating OR nurse. This handoff should include patient verification using two patient identifiers, age, weight, fetal diagnosis, allergies, relevant past medical and surgical history, medications, immediate concerns, peripheral access, and verification of informed surgical consent.

Within the OR, members of the fetal surgery, anesthesia, and nursing teams will have set up the room specifically to ensure all instruments and equipment are sterile and in working order prior to arrival of the patient. Operating room nursing and anesthesia staff collaborate to ensure the least amount of anesthesia time and efficiency of operations, so attention to detail is paramount. An initial instrument count including sharps and sponges is performed by the fetal surgery scrub and circulating nurses. The room should be set up with the ability to accommodate an emergency cesarean section if this becomes necessary.

Preoperative Preparation

Every fetal procedure requires a significant amount of specialized equipment and supplies. To ensure everything needed for each procedure is ready and available, specialized pick sheets or preference cards are maintained for each procedure by the Fetal Surgery OR Nurse and attending fetal surgeon. These lists ensure that the appropriate items are selected and available for each procedure as not having a pertinent item could be catastrophic to the patients. These pick sheets or preference cards should be updated in real time so nothing is forgotten and preparation for the next such case is pristine. In addition, educational checklists or job aids for each procedure and specialized equipment should be created and updated in real time so that they are always ready and available for an impending case. Resources that can be referenced are helpful for the entire team and ensure consistency.

For candidates undergoing an EXIT procedure, the case is picked and kept in a convenient spot as soon as the fetus is of viable gestation. Should the mother of such a fetus present to the hospital in active labor, the EXIT procedure must be performed expeditiously. In such scenarios, having the equipment and supplies ready saves precious time as the specialized team is called in and the procedure is set up. During these emergent life-threatening instances, teamwork is of the utmost importance. Not one specialty subset of staff can perform appropriately without another.

Intraoperative Phase

Once the patient is brought into the OR, there is a sign-in with the nursing and anesthesia teams identifying the appropriate patient using two patient identifiers, and stating/confirming the patient's weight and allergies as well as the procedure to be performed. The American Society of Anesthesiologists (ASA) physical status, hypothermia risk, airway issues, deep vein thrombosis (DVT) prophylaxis, and preoperative antibiotics to be administered within one hour of the surgical procedure are also confirmed. The patient is then transferred to the OR bed. At this time, all pertinent monitors are applied (e.g. electrocardiogram, blood pressure and oxygen saturation monitors). A bump is placed under the patient's right flank and hip, to relieve compression of the inferior vena cava. Sequential compression device (SCD) stockings are applied to both legs. Gel positioning rolls are placed under both of the patient's knees and ankles to aid in comfort and decrease the risk of pressure ulcers. A safety strap is applied across the patient's thighs. An ultrasound is performed to confirm fetal viability, fetal position, and placental location to identify optimal hysterotomy placement.[21]

A "time out" prior to the procedure includes introduction of all staff members in the room, confirmation of the procedure to be performed, the patient's name, weight, allergies, antibiotics given, fire risk, blood products available if necessary, and the essential imaging needed during the procedure.

Intraoperative Phase: Open and EXIT Procedures

Anesthetic management requires an anesthesiologist or an anesthesia team skilled in both obstetric and fetal anesthesia.[22–24] The anesthesiologist will intubate the pregnant patient and begin general anesthesia protocols, as discussed elsewhere in the text. General anesthesia is critical for uterine relaxation so that the procedure may be performed with minimal risk of a placental abruption which may result in termination of the procedure. An additional venous line, arterial line, and nasogastric tube will also be placed by the anesthesiologist. Once the patient is anesthetized, the circulating nurse will insert a bladder catheter and place an electrocautery pad on the patient to provide appropriate electrosurgical grounding. Emergency cesarean section instruments and supplies should be in the room during open fetal surgery when the fetus is at a viable gestational age should there be any complications that would necessitate the immediate delivery of the fetus.

The surgical team (pediatric surgery, MFM, fetal cardiologist, and depending upon procedure, the pediatric neurosurgeon) in appropriate OR attire, scrub and don sterile gowns and gloves. Location of various team members at the OR table alternate depending on the procedure and their role in the procedure (Table 4.1). For example, the neurosurgeon

Table 4.1 Clinical team requirements for fetal interventions

	Fetoscopy	Open fetal surgery	EXIT	C-section to resection
Team	• Anesthesiologist (sedation)	• Anesthesiologist (general anesthesia)	• 2 Anesthesiologists (general anesthesia)	• 2 Anesthesiologists (general anesthesia)
	• Sonographer	• Sonographer	• Sonographer	• Sonographer
	• 2 MFMs	• 1 MFM	• 1 MFM	• 1 MFM
	• 1 circulator	• 1 circulator	• 2 circulators	• 2 circulators
	• 1 scrub person	• 1 scrub person	• 2 scrub persons	• 2 scrub persons
	• 1 APN	• 1 float OR RN	• 1 float OR RN	• 1 float OR RN
	• 1 Special Delivery Unit (SDU) RN	• 1 APN	• 1 APN	• 1 APN
		• 1+Fetal Surgeon	• 2 Fetal Surgeons	• 2 Fetal Surgeons
		• NICU staff (viable fetus)	• NICU staff	• NICU staff
		• Cardiologist and cardiology sonographer	• Cardiologist and cardiology sonographer	• Cardiologist and cardiology sonographer
		• SDU RN	• SDU RN	• SDU RN

will enter the sterile field once the fetal MMC is exposed or the fetal cardiologist will step out once the procedure is completed. The MFM is responsible for identifying uterine placental margins via sterile ultrasound, ensuring anesthetic management has resulted in a relaxed uterus and continuing to assess any maternal issues. After the laparotomy is performed, the uterus is exposed and a sterile intraoperative ultrasound is performed to determine the margins of the placenta and the appropriate location for uterine incision so as to avoid the placenta. Once the hysterotomy is made, a Level 1 infusion system is used to infuse warm lactated Ringer's solution into the uterus to keep the fetus buoyant during the procedure and avoid cord compression. The perinatal APN or another designated person typically ensures the Level 1 infusion system is flowing as directed by the MFM or Fetal Surgeon in the field.

Continuous fetal echocardiography is performed by a fetal cardiologist throughout the procedure as a result of myocardial depression related to anesthesia.[14] Throughout the procedure, it is important to monitor the fetal heart rate, and any deterioration or change in fetal echo. Fetal echocardiography changes can signal to the anesthesiologist that blood, crystalloid, or atropine may be required for the fetus.[15] The fetus is given an intramuscular injection of fentanyl, vecuronium, and at times atropine, in addition to the transplacental anesthesia from the mother. During an EXIT procedure,[25–27] a peripheral intravenous (IV) line is placed in the fetus, allowing for preloading with blood and/or enhancing intravascular volume to help minimize cardiovascular consequences. In rare circumstances, venous access will be placed in a fetus during an open fetal surgery case if there is an emergent need for blood or volume during the procedure. At the conclusion of an open fetal surgery procedure, an antibiotic prepared by the OR nurse and provided to the surgeon, is infused into the uterus, the uterus is closed in two layers and the omentum is tacked over the uterine incision in an attempt to form an increased protection barrier and promote healing of the hysterotomy site. At the completion of the procedure, a clear plastic dressing is applied to the patient's incision to accommodate the need for frequent ultrasounds over the next few days.[21]

At the end of the procedure, the MFM specialist performs an ultrasound to evaluate fetal well-being and amniotic fluid level. Magnesium sulfate is started by the anesthesiologist to preempt preterm labor, and also an infusion of local anesthetic into the previously placed epidural catheter for postoperative pain management. The circulating and scrub nurse complete an instrument, sponge, and sharps count at the closure of the uterus and at the closure of the abdominal cavity. A sponge and sharps count is completed at the closure of skin.

If the postoperative fetal heart rate is appropriate and the fetus is stable, the anesthesiologist begins the emergence process, extubates the patient's trachea, and provides supplemental oxygen. Communication between the surgical, obstetric, anesthesia, and nursing teams is essential as emergence from anesthesia is initiated. A final ultrasound is performed after extubation of the mother's trachea, to verify that the fetus has remained stable following closure of the uterus and abdomen. The patient is then transferred to a postoperative bed and transported to the Level I recovery unit on L&D. Lateral transfer devices help make the transfer from OR bed to postoperative bed safe for patient and staff. Subsequent monitoring and care is provided by an experienced L&D nurse as well as an obstetrician experienced in postoperative care of fetal surgery patients together with the MFM specialists.

Intraoperative Phase: Fetoscopic and Ultrasound Guided Procedures

Ultrasound guided and minimally invasive fetoscopic procedures are listed in Table 4.2. While these procedures may be less invasive than open fetal surgery and the EXIT procedure, care of the mother and fetus cannot be minimized.[28] Fewer specialty team members and equipment are required for these procedures as well. MFM, circulating nurse, scrub person, ultrasound technician, anesthesiologist, and Perinatal APN are present for these cases (Table 4.1).

Patients undergoing these types of procedure receive conscious sedation as well as a local anesthetic at the operative trocar insertion sites. The mother receives oxygen via nasal cannula to maintain appropriate oxygenation throughout the procedure. During these procedures, it is extremely important for all team members to remember the woman is awake but sedated and can hear what is being said. Emergency cesarean section instruments and supplies need to be easily available in the room when the fetus is at a viable gestational age should there be any complications that would necessitate the immediate delivery of the fetus.

The circulating nurse ensures the safety of staff and patient during these procedures by following appropriate safety protocols. This includes applying four electrocautery pads during radiofrequency ablation (RFA) or providing laser goggles and laser safety techniques during any laser procedures as appropriate.

Postoperative Phase

Open Fetal Surgery

Following an open fetal surgical procedure, the pregnant patient is recovered in a Phase I recovery area, typically an L&D unit able to provide this level of care. One obstetric RN is assigned to a recovering fetal surgery patient for the first 24–48 hours. Control of preterm labor and pain management is critical during this time. Preterm labor is a major risk factor after open fetal surgery, so the patient is started on tocolytic medications in an attempt to prevent preterm labor and subsequent delivery. The patient is usually in the hospital for approximately four days postoperatively. Once discharged, the patient is instructed to remain on strict bed rest for three weeks. Weekly follow-up ultrasounds and prenatal visits are performed by maternal fetal medicine specialists. The patient is delivered via cesarean section at 37 weeks' gestation or earlier in the event of uncontrolled preterm labor or rupture of membranes resulting in chorioamnionitis.[29] In addition, any future pregnancies will need to be delivered by cesarean section before the onset of active labor to prevent scar dehiscence or rupture.

Cesarean Section to Immediate Neonatal Resection

Mothers of fetuses with significant fetal diagnoses which may benefit from mid-gestation intervention may decline an EXIT procedure if indicated or may not be medically stable enough to undergo the procedure. In these instances, immediate access to the fetus/neonate following delivery may improve outcome. The multidisciplinary team may suggest the possibility of a low-hysterotomy cesarean section to immediate neonatal resection. During this scenario, the mother will have a controlled, planned cesarean section while the neonatology team and an adjacent OR team for the neonatal surgery are arranged in advance of the procedure. Depending on the OR setup, once delivered via cesarean section, the neonate is taken to the adjacent OR

Table 4.2 Types of fetal interventions

Fetoscopy/ultrasound guided	Open fetal surgery	EXIT	C-section to resection
Vesico/thoraco-amniotic shunt	Myelomeningocele repair	Cervical teratoma	Airway/debulking of giant neck mass
Selective laser photocoagulation	Lung lesion lobectomy	Airway/debulking	Lung lesion lobectomy
Radio frequency ablation (RFA)	Sacrococcygeal teratoma (SCT) debulking	Lung lesion lobectomy	SCT debulking
Bipolar umbilical cord coagulation	Pericardial teratoma removal	SCT debulking	
Amniotic band release		Hypertrophic left heart syndrome(HLHS) with intact ventricular septum	
Fetal endoluminal tracheal obstruction (FETO)			
Fetal blood sampling/intrauterine transfusion			
Cardiac balloor valvuloplasty and stent placement			
In-utero hematopoietic stem cell transplant			

where the infant is stabilized and subsequently undergoes surgery. Alternatively, if the neonate is not medically stable after delivery, the neonate is immediately prepared for surgery on arrival to the adjacent OR. Endotracheal intubation, venous access placement, patient preparation with antiseptic solution and surgery are started immediately. Care for the mother and the neonate in this scenario is equivalent to the care of a mother undergoing a cesarean section and that of a neonate undergoing general surgery.

Fetoscopic Surgery

Pregnant patients undergoing fetoscopic procedures are typically discharged within 23 hours following the procedure. They return one week later for a sonographic assessment by their MFM and in all cases where the patient is stable, she may return home, except in the case of fetal endotracheal occlusion (FETO).[30] Undergoing FETO will require that the mother remain within 10 minutes distance of the FTC (per our fetal center protocol) in the event that the balloon placed fetoscopically requires urgent removal because of impending imminent delivery by the Fetal Surgery team. Having a 24/7 team prepared for everything from a fetoscopic balloon removal to an EXIT procedure is essential for any FTC performing these procedures.

Other Considerations

Communication

As noted from the disparate training and preparation, team roles are complex and varied, dependent on patient population and types of interventions. The multidisciplinary team is prepared in their particular specialty areas and expected to integrate this knowledge with other members of the team. Another challenge is the nature of the interventions in an occasionally tense, high-stakes, OR environment. A key point is ensuring this diverse team remains in constant communication. Strategies to overcome communication barriers include weekly multidisciplinary fetal patient review conferences, computerized programmatic database, standardized order sets, on-call protocols for the different fetal procedures, team meetings prior to fetal interventions, fetal call schedule in the respective disciplines, sharing of research in the various interdisciplinary professional meetings, and simulation.

Oversight and Ethics

Any FTC performing fetal interventions that constitute innovative and/or experimental work must adhere to institutional review board standards and establish an independent multidisciplinary oversight committee. The goal of both is to provide a pregnant woman additional protection to ensure they have been appropriately counseled about a proposed procedure and that ethical and regulatory standards are met. These committee members should not be involved in fetal care decisions, but have a knowledge of the patient population. These individuals offer the pregnant woman additional protection to ensure proper and ethical standards are met and resolve any subspecialty conflicts.[31,32]

Simulation

Fetal surgery is a high-risk, low-volume procedure requiring multidisciplinary teams using specialized skills and precise communication. The use of simulation among the entire multidisciplinary team (surgery, anesthesia, cardiology, maternal-fetal medicine, and nursing) encourages team building within this specialized team while also offering the opportunity to learn and practice essential skills in a risk-free environment. Scenarios for simulation may be developed that allow further refinement of the team's response to an emergent situation, the ability to practice a new procedure, provide for educational needs and for onboarding of new staff members to the team, and also allow for development of teamwork among the specialized multidisciplinary team. To be successful, the entire team must participate and treat the simulation as realistically as possible, while also providing the appropriate time needed to simulate all necessary steps or procedures. Furthermore, a postsimulation discussion is important for the entire team to discuss the positive and negative aspects of the simulation. This time can also be used to critically evaluate the need for changes or improvements. Problem solving is the best way to initiate these changes or improvements.

Operating Room

Advances in technology have increased the ability for the multidisciplinary team to learn from and update practice in management of these fetal cases. The use of boom and in-light cameras enables each surgery to be recorded and the OR is set up and tested prior to each procedure for the functionality of this technology. These surgeries can be reviewed for training or research purposes. Critical to any excellent operation is the assurance of stellar OR standards. Specialists providing laser intervention should undergo laser training and competency demonstration.

Long-Term Follow-Up

The multidisciplinary team at a FTC where fetal interventions are performed should extend over the course of the mother and child's life. Subspecialty follow-up programs such as a Spina Bifida Program,[33] Single Ventricle Program,[34] Pulmonary Hypoplasia Program,[35] and Palliative Care and Bereavement Program[19] play an essential role in describing the outcomes of fetal surgical interventions, how best to counsel prospective parents, and measuring developmental and neurocognitive outcomes. Similarly, maternal outcomes are equally important and should be followed over the long term.[36] Outcome information must be shared in peer-reviewed journals, and at national and international conferences. Clearly, establishing and maintaining long-term follow-up programs can be costly, but even more costly is not knowing the long-term effect of a particular intervention nor providing the family with accurate counseling.

Conclusion

An experienced FTC team can improve neonatal outcome by determining the best prenatal surveillance, intervention, and delivery technique for a pregnant patient whose fetus has an anomaly. FTCs should develop regional Centers of Excellence with high patient volumes. Clearly, a FTC requires a large amount of resources and should be undertaken only when expertise and patient volume can be supported. The multidisciplinary team extends to administrative and finance representatives from the hospital as well as insurers. The notion of taking care of a patient from gestation to graduation should be the hallmark of an excellent FTC.

References

1. Harrison MR, Evans ME, Adzick NS. eds: Professional considerations in fetal treatment. *The Unborn Patient* 3rd Ed. 3–9. Philadelphia: WB Saunders; 2001.

2. Harrison MR. Fetal Surgery: trials, tribulations and turf. *J Pediatr Surg.* 2003;**38**:275–282.

3. American College of Obstetricians and Gynecologists Committee Opinion. Maternal-fetal intervention and fetal care centers. *Obstet Gynecol.* 2011;**118**:405–410.

4. Howell LJ, Johnson MP, Adzick NS. Creating a state of the art center for fetal diagnosis and treatment: Importance of a multidisciplinary approach. *Prog Pediatr Cardiol.* 2006;**22**:121–127.

5. Howell LJ, Adzick NS. The essentials of a fetal therapy center. *Semin Perinatol.* 1999;**23**:535–540.

6. Howell LJ, Adzick NS. Establishing a Fetal Therapy Center: Lessons Learned. *Semin Pediatr Surg.* 2003;**12**:209–217.

7. Moon-Grady AJ, Baschat A, Cass D, et al. Fetal treatment 2017: the evolution of fetal therapy centers – a joint opinion from the International Fetal Medicine and Surgical Society (IFMSS) and the North American Fetal Therapy Network (NAFTNet). *Fetal Diagn Ther.* 2017;**42**:241–248.

8. Johnson MP. The North American Fetal Therapy Network (NAFTNet): a new approach to collaborative research in fetal diagnosis and therapy. *Semin Fetal Neonatal Med.* 2010;**15**: 52–57.

9. Moise KJ, Moldenhauer JS, Bennett KA, et al. Current selection criteria and perioperative therapy used for fetal myelomeningocele surgery. *Obstet Gynecol.* 2016;**127**(3):593–597.

10. Guidelines for Perinatal Care. 8th Edition. American Academy of Pediatrics and American College of Obstetricians and Gynecologists; 2017.

11. Crombleholme TM, D'Alton M, Cendron M, et al. Prenatal diagnosis and the pediatric surgeon: the impact of prenatal consultation on perinatal management. *J Pediatr Surg.* 1996;**31**:156–163.

12. Coleman BG, Adzick NS, Crombleholme TM, et al. Fetal therapy state of the art. *J Ultrasound Med.* 2002;**21**:1257–1288.

13. Didier RA, DeBari SE, Oliver ER, et al. Secondary imaging findings in prenatal diagnosis and characterization of congenital diaphragmatic hernia: abnormal orientation of vascular structures and gallbladder position. *J Ultrasound Med.* 2019;**38**:1449–1456.

14. Keswani SG, Crombleholme TM, Rychik J, et al. Impact of continuous intraoperative monitoring on outcomes in open fetal surgery. *Fetal Diagn Ther.* 2005;**20**:316–320.

15. Rychik J, Cohen D, Tran KM, et al. The role of echocardiography in the intraoperative management of the fetus undergoing myelomeningocele repair. *Fetal Diagn Ther.* 2015;**37**:172–178.

16. Miquel-Verges F, Woods SL, Aucott SW, et al. Prenatal consultation with a neonatologist for congenital anomalies: parental perceptions. *Pediatrics.* 2009;**124**: e573–e579.

17. Besuner P, Imhoff S. The fetal patient: coordinated care for families. *Newborn Infant Nurs Rev.* 2007;7:211–215.

18. Adzick NS, Thom EA, Spong CY, et al. A randomized trial of prenatal versus postnatal repair of myelomeningocele. *N Engl J Med.* 2011;**364**(11):993–1004.

19. Cole JCM, Moldenhauer JS, Jones TR, et al. A proposed model for perinatal palliative care. *J Obstet Gynecol Neonatal Nurs.* 2017;**46**(6):904–911. Doi: 10.1016/j.jogn.2017.01.014.

20. Cole JCM, Olkkola M, Zarrin H, et al. Universal postpartum mental health screening for parents of newborns with prenatally diagnosed birth defects. *J Obstet Gynecol Neonatal Nurs.* 2018;**47**(1):84–93. Doi: 10.1016/j.jogn.2017.04.131.

21. Adzick NS. Open fetal surgery for life-threatening fetal anomalies. *Semin Fetal Neonatal Med.* 2010;**15**:1–8.

22. Lin EE, Tran KM. Anesthesia for fetal surgery. *Semin Pediatr Surg.* 2013;**22**:50–55.

23. Sviggum HP, Kodali BS. Maternal anesthesia for fetal surgery. *Clin Perinatol.* 2013;**40**:413–427.

24. Brusseau R, Mizarhi-Arnaud A. Fetal anesthesia and pain management for intrauterine therapy. *Clin Perinatol.* 2013;**40**:429–442.

25. Oliveira E, Pereira P, Retroz C, et al. Anesthesia for EXIT procedure (ex utero intrapartum treatment) in congenital cervical malformation – a challenge to the anesthesiologist. *Braz J Anesthesiol.* 2015;**65**:529–533.

26. Braden A, Maani C, Nagy C. Anesthetic management of an ex utero intrapartum treatment procedure: a novel balanced approach. *J Clin Anesth.* 2016;**31**:60–63.

27. Helfer DC, Clivatti J, Yamashita AM, et al. Anesthesia for ex utero intrapartum treatment (EXIT procedure) in fetus with prenatal diagnosis of oral and cervical malformations: case reports. *Rev Bras Anestesiol.* 2012;**62**:411–423.

28. Saracoglu A, Saracoglu KT, Alatas I, Kafali H. Secrets of anesthesia in fetoscopic surgery. *Trends Anesth Crit Care.* 2015;**5**:179–183.

29. Wilson RD, Johnson MP, Crombleholme TM, et al. Chorioamniotic membrane separation following open fetal surgery: Pregnancy outcome. *Fetal Diagn Ther.* 2003;**18**:314–320.

30. Deprest J, Brady P, Nicolaides K, et al. Prenatal management of the fetus with isolated congenital diaphragmatic hernia in the era of the TOTAL trial. *Semin Fetal Neonatal Med.* 2014;**19**:338–348.

31. Ville Y. Fetal therapy: practical ethical considerations. *Prenat Diagn.* 2011;**31**:621–627.

32. Johnson A, Luks FI. A cautionary note on new fetal interventions. *Obstet Gynecol.* 2014;**2**:411–415.

33. Moldenhauer JS, Soni S, Rintoul NE, et al. Fetal myelomeningocele repair: the post-MOMS experience at the Children's Hospital of Philadelphia. *Fetal Diagn Ther.* 2014;**37**:235–240.

34. Goldberg DJ, Dodds K, Rychik J. New concepts: development of a survivorship programme for patients with a functionally univentricular heart. *Cardiol Young.* 2011;**2**:77–79.

35. Danzer E, Hoffman C, D'Agostino JA, et al. Neurodevelopmental outcomes at 5 years of age in congenital diaphragmatic hernia. *J Pediatr Surg.* 2017;**52**(3):437–443. doi: 10.1016/j.jpedsurg.2016.08.008.

36. Wilson RD, Johnson MP, Flake AW, et al. Reproductive outcomes after pregnancy complicated by maternal-fetal surgery. *Am J Obstet Gynecol.* 2004;**191**:1430–1436.

Chapter 5

Intrauterine Transfusion

Saul Snowise and Ranu Jain

Background

The history of fetal and neonatal anemia resulting from alloimmunization, better known as hemolytic disease of the fetus and newborn (HDFN), is a lesson in how modern medicine can both treat and prevent serious perinatal morbidity and mortality. In the 1950s, HDFN resulted in stillbirths in 15% of affected patients.[1] Today, serial intrauterine transfusions (IUT) for the treatment of severe HDFN result in survival in over 90% of cases. Additionally, medical therapies such as the administration of Rhesus immunoglobulin (RhIg), plasmapheresis, and intravenous immunoglobulin (IVIG) treatment have decreased the incidence and severity of HDFN.

Liley[2] was the first to report in 1963, on the successful intraperitoneal fetal transfusion of donor red blood cells for treatment of severely affected fetuses that were too premature for delivery.[2] This was followed by the work of Rodeck who was the first to report in 1981 on the successful intravascular approach to fetal transfusions, which is the current cornerstone of modern therapy for severely affected fetuses with HDFN.[3]

The incidence of HDFN ranges from 1/300–1/600 live births[4] and despite the improvement in outcomes, intravascular fetal transfusion remains a highly technical procedure. The average diameter of the umbilical vein ranges from 3 mm at 18 weeks to 7 mm at 34 weeks.[5] Placing a 20–22 gauge needle into such a small target via the maternal abdomen with respiratory movements, through a contractile uterus, and adjacent to an active fetus requires a skilled operator and appropriate sedation and/or anesthesia to relax both the maternal and fetal patient.

This chapter will address the appropriate patient selection, technique, and anesthetic approach to intrauterine fetal transfusion necessary to minimize complications and maximize maternal, fetal, and also neonatal outcomes.

Epidemiology

Fetal red blood cells express antigens by 30 days of gestation, half of these are paternally derived and may be foreign to the maternal immune system. Exposure of a Rhesus D negative mother to paternal antigen can result in alloimmunization and the production of maternal antibodies that cross the placenta, mark fetal red blood cells for destruction, and ultimately result in HDFN.

Spontaneous feto-maternal hemorrhage does occur in almost all pregnancies, with an increasing frequency and volume as gestation progresses.[6] Antepartum hemorrhage during or prior to birth is thought to be the primary cause of feto-maternal hemorrhage, but a list of potential precipitating events is shown in Table 5.1.

Table 5.1 Potential causes of alloimmunization

Unprovoked	Provoked
Idiopathic-spontaneous	Termination of pregnancy
Delivery	Amniocentesis
Spontaneous abortion	Chorionic villus sampling
Ectopic pregnancy	Cordocentesis
Abruption	External cephalic version
Antepartum hemorrhage	Fetal intervention – fetoscopy, shunt, drainage
	Trauma
	Manual removal of placenta

Table 5.2 Prevalence of Rh (D)-negative blood type in different ethnic populations

Ethnicity	% Rh(D)-negative
Basque	30–35
White – North American and European	15
African-American	8
African	4–6
Indian	5
Native North American/Inuit Eskimo	1–2
Japanese	0.3
Thai	0.3
Chinese	0.3

The likelihood of an antibody causing HDFN is dependent on the amount and type of antibody produced, the transport of the antibody across the placenta to the fetus, and the fetal response to the antibody. The antibodies most associated with HDFN are Rh (D), Rh (c), and Kell, but other antibodies, such as Rh (e), Rh (E), Duffy, and Kidd, have also been shown to be associated with moderate to severe HDFN. The prevalence of Rh (D) negative individuals varies greatly with about 1/3 of the Basque population being Rh (D) negative, but only 0.3% of the Chinese population being affected[7] (Table 5.2). The relative incidence of Rh (D) alloimmunization has decreased with the routine administration of Rh (D) immunoglobulin to Rh (D) negative mothers. A prospective study of 300,000 women in the Netherlands, showed that the antibodies most commonly associated with HDFN in decreasing order, were anti-E, anti-D, anti-Kell, and anti-c antibodies.[8]

Patient Selection

Diagnosis

All pregnant patients with a positive indirect Coombs test are at risk for HDFN. In this test maternal plasma is incubated with indicator red blood cells with a known antigenicity. The red blood cells are then washed and suspended in antihuman globulin, or Coombs serum. Cells coated with maternal antibody will agglutinate, and the visualization of this clumping is considered a positive test. The maternal plasma is then diluted successively to determine the level of antibody response. This is reported as the reciprocal of the last dilution tube that demonstrates evidence of visual clumping. For example, a titer of 32 is equivalent to the disappearance of clumping at a 1:64 dilution of the maternal plasma.

The American Association of Blood Banks (AABB) recommends screening of all pregnant women for maternal antibodies at the first prenatal visit and for all women without evidence of alloimmunization to have a repeat screening later in the gestation. The American Board of Obstetrics and Gynecology states that follow-up screening for maternal antibodies should be left at the discretion of the treating physician.

Determination of Fetal Risk

Once a positive maternal titer has been established further tests should be undertaken to establish the fetal risk of developing HDFN. Paternal zygosity testing should first be undertaken to see if the father carries the offending antigen, and if he does, to evaluate if he is homozygous or heterozygous for the antigen. If the paternal testing is negative for the antigen, no further evaluation of the pregnancy with regards to alloimmunization is needed. If paternity testing demonstrates the father is homozygous for the antigen of interest, the fetus is definitely at risk of developing HDFN and should be followed later as described below. The most challenging scenario is if paternity testing demonstrates heterozygosity for the antigen of interest, resulting in a 50% chance that the fetus carries the antigen of interest. In this case the options for determination of fetal antigen status and subsequent risk are either obtaining cell-free DNA (cfDNA) testing if available or performing amniocentesis for the direct evaluation of fetal cells.

Testing for fetal Rh (D) status can be evaluated by fetal cfDNA sequences in the maternal plasma with a 99.1% sensitivity for detection of the fetal Rh (D) status. Testing should be performed after 10 weeks' gestation to ensure an adequate fetal fraction of cfDNA and combinations of assays for the detection of exons 4, 5, 7, and 10 on the Rh (D) gene are recommended.[9-14] In the absence of these exons the fetus can be assumed to be Rh (D) negative and no further testing is required. Currently in the United States cfDNA testing for fetal antigen status is only available for Rh (D) status, but assays for Kell, Rh (E), Rh (C), and Rh (c) fetal blood typing are available in Europe.[15-17] The importance of any test screening for alloimmunization is that a false-negative diagnosis, or reporting of a Rh (D) positive fetus as Rh (D) negative, should be low. A recent prospective observational study in Rh (D) negative patients demonstrated a false-positive rate of 1.54% (95% CI 0.42–5.44%) in the accurate identification of the fetal Rh (D) status. On review the single false-negative result in this study was noted to result from an error in the labeling of samples and not from any inaccuracy in the test.[18]

In situations where cfDNA testing is not available, polymerase chain reaction (PCR) of uncultured amniocytes obtained from an amniocentesis can be used to determine the fetal antigen status. A transplacental approach to obtain fluid should be avoided if possible as this may stimulate the maternal immune response and increase the severity of alloimmunization.[19] In addition, chorionic villus biopsy should be avoided for fetal genotype testing because of similar concerns. While the timing of an amniocentesis in this situation can be dependent on patient and physician preferences, it can also be performed at a later time when a "critical titer" is reached. The critical titer, when detected, is the suggested timing to initiate direct fetal monitoring for possible anemia. If the information obtained from the amniocentesis demonstrates that the fetus is not at risk for HDFN, then unnecessary screening and possible intervention can be prevented.

Of importance, it should be noted that erroneous identification of paternity occurs in 2–5% of all pregnancies[20] and this topic should be addressed cautiously not only to avoid offending the patient, but also to ensure correct risk stratification for the fetus.[21]

Screening for Anemia

Once a fetus has been determined to be at risk for HDFN, monitoring with serial maternal antibody titers should be initiated. Maternal antibody titers should be repeated at least monthly and repeated within shorter intervals when rising titers are detected. The same laboratory should be used to ensure consistent results.

The critical titer is defined as the maternal antibody titer at which the fetus is at risk of developing severe anemia and possibly hydrops. It is at this time that interrogation with fetal ultrasound should be initiated. Most institutions use a critical titer of either 16 or 32 for red cell alloimmunization cases other than those secondary to anti-Kell. Because of the erythroid precursor suppression that occurs with Kell alloimmunization, a critical titer of eight should prompt the initiation of fetal observation.[22–24] If the fetal blood type has not been determined, amniocentesis or cfDNA for the confirmation of the fetal blood type should be considered when a critical titer level is reached as titers can rise even when the fetus is antigen negative.

Ultrasound surveillance for fetal anemia is based on interrogation of the <u>m</u>iddle <u>c</u>erebral <u>a</u>rtery <u>p</u>eak <u>s</u>ystolic <u>v</u>elocity (MCA-PSV) as it is a sensitive indicator of fetal anemia from any cause.[25–30] The theory behind its accuracy in predicting anemia severity is that the anemic fetus preserves the brain by increasing cerebral blood flow, this in turn results in an increased velocity of flow through the cerebral vessels. In the seminal study comparing MCA-PSV measurements to fetal blood sampling, Mari et al. demonstrated that an MCA level > 1.5 MoM (multiples of the median), predicted moderate or severe anemia with a sensitivity of 100% (95% CI 86–100%) with or without hydrops, with a false-positive rate of 12%.[26] Since then, MCA-PSV has become widely accepted as the diagnostic tool to detect fetal anemia.

In first affected pregnancies MCA-PSV testing should be initiated at 20 weeks, (18 weeks if Kell alloimmunization), and should be performed every one to two weeks based on the maternal antibody titer and the previous MCA-PSV value.[26] The technique for obtaining the MCA-PSV is important. The fetus should be in a quiescent state as activity can falsely elevate the result.[31,32] In addition, the Doppler angle of interrogation should be as close to zero degrees as possible, although angle correction can be used up to 30 degrees with good correlation with the true velocity.[33] Finally, the Doppler cursor should be as close as possible to the origin of the MCA from the carotid siphon. (Figure 5.1). MCA-PSV values that remain below 1.5 MoM are consistent with the absence of moderate to severe fetal anemia and no intervention is necessary. The MCA-PSV increases throughout gestation, and calculators to determine the MoM are available at www.perinatology.com.

For second affected pregnancies, anemia may occur as early as 15 weeks.[34] In at risk pregnancies with a previous need for Intra uterine transfusion (IUT), postnatal exchange transfusion, or a history of a perinatal loss secondary to HDFN, early evaluation in an

(a)

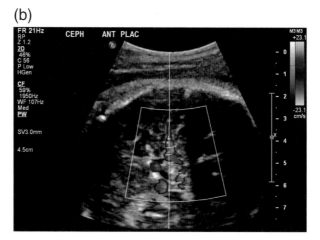

(b)

(c)

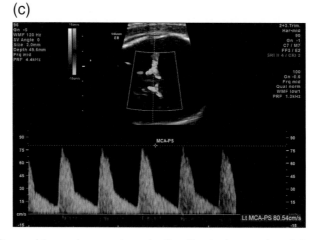

Figure 5.1 (a) Ultrasound image demonstrating color flow Doppler interrogation of the Circle of Willis. (b) Ultrasound image showing the optimal method for obtaining a middle cerebral artery peak systolic velocity (MCA-PSV) Doppler. The pulsed wave Doppler cursor is placed at the origin of the MCA, off the carotid siphon with a close to 0 degree angle of interrogation. (c) Ultrasound image showing the optimal method for obtaining a MCA-PSV Doppler. The MCA spectral tracing demonstrates a uniform MCA-PSV trace. The highest peak on the spectral Doppler tracing is used to determine the MCA-PSV.
Images courtesy of Minneapolis Perinatal Physicians-Midwest Fetal Care Center.

Table 5.3 Nomogram of predicted MCA PSV at the 5th, 10th, 50th 90th, and 95th percentiles and 1.5 MoM for 11–18 weeks' gestational age

GA, wk.	MCA PSV, cm/s					
	5th	10th	50th	90th	95th	1.5 MoM
11	3.2	5.2	10.7	15.2	19.5	16.1
12	4.5	6.5	12.1	16.9	21.2	18.2
13	5.8	7.8	13.6	18.5	22.8	20.3
14	7.1	9.0	15.0	20.2	24.5	22.4
15	8.4	10.3	16.4	21.8	26.1	24.5
16	9.8	11.5	17.8	23.4	27.7	26.7
17	11.1	12.8	19.2	25.1	29.4	28.8

Adapted from Tongsong et al. *J Ultrasound Med.* 2007;26:1013–1017.

experienced, qualified center with the initiation of weekly MCA-PSV Dopplers from as early as 15 weeks should be considered. As the above MCA calculators only have values from 18 weeks' gestation, Tongsong et al.[35] have published data on early normal MCA-PSV measurements in prenatal patients being screened for fetal anemia secondary to alpha thalassemia (Table 5.3).[35]

Pre-Procedure

Timing

An MCA-PSV measurement greater than 1.5 MoM after 18 weeks and before 35 weeks' gestation should initiate fetal blood sampling with the intention to transfuse with blood if fetal anemia is confirmed. Before 18 weeks the fetal vessels are too small to allow reliable access and after 35 weeks' gestation, delivery is preferred to fetal blood sampling because of the risk-benefit ratio in favor of delivery compared to prematurity.[36] For cases of early onset fetal anemia, that is earlier than 18 weeks' gestation, intraperitoneal transfusion is a treatment option and is discussed later.

Setting and Staff

Fetal blood sampling and IUT should be undertaken adjacent to, or in an operating theater once a viable gestation is attained, to allow for delivery if necessary. A maternal-fetal medicine specialist or another qualified physician with experience in fetal transfusion should lead the team. The staff should also include an experienced sonographer, one to two nurses, and an assistant physician or physician's assistant to manage the delivery of the blood products.[37–40] Direct access to an automated hemocytometer to rapidly determine the fetal levels of hemoglobin and hematocrit is optimal to minimize the intervention time. Depending on the center where the transfusion occurs, blood bank staff may run the hemocytometer and the anesthesiologist managing maternal sedation may also be responsible for setting up the fetal blood and managing delivery to the surgical field. Regardless of the gestational age or location, an aseptic technique should be used.

Maternal Preparation

For fetuses with a nonviable gestation, no specific maternal therapy is indicated. Prophylactic antibiotic consisting of 1–2 g of a first generation cephalosporin is administered one hour prior to the procedure in some centers, although there is no evidence that this reduces the risk of infection.[39,41–43] For viable fetuses, a neonatology consultation should be obtained and betamethasone should be administered, ideally greater than 48 hours prior to the procedure. The mothers should also be fasted if the decision is to proceed with cesarean delivery in the setting of fetal distress unresponsive to intrauterine resuscitation. Tocolytic medications, such as terbutaline 0.25 mg or indomethacin, may also be administered to reduce uterine contractility.

Blood Preparation

All donor units of red blood cells are cross-matched to maternal blood to prevent the risk of sensitization to new antibodies. It is advisable to perform an extended cross-match as this has been shown to drastically reduce the likelihood of the production of new antibodies to the Duffy, Kidd, and S antigens.[44] Donor units should be less than seven days old to maximize 2,3-diphosphoglycerate levels,[45] irradiated to prevent graft-versus-host reaction,[46] and also be cytomegalovirus (CMV) negative or at the minimum, leukodepleted, to reduce the risk of CMV infection if CMV negative blood is not available. The blood must also be washed and concentrated to a final hematocrit of 75–85% to minimize the volume administered to the fetus. Maternal donor units can be considered for fetal transfusion if the patient has a pre-donation hemoglobin above 12.5 g/dL and all other prerequisites for autologous donation are met. Maternal donor units reduce the likelihood of new sensitizations, may have a longer half-life, and may be especially helpful in the case of rare antibodies, but they should be used cautiously as there is evidence that they are associated with worse pregnancy outcomes.[47–49]

Anesthesia

Maternal

The mother undergoes numerous physiological changes during pregnancy including changes to the gastrointestinal, pulmonary, cardiovascular, and central nervous systems that are of great importance to the anesthesiologist.[50–52]

As the uterus enlarges, the gastroesophageal junction is shifted superiorly and posteriorly resulting in progressively increased gastroesophageal incompetence and an increased risk of reflux. The pylorus is also displaced and gastric emptying is delayed. Compounding these changes, gastrin is secreted by the placenta resulting in an increased acid content in the stomach. As a result of all these changes the pregnant patient is at increased risk of aspiration of gastric contents and should always be considered to have a full stomach.

Maternal cardiovascular changes must also be considered when taking care of a pregnant patient. Maternal plasma volume increases by 50% by 28–30 weeks' gestation in singleton pregnancies. Maternal heart rate and cardiac output increase correspondingly from very early in gestation. The increased plasma volume associated with the decreased protein production in pregnancy results in a decrease in oncotic pressures which make the pregnant patient vulnerable to fluid retention and pulmonary edema. As a result of compression of the inferior vena cava by the enlarging uterus, especially after 20–24 weeks' gestation, the pregnant patient can experience supine hypotension syndrome via decreased cardiac return when lying flat on their back. This compression can in turn cause fetal hypoxia. The resulting drop in systemic venous return causes a decrease in uterine perfusion and an increase in uterine venous pressure. The gravid uterus can also cause direct compression of the aorta that can further decrease uterine perfusion pressure by direct compression of the uterine blood flow. Left uterine displacement can minimize the effects of aorto-caval compression and should be standard positioning for all pregnant patients on the operating table. This can be accomplished with a wedge under the patient's right flank, tilting of the operating table, or use of both interventions.

Maternal respiratory changes in pregnancy include an increase in minute ventilation by 50% and an increased oxygen consumption which is required to meet the increased metabolic demands of pregnancy. The functional residual capacity decreases by 20% making the pregnant patient susceptible to hypoxia. The increase in minute ventilation results in a mild respiratory alkalosis with a $PaCO_2$ of 3.7–4.3 kPa (28–32 mmHg), which is compensated for by increased renal excretion of bicarbonate.

While general anesthesia will only be required for an emergent cesarean delivery for a viable fetus in distress, the physician needs to be aware that overzealous ventilation can decrease the $PaCO_2$, resulting in a left shift of the oxyhemoglobin curve, and a reduction in oxygen availability to the fetus. Secondary to the increased maternal plasma volume, mucosal capillary engorgement may be present and can create difficulty with intubation of the trachea.

Prior to taking a patient to the operating theater, a complete preoperative history and physical examination of the mother should be performed as well as a baseline blood chemistry and complete blood count.

Intrauterine blood transfusion is performed under maternal local or neuraxial anesthesia, with or without intravenous sedation. General anesthesia is rarely required.

The anesthetic plan is discussed with the patient; this includes monitored anesthetic care and if required, as in the case for emergent cesarean delivery, a general anesthetic. The anesthetic considerations also include the anticipated patient position, and surgeon and patient preference. Preoperative medications should include H-2 blockers and citric acid/sodium citrate to neutralize gastric contents.

The patient is monitored with standard ASA (American Society of Anesthesia) monitors and the fetal heart rate (FHR) is assessed before moving the patient to the operating theater and also continuously during the case using ultrasound. Intraoperative intravenous sedation with remifentanil 0.08–1 mcg/kg/min has been used very effectively with the addition of longer acting opioids, for example fentanyl or sedatives such as midazolam as required by the patient. Intravenous dexmedetomidine loading dose and infusions can also be considered for these procedures. Intravenous sedatives and neuraxial blocks do not provide uterine relaxation but this is rarely required for this procedure. Intravenous fluids should be minimal during this procedure as it is a closed procedure and blood loss is negligible. Perioperative tocolytics may also be administered to the mother so fluid administration should be less than 750 mL to prevent postoperative pulmonary edema. Vasopressors such as phenylephrine and ephedrine should be readily available to maintain hemodynamics if required.

Fetal

Although maternal anesthetics may cross the placenta and have some effect on the fetus, separate anesthesia for the fetus is paramount in reducing the risk of complications during a fetal blood transfusion. A muscle relaxant, delivered either intramuscularly or intravenously, should be administered to the fetus in all cases.[37,53] The intravenous route is preferred as the effect is almost immediate and occurs through the intravascular access established for the fetal blood sampling and transfusion procedure. Relaxation of the fetus reduces the risk of needle dislodgement from fetal movement and has also been shown to decrease the incidence of FHR changes by 80%.[54] Atracurium (0.4 mg/kg) and vecuronium (0.1 mg/kg) are the muscle relaxants most commonly utilized.[49,55–57] Where available, pancuronium (0.1 mg/kg) is also an option, but this has been associated with fetal cardiovascular side effects.[58] Fetal nociception is present from 24–28 weeks' gestation, and medication to reduce any fetal pain or stress response should be considered.[59] Therefore fentanyl (2–10 µg/kg) can be administered to the fetus in combination with the muscle relaxant of choice. Some practitioners also add atropine 20 µg/kg. All these medications are typically administered to the fetus together in a single syringe. There is no evidence, however, to demonstrate a reduction in the fetal stress response with these medications and some believe that the stress response noted during intrauterine fetal transfusion is secondary to volume expansion and independent of the needle insertion.[60,61]

Procedure

Fetal Access Site

The goal of fetal transfusion is to obtain intravascular access, preferably through a vein. Access to the fetal circulation via the umbilical artery is associated with an increased risk of spasm, subsequent fetal bradycardia,[54,62] and an increased risk of other complications that will be discussed later.[53,54] The exact site of intravenous access depends on gestational age, fetal and placental position, the presence or absence of ascites, and operator preference.

The most common access sites are the placental cord insertion, the intrahepatic portion of the umbilical vein, a "free" loop of cord, and the fetal intraperitoneal space. In extreme circumstances intravascular access via the intracardiac approach has been performed.[53] The placental cord insertion and intrahepatic portion of the fetal umbilical vein have been shown to be the safest points of access.[40,43,53,63,64] Centers in North America tend to prefer the placental cord insertion site, especially in the case of an anterior placenta, while most European centers use the intrahepatic approach secondary to similar or lower reported fetal loss rates compared to transfusion via the placental cord insertion,[54,65] lower rates of fetal bradycardia, and the fact that any bleeding associated with the procedure is likely to be reabsorbed via the fetal peritoneal cavity.[65,66] Arguments against the intrahepatic approach are that it is more dependent on fetal position, there is an increased potential for fetal pain with subsequent increased levels of noradrenaline, beta endorphin, and cortisol,[67] and an increased risk of fetal trauma.

When access to the placental cord insertion is not possible, a free loop of cord, the intraperitoneal approach, or rarely the intracardiac approach are alternative sites of intravascular access. In late gestation, depending on the fetal position and placental cord insertion site, a free-floating loop of cord may be the only point of access. Use of a free-loop is associated with a three-fold increase in rates of perinatal loss and also fetal bradycardia leading to an emergency cesarean.[54] If a free loop of cord is the only choice, it is suggested that the loop selected is anteriorly adjacent to the uterine wall or against the fetal body to prevent movement of the cord away from the needle during insertion. The use of a 22-gauge needle should also be considered as this may facilitate entry into the cord more easily than a larger 20-gauge needle.

Intraperitoneal transfusion (IPT) is an option with benefits in numerous clinical scenarios. The blood transfused into the fetal peritoneal cavity is absorbed by the subdiaphragmatic lymphatics and the thoracic duct.[68] Intravenous transfusion is clearly superior to IPT, especially in cases of fetal hydrops where the lymphatic function appears to be compromised.[69–72] Intraperitoneal transfusion, however, can be beneficial in cases of fetal anemia which present prior to 18 weeks when vascular access is severely limited. Fox et al.[73] reported on six high-risk pregnancies with alloimmunization, four with previous perinatal losses, who were treated with biweekly intraperitoneal transfusions initiated at 15 weeks' gestation. A total red cell volume of 5 mL of packed red blood cells (RBCs) was transfused up to 18 weeks' gestation and 10 mL was transfused thereafter. Four of the patients also received intravenous immunoglobulin G (IVIG) 0.8 g/kg/week. They reported fetal survival in five of the six gestations.[73] Intraperitoneal transfusion has also shown to be beneficial in a combined approach with intravenous transfusion.[74] Placement of packed RBCs into the fetal peritoneal cavity at the time of intravenous transfusion provides a more stable fetal hematocrit between procedures. The resulting slower decline in hematocrit allows for a longer interval between procedures.[74,75]

Intracardiac transfusion is the final route for consideration when trying to obtain intravenous fetal access. This should be considered a salvage procedure in hydropic fetuses at early gestations where intravenous access through more established routes has been unsuccessful. There are small case series and case reports demonstrating the effectiveness of intracardiac transfusion in this setting.[76,77]

Volume to Transfuse

The total volume of RBCs to transfuse is dependent on the gestational age, the fetal size, the initial fetal hematocrit, and the hematocrit of the RBCs to be transfused. The normal fetal hematocrit increases as gestation progresses ranging from 37 ± 4% at 17 weeks to 43 ± 7% at term.[78] The target final hematocrit should be about 45% in almost all cases.[37,43,55,79] Exceptions to this are fetuses less than 24 weeks with severe anemia (Hct < 10%). The transfused RBC volume in these cases should be limited to prevent cardiovascular strain resulting from a sudden increase in blood viscosity. The final hematocrit should not be increased by more than four-fold over the initial value.[78] A repeat procedure in 48 hours is undertaken in these cases to achieve the usual target fetal hematocrit. In all cases supraphysiologic hematocrit values (50–60%) should be avoided as this can result in an increased incidence of complications.[80,81]

For intravascular transfusion, and assuming the hematocrit of the donor unit is approximately 75–80%, simply multiplying the fetal weight in grams by a coefficient of 0.02 will indicate the volume in milliliters (mL) of donor RBCs to be transfused to increase the fetal hematocrit by 10%.[82]

An additional formula is:

Volume transfused (mL) = [volume of fetoplacental unit (mL) × (final Hct − initial Hct)]/ Hct of transfused blood. The fetoplacental volume = 1.046 + EFW (g) × 0.14.[83] This formula is useful in calculating the final fetal Hct when a final fetal blood sample cannot be obtained.

For IPT, the limiting factor is the resulting increase in intra-abdominal pressure. At 30 weeks the appropriate volume to transfuse into the intraperitoneal space is 100 mL. By adding or subtracting 10 mL for every week of gestation above or below 30 weeks, the volume to place into the peritoneal cavity can be easily determined. For example, the volume for IPT at 29 weeks is 90 mL and the volume at 31 weeks is 110 mL.[84]

Technique

After mapping of the uterus, placental location, placental cord insertion, and fetal lie, continuous ultrasound should be used to guide the placement of a 20- or 22-gauge needle into the planned entry site. There are no data correlating needle size to complications, but we suggest using a 22-gauge needle until 22 weeks' gestation and a 20-gauge needle after that point.[37–40,42]

Once intravenous access is obtained, a sample of fetal blood should be obtained for determination of the initial hematocrit and reticulocyte count. Immediately after collection of the initial blood sample, injection of a combination of medication including a muscle relaxant e.g. vecuronium (0.4 mg/kg) and fentanyl (5–10 mcg/kg), should be administered with visualization of the injected fluid seen coursing through the umbilical vein. Additional confirmation of needle placement is by continued blood flow into the syringe with negative pressure after completion of the medication delivery. After obtaining the initial sample, and administration of the fetal medications, a slow transfusion of donor RBCs should be performed while awaiting the initial fetal Hct result. A closed system for the donor RBCs should be used with sufficient sterile intravenous blood tubing connected to a 20cc syringe via a three-way stop-cock. The line should be cleared of all air prior to the procedure and it is recommended to have a second assistant so the needle operator can focus solely on the needle and vessel. It is important for someone to visually monitor the donor RBC bag and prevent it from emptying so air does not enter the system during the procedure. Intermittent FHR monitoring should also be performed during transfusion of the donor RBCs. This can be accomplished by placing the pulsed-wave Doppler gate on the adjacent umbilical artery, or by looking directly at the fetal heart during pauses in the transfusion to refill the 20cc syringe. If fetal blood is noted to stop streaming through the umbilical vein at any point during the procedure, the FHR should be assessed as bradycardia can signify decreased myocardial function and resultant decreased fetal cardiac output. Decreased myocardial function can also be confirmed by decreased movement of the atrioventricular valves.

If fetal bradycardia occurs, the transfusion should be stopped and the FHR monitored. If there is no resolution of the bradycardia in 30–60 seconds, the needle should be removed and the mother placed in the left lateral position. If the FHR abnormality persists and there is evidence of depressed myocardial function for greater than three minutes, delivery should be considered if the fetus is of viable gestational age.

After completing the transfusion of the appropriate RBC volume, a final fetal blood sample should be drawn to determine the final fetal Hct and a Kleihauer-Betke stain should be sent. A rapid determination of the fetal hematocrit will give reassurance that the desired target hematocrit has been attained prior to removal of the needle. The final Kleihauer-Betke stain result will help to determine the interval until the next transfusion. A Kleihauer-Betke sample demonstrating mostly transfused adult RBCs, with minimal fetal RBCs, signifies that fetal hematopoiesis has been suppressed and indicates that the interval period between procedures can be extended as the rate of fetal Hct decline will be slower. The result of the reticulocyte count from the initial sample can also give further clarification on the fetal hematopoietic status.

After completion of the procedure the patient is monitored until regular fetal movement is noted either by the patient or by ultrasound. In patients at gestational ages past the point of viability, a reassuring nonstress test (NST) is recommended prior to discharging the patient home. All patients should have a postoperative scan as most fetal losses occur within 24 hours of the procedure.

Timing of Subsequent Procedures

The goal of subsequent transfusions is to maintain the fetal Hct above 25%, but the timing of when to perform these procedures is an area of ongoing debate and research. Continued transfusions are necessary secondary to the shorter life span of adult RBCs in the fetal circulation and the increased vascular volume of the growing fetus in the setting of depressed fetal hematopoiesis.[85–87] Some practitioners use empiric intervals based on previous experience: seven to ten days between the first two transfusions, two to three weeks between the second and third transfusions, and three to four weeks between subsequent procedures.

Another method of establishing the intertransfusion interval is based on the theoretical expected decline in the fetal hemoglobin (Hgb) between procedures. An expected rate of decline in Hgb from the final fetal Hgb value obtained at the time of transfusion can be estimated based on the number of transfusions undertaken to that point. A rate of Hgb decline of 0.4 mg/dL/day can be expected between the first and second transfusions, 0.3 mg/dL/day after the second IUT, and 0.2 mg/dL/day after the third IUT. These rates of decline can be used to estimate the intertransfusion interval necessary to prevent the development of severe anemia in the fetus.[88] These values correspond roughly to a decline in Hct of 1% a day. The exception to this is if fetal hydrops is present, as the rate of decline in the fetal Hct has been shown to be accelerated at 1.88%/day compared to 1.08%/day if hydrops is not present.[68]

Other physicians prefer to use the MCA-PSV to determine the timing of subsequent transfusions. There is concern about the ability of the MCA-PSV to accurately diagnose moderate to severe fetal anemia. These concerns have arisen secondary to the inherent rheologic differences between adult and fetal RBCs. Compared to fetal RBCs, adult RBCs are larger, less rigid, and have a different oxygen carrying capacity. Additionally, there is an improvement in fetal hemodynamics and improved oxygen delivery to peripheral tissues after performing a fetal transfusion. Detti et al.[89] evaluated the accuracy of using the MCA-PSV for the evaluation of moderate to severe fetal anemia between the first and second IUTs. They demonstrated that a threshold of 1.69 MoM predicted all cases of severe anemia with a false-positive rate of only 6%.[89] A recent multicenter, randomized trial evaluated the MCA-PSV as a predictor of the need for subsequent fetal transfusion compared to using the predicted daily decrease in fetal Hct as described earlier. The investigators randomized 71 women to either serial MCA-PSV with transfusion for upward trending values greater than 1.5 MoM or to timing of transfusion based on an expected 1% per day decrease in Hct. They found no statistical differences in mean Hgb at birth (MCA-PSV group 103.6 ± 38.2 g/dL, Fetal Hct group 120.3 ± 31.4 g/dL; adjusted mean difference – 15.6; 95% CI -32.4 to 1.3; p=0.070).[90]

Complications

Procedural

The most common complications associated with IUT are fetal bradycardia and bleeding with rare cases of rupture of membranes, preterm delivery, and infection.[91] The risks from transfusion are not consistent across gestation. Transfusions in fetuses of earlier gestation are associated with increased risks secondary to the presence of more severe disease and the increased technical challenges associated with earlier gestation fetuses. There is a reported four-fold increase in the risk of perinatal death and decreased overall survival when an intravascular transfusion is performed before 20–22 weeks' gestation.[92–94] In these early cases, consideration for IPT to buy time until intravenous transfusion is technically more feasible should be considered.[40,79] Although beyond the scope of this chapter, the utility of immune modulation with IVIG should also be considered in patients with a history of severe disease. In early-onset, severe alloimmunization cases, immunomodulation, consisting of plasmapheresis followed by weekly IVIG has been shown to be effective in delaying the gestational age at which fetal transfusions need to be initiated, resulting in overall improved fetal survival.[79,95]

Zwiers et al.[53] reported on the complications from a single series of 1,678 intravascular transfusions in 589 fetuses from a single institution including umbilical vein (n=798), intrahepatic (n=552), umbilical artery (n=24), and IPT (n=5). The total complication rate was 3.1%, with transient bradycardia being the single most common complication. The authors found gestational age to be an independent predictor of poor outcomes with a procedural loss rate of 5.6% before 20 weeks versus an overall procedural loss rate of 0.9%. The presence of fetal hydrops was also strongly associated with increased risks. Transfusion in hydropic fetuses was associated with a complication rate of 3.8% and procedure-related death rate of 2.5% versus non-hydropic fetuses (2.9% and 1.4%, respectively).[53]

Other factors that have been shown to increase the risks of complications during intravascular transfusions include the absence of muscle relaxant administration to the fetus for the procedure,[54] use of a free loop of cord,[43,54] operator experience,[43,96] and an increased severity of anemia.[41]

Safety data on IPT have also been reported. Watts et al.[97] described 77 IPT without any deaths, need for urgent delivery, or long-term sequelae. They did, however, report two colon infusions, two retroperitoneal transfusions, and one abdominal wall hematoma.[97]

Long-Term

Neonates that have undergone IUT have an increased risk of requiring "top up" transfusions secondary to the aforementioned decreased hematopoiesis that accompanies serial transfusions. This is further exacerbated by the persistence of maternal antibodies in the neonatal circulation.[98,99] Roughly 50% of neonates will require a top up transfusion by one month of age.[99] Delayed cord clamping at time of delivery is recommended to help increase the fetal Hgb in neonates who have undergone serial transfusions.[100]

The development of new maternal antibodies also poses long-term risks to future pregnancies with 19–26% of patients developing new antibodies from the donor RBCs. Expanded screening as described earlier may beneficially impact this issue.

Outcomes

Excellent neonatal outcomes are reported in high-volume centers with overall survival rates of 94% for non-hydropic fetuses and 74% for hydropic fetuses.[49] The largest single series in the literature is the previously referenced study by Zwiers et al.[53] The total 1,678 procedures performed between 1988 and 2014 included 798 transfusions via the umbilical vein at the cord insertion, 552 via the intrahepatic umbilical vein, 280 via the transamniotic umbilical vein (insertion at posterior placenta or free loop), 24 via the umbilical artery, 10 intraperitoneal, and one intracardiac transfusion.[53] The authors reported a 93% overall survival rate that decreased to 78% when hydrops was present. The overall perinatal loss rate decreased over the course of the study period from 1.6% per procedure in the first half, to 0.6% from 2001 onwards.

The Long-term neurodevelopmental outcome after intrauterine transfusion for hemolytic disease of the fetus/newborn (LOTUS) trial,[101] evaluated 451 fetuses who underwent 1,284 transfusions over the course of 20 years. At eight years of age they noted the presence of an isolated severe developmental delay in 1.7% of subjects who underwent a transfusion that was similar to the general population. The investigators also detected a higher level of cerebral palsy (0.7%) in the study population and noted that severe hydrops was also associated with a higher rate of neurodevelopmental impairment.[101]

References

1. Fairweather DV, Tacchi D, Coxon A, et al. Intrauterine transfusion in Rh-isoimmunization. *Br Med J.* 1967;4:189–194.

2. Liley AW. Intrauterine transfusion of foetus in haemolytic disease. *Br Med J.* 1963;2:1107–1109.

3. Rodeck CH, Kemp JR, Holman CA, et al. Direct intravascular fetal blood transfusion by fetoscopy in severe Rhesus isoimmunization. *Lancet.* 1981;1:625–627.

4. Hendrickson JE, Delaney M. Hemolytic disease of the fetus and newborn: modern practice and future investigations. *Transfus Med Rev.* 2016;30:159–164.

5. Weissman A, Jakobi P, Bronshtein M, Goldstein I. Sonographic measurements of the umbilical cord and vessels during normal pregnancies. *J Ultrasound Med.* 1994;13:11–14.

6. Medearis AL, Hensleigh PA, Parks DR, Herzenberg LA. Detection of fetal erythrocytes in maternal blood post partum with the fluorescence-activated cell sorter. *Am J Obstet Gynecol.* 1984;148:290–295.

7. Zipursky A, Paul VK. The global burden of Rh disease. *Arch Dis Child Fetal Neonatal Ed.* 2011;96(2):F84–85.

8. Koelewijn JM, Vrijkotte TG, van der Schoot CE, et al. Effect of screening for red cell antibodies, other than anti-D, to detect hemolytic disease of the fetus and newborn: a population study in the Netherlands. *Transfusion.* 2008;48:941–952.

9. Bombard AT, Akolekar R, Farkas DH, et al. Fetal RHD genotype detection from circulating cell-free fetal DNA in maternal plasma in non-sensitized RhD negative women. *Prenat Diagn.* 2011;31:802–808.

10. Daniels G, van der Schoot CE, Olsson ML. Report of the First International Workshop

on molecular blood group genotyping. *Vox Sang.* 2005;**88**:136–142.

11. Pirelli KJ, Pietz BC, Johnson ST, et al. Molecular determination of RHD zygosity: predicting risk of hemolytic disease of the fetus and newborn related to anti-D. *Prenat Diagn.* 2010;**30**:1207–1212.

12. Singleton BK, Green CA, Avent ND, et al. The presence of an RHD pseudogene containing a 37 base pair duplication and a nonsense mutation in Africans with the Rh D-negative blood group phenotype. *Blood.* 2000;**95**:12–18.

13. Tynan JA, Angkachatchai V, Ehrich M, et al. Multiplexed analysis of circulating cell-free fetal nucleic acids for noninvasive prenatal diagnostic RHD testing. *Am J Obstet Gynecol.* 2011;**204**:251.e1–6.

14. Wikman AT, Tiblad E, Karlsson A, et al. Noninvasive single-exon fetal RHD determination in a routine screening program in early pregnancy. *Obstet Gynecol.* 2012;**120**:227–234.

15. Finning K, Martin P, Summers J, Daniels G. Fetal genotyping for the K (Kell) and Rh C, c, and E blood groups on cell-free fetal DNA in maternal plasma. *Transfusion.* 2007;**47**:2126–2133.

16. Gutensohn K, Muller SP, Thomann K, et al. Diagnostic accuracy of noninvasive polymerase chain reaction testing for the determination of fetal rhesus C, c and E status in early pregnancy. *BJOG.* 2010;**117**:722–729.

17. Li Y, Finning K, Daniels G, et al. Noninvasive genotyping fetal Kell blood group (KEL1) using cell-free fetal DNA in maternal plasma by MALDI-TOF mass spectrometry. *Prenat Diagn.* 2008;**28**:203–208.

18. Moise KJ, Jr., Gandhi M, Boring NH, et al. Circulating cell-free DNA to determine the fetal RHD status in all three trimesters of pregnancy. *Obstet Gynecol.* 2016;**128**:1340–1346.

19. Moise KJ, Jr., Carpenter RJ, Jr. Increased severity of fetal hemolytic disease with known rhesus alloimmunization after first-trimester transcervical chorionic

villus biopsy. *Fetal Diagn Ther.* 1990;**5**:76–78.

20. Le Roux MG, Pascal O, Andre MT, et al. Non-paternity and genetic counselling. *Lancet.* 1992;**340**:607.

21. Rothenberg JM, Weirermiller B, Dirig K, et al. Is a third-trimester antibody screen in Rh+ women necessary? *Am J Manag Care.* 1999;**5**:1145–1150.

22. Bowman JM, Pollock JM, Manning FA, et al. Maternal Kell blood group alloimmunization. *Obstet Gynecol.* 1992;**79**:239–244.

23. McKenna DS, Nagaraja HN, O'Shaughnessy R. Management of pregnancies complicated by anti-Kell isoimmunization. *Obstet Gynecol.* 1999;**93**:667–673.

24. van Wamelen DJ, Klumper FJ, de Haas M, et al. Obstetric history and antibody titer in estimating severity of Kell alloimmunization in pregnancy. *Obstet Gynecol.* 2007;**109**:1093–1098.

25. Mari G. Middle cerebral artery peak systolic velocity: is it the standard of care for the diagnosis of fetal anemia? *J Ultrasound Med.* 2005;**24**:697–702.

26. Mari G, Deter RL, Carpenter RL, et al. Noninvasive diagnosis by Doppler ultrasonography of fetal anemia due to maternal red-cell alloimmunization. Collaborative Group for Doppler Assessment of the Blood Velocity in Anemic Fetuses. *N Engl J Med.* 2000;**342**:9–14.

27. Moise KJ, Jr. The usefulness of middle cerebral artery Doppler assessment in the treatment of the fetus at risk for anemia. *Am J Obstet Gynecol.* 2008;**198**(161).e1–4.

28. Oepkes D, Seaward PG, Vandenbussche FP, et al. Doppler ultrasonography versus amniocentesis to predict fetal anemia. *N Engl J Med.* 2006;**355**:156–164.

29. Pretlove SJ, Fox CE, Khan KS, Kilby MD. Noninvasive methods of detecting fetal anaemia: a systematic review and meta-analysis. *BJOG.* 2009;**116**:1558–1567.

30. van Dongen H, Klumper FJ, Sikkel E, Vandenbussche FP, Oepkes D. Non-invasive tests to predict fetal anemia in Kell-alloimmunized pregnancies. *Ultrasound Obstet Gynecol.* 2005;25:341–345.

31. Sallout BI, Fung KF, Wen SW, Medd LM, Walker MC. The effect of fetal behavioral states on middle cerebral artery peak systolic velocity. *Am J Obstet Gynecol.* 2004;**191**:1283–1287.

32. Shono M, Shono H, Ito Y, et al. The effect of behavioral states on fetal heart rate and middle cerebral artery flow-velocity waveforms in normal full-term fetuses. *Int J Gynaecol Obstet.* 1997;**58**:275–280.

33. Ruma MS, Swartz AE, Kim E, et al. Angle correction can be used to measure peak systolic velocity in the fetal middle cerebral artery. *Am J Obstet Gynecol.* 2009;**200**:397. e1-3.

34. MacKenzie IZ, MacLean DA, Fry A, Evans SL. Midtrimester intrauterine exchange transfusion of the fetus. *Am J Obstet Gynecol.* 1982;**143**:555–559.

35. Tongsong T, Wanapirak C, Sirichotiyakul S, et al. Middle cerebral artery peak systolic velocity of healthy fetuses in the first half of pregnancy. *J Ultrasound Med.* 2007;**26**:1013–1017.

36. Klumper FJ, van Kamp IL, Vandenbussche FP, et al. Benefits and risks of fetal red-cell transfusion after 32 weeks gestation. *Eur J Obstet Gynecol Reprod Biol.* 2000;**92**:91–96.

37. van Kamp IL, Klumper FJ, Meerman RH, et al. Treatment of fetal anemia due to red-cell alloimmunization with intrauterine transfusions in the Netherlands, 1988–1999. *Acta Obstet Gynecol Scand.* 2004;**83**:731–737.

38. Guilbaud L, Garabedian C, Cortey A, et al. In utero treatment of severe fetal anemia resulting from fetomaternal red blood cell incompatibility: a comparison of simple transfusion and exchange transfusion. *Eur J Obstet Gynecol Reprod Biol.* 2016;**201**:85–88.

39. Society for Maternal-Fetal Medicine. (SMFM) Clinical Guideline #8: the fetus at risk for anemia–diagnosis and management. *Am J Obstet Gynecol.* 2015;**212**:697–710.

40. Tiblad E, Kublickas M, Ajne G, et al. Procedure-related complications and perinatal outcome after intrauterine transfusions in red cell alloimmunization in Stockholm. *Fetal Diagn Ther.* 2011;**30**:266–273.

41. Osanan GC, Silveira Reis ZN, Apocalypse IG, et al. Predictive factors of perinatal mortality in transfused fetuses due to maternal alloimmunization: what really matters? *J Maternal Fetal Neonatal Med.* 2012;**25**:1333–1337.

42. Deka D, Dadhwal V, Sharma AK, et al. Perinatal survival and procedure-related complications after intrauterine transfusion for red cell alloimmunization. *Arch Gynecol Obstet.* 2016;**293**:967–973.

43. Johnstone-Ayliffe C, Prior T, Ong C, et al. Early procedure-related complications of fetal blood sampling and intrauterine transfusion for fetal anemia. *Acta Obstet Gynecol Scand.* 2012;**91**:458–462.

44. Schonewille H, Prinsen-Zander KJ, Reijnart M, et al. Extended matched intrauterine transfusions reduce maternal Duffy, Kidd, and S antibody formation. *Transfusion.* 2015;**55**:2912–2919; quiz 1.

45. Fung M. *Technical Manual of the American Association of Blood Banks*, 18th ed., Bethesda, Maryland: American Association of Blood Banks; 2014.

46. el-Azeem SA, Samuels P, Rose RL, et al. The effect of the source of transfused blood on the rate of consumption of transfused red blood cells in pregnancies affected by red blood cell alloimmunization. *Am J Obstet Gynecol.* 1997;**177**:753–757.

47. Gonsoulin WJ, Moise KJ, Jr., Milam JD, et al. Serial maternal blood donations for intrautcrinc transfusion. *Obstet Gynecol.* 1990;**75**:158–162.

48. Bleile MJ, Rijhsinghani A, Dwyre DM, Raife TJ. Successful use of maternal blood in the management of severe hemolytic disease of the fetus and newborn due to

anti-Kp(b). *Transfus Apher Sci.* 2010;**43**:281–283.

49. Schumacher B, Moise KJ, Jr. Fetal transfusion for red blood cell alloimmunization in pregnancy. *Obstet Gynecol.* 1996;**88**:137–150.

50. Gaiser RR, Kurth CD. Anesthetic considerations for fetal surgery. *Semin Perinatol.* 1999;**23**:507–514.

51. Okamoto M, Walewski JL, Artusio JF, Jr., Riker WF, Jr. Neuromuscular pharmacology in rat neonates: development of responsiveness to prototypic blocking and reversal drugs. *Anesth Analg.* 1992;**75**:361–371.

52. Shearer ES, Fahy LT, O'Sullivan EP, Hunter JM. Transplacental distribution of atracurium, laudanosine and monoquaternary alcohol during elective caesarean section. *Br J Anaesth.* 1991;**66**:551–556.

53. Zwiers C, Lindenburg ITM, Klumper FJ, et al. Complications of intrauterine intravascular blood transfusion: lessons learned after 1678 procedures. *Ultrasound Obstet Gynecol.* 2017;**50**:180–186.

54. Van Kamp IL, Klumper FJ, Oepkes D, et al. Complications of intrauterine intravascular transfusion for fetal anemia due to maternal red-cell alloimmunization. *Am J Obstet Gynecol.* 2005;**192**:171–177.

55. Moise KJ, Jr. Management of rhesus alloimmunization in pregnancy. *Obstet Gynecol.* 2002;**100**:600–611.

56. Moise KJ, Jr., Deter RL, Kirshon B, et al. Intravenous pancuronium bromide for fetal neuromuscular blockade during intrauterine transfusion for red-cell alloimmunization. *Obstet Gynecol.* 1989;**74**:905–908.

57. Leveque C, Murat I, Toubas F, et al. Fetal neuromuscular blockade with vecuronium bromide: studies during intravascular intrauterine transfusion in isoimmunized pregnancies. *Anesthesiology.* 1992;**76**:642–644.

58. Mouw RJ, Klumper F, Hermans J, et al. Effect of atracurium or pancuronium on the anemic fetus during and directly after

intravascular intrauterine transfusion. A double blind randomized study. *Acta Obstet Gynecol Scand.* 1999;**78**:763–767.

59. Fisk NM, Gitau R, Teixeira JM, et al. Effect of direct fetal opioid analgesia on fetal hormonal and hemodynamic stress response to intrauterine needling. *Anesthesiology.* 2001;**95**:828–835.

60. Adama van Scheltema PN, Borkent S, Sikkel E, et al. Fetal brain hemodynamic changes in intrauterine transfusion: influence of needle puncture site. *Fetal Diagn Ther.* 2009;**26**:131–133.

61. Adama van Scheltema PN, Pasman SA, Wolterbeek R, et al. Fetal stress hormone changes during intrauterine transfusions. *Prenat Diagn.* 2011;**31**:555–559.

62. Weiner CP, Wenstrom KD, Sipes SL, Williamson RA. Risk factors for cordocentesis and fetal intravascular transfusion. *Am J Obstet Gynecol.* 1991;**165**:1020–1025.

63. Pasman SA, Claes L, Lewi L, et al. Intrauterine transfusion for fetal anemia due to red blood cell alloimmunization: 14 years experience in Leuven. *Facts Views Vis Obgyn.* 2015;**7**:129–136.

64. Sainio S, Nupponen I, Kuosmanen M, et al. Diagnosis and treatment of severe hemolytic disease of the fetus and newborn: a 10-year nationwide retrospective study. *Acta Obstet Gynecol Scand.* 2015;**94**:383–390.

65. Nicolini U, Santolaya J, Ojo OE, et al. The fetal intrahepatic umbilical vein as an alternative to cord needling for prenatal diagnosis and therapy. *Prenat Diagn.* 1988;**8**:665–671.

66. Nicolini U, Nicolaidis P, Fisk NM, et al. Fetal blood sampling from the intrahepatic vein: analysis of safety and clinical experience with 214 procedures. *Obstet Gynecol.* 1990;**76**:47–53.

67. Giannakoulopoulos X, Sepulveda W, Kourtis P, et al. Fetal plasma cortisol and beta-endorphin response to intrauterine needling. *Lancet.* 1994;**344**:77–81.

68. Lobato G, Soncini CS. Fetal hydrops and other variables associated with the fetal

hematocrit decrease after the first intrauterine transfusion for red cell alloimmunization. *Fetal Diagn Ther.* 2008;**24**:349–352.

69. Harman CR, Bowman JM, Manning FA, Menticoglou SM. Intrauterine transfusion–intraperitoneal versus intravascular approach: a case-control comparison. *Am J Obstet Gynecol.* 1990;**162**:1053–1059.

70. Lewis M, Bowman JM, Pollock J, Lowen B. Absorption of red cells from the peritoneal cavity of an hydropic twin. *Transfusion.* 1973;**13**:37–40.

71. Creasman WT, Duggan ER, Lund CJ. Absorption of transfused chromium-labeled erythrocytes from the fetal peritoneal cavity in hydrops fetalis. *Am J Obstet Gynecol.* 1966;**94**:586–588.

72. Taylor WW, Scott DE, Pritchard JA. Fate of compatible adult erythrocytes in the fetal peritoneal cavity. *Obstet Gynecol.* 1966;**28**:175–181.

73. Fox C, Martin W, Somerset DA, et al. Early intraperitoneal transfusion and adjuvant maternal immunoglobulin therapy in the treatment of severe red cell alloimmunization prior to fetal intravascular transfusion. *Fetal Diagn Ther.* 2008;**23**:159–163.

74. Moise KJ, Jr., Carpenter RJ, Jr., Kirshon B, et al. Comparison of four types of intrauterine transfusion: effect on fetal hematocrit. *Fetal Ther.* 1989;**4**:126–137.

75. Nicolini U, Kochenour NK, Greco P, et al. When to perform the next intra-uterine transfusion in patients with Rh allo-immunization: combined intravascular and intraperitoneal transfusion allows longer intervals. *Fetal Ther.* 1989;**4**:14–20.

76. Mackie FL, Pretlove SJ, Martin WL, et al. Fetal intracardiac transfusions in hydropic fetuses with severe anemia. *Fetal Diagn Ther.* 2015;**38**:61–64.

77. Allaf MB, Matha S, Chavez MR, Vintzileos AM. Intracardiac fetal transfusion for parvovirus-induced hydrops fetalis: a salvage procedure. *J Ultrasound Med.* 2015;**34**:2107–2109.

78. Radunovic N, Lockwood CJ, Alvarez M, et al. The severely anemic and hydropic isoimmune fetus: changes in fetal hematocrit associated with intrauterine death. *Obstet Gynecol.* 1992;**79**:390–393.

79. Papantoniou N, Sifakis S, Antsaklis A. Therapeutic management of fetal anemia: review of standard practice and alternative treatment options. *J Perinat Med.* 2013;**41**:71–82.

80. Dildy GA, Smith LG, Moise KJ, et al. Porencephalic cyst: a complication of fetal intravascular transfusion. *Am J Obstet Gynecol.* 1991;**165**:76–78.

81. Drew JH, Guaran RL, Cichello M, Hobbs JB. Neonatal whole blood hyperviscosity: the important factor influencing later neurologic function is the viscosity and not the polycythemia. *Clin Hemorheol Microcirc.* 1997;**17**:67–72.

82. Giannina G, Moise KJ, Dorman K. A simple method to estimate volume for fetal intravascular transfusions. *Fetal Diagn Ther.* 1998;**13**:94–97.

83. Mandelbrot L, Daffos F, Forestier F, et al. Assessment of fetal blood volume for computer-assisted management of in utero transfusion. *Fetal Ther.* 1988;**3**:60–66.

84. Bowman JM. The management of Rh-Isoimmunization. *Obstet Gynecol.* 1978;**52**:1–16.

85. Egberts J, van Kamp IL, Kanhai HH, et al. The disappearance of fetal and donor red blood cells in alloimmunised pregnancies: a reappraisal. *Br J Obstet Gynaecol.* 1997;**104**:818–824.

86. Lobato G, Soncini CS. Fetal hematocrit decrease after repeated intravascular transfusions in alloimmunized pregnancies. *Arch Gynecol Obstet.* 2007;**276**:595–599.

87. Mari G, Detti L, Oz U, et al. Accurate prediction of fetal hemoglobin by Doppler ultrasonography. *Obstet Gynecol.* 2002;**99**:589–593.

88. Scheier M, Hernandez-Andrade E, Fonseca EB, Nicolaides KH. Prediction of severe fetal anemia in red blood cell alloimmunization after previous

intrauterine transfusions. *Am J Obstet Gynecol.* 2006;**195**:1550–1556.

89. Detti L, Oz U, Guney I, et al. Doppler ultrasound velocimetry for timing the second intrauterine transfusion in fetuses with anemia from red cell alloimmunization. *Am J Obstet Gynecol.* 2001;**185**:1048–1051.

90. Dodd JM, Andersen C, Dickinson JE, et al. Fetal MCA Doppler to time intrauterine transfusions in red cell alloimmunisation: A randomised trial. *Ultrasound Obstet Gynecol.* 2018;**51**:306–312.

91. Zwiers C, van Kamp I, Oepkes D, Lopriore E. Intrauterine transfusion and non-invasive treatment options for hemolytic disease of the fetus and newborn – review on current management and outcome. *Expert Rev Hematol.* 2017;**10**:337–344.

92. Canlorbe G, Mace G, Cortey A, et al. Management of very early fetal anemia resulting from red-cell alloimmunization before 20 weeks of gestation. *Obstet Gynecol.* 2011;**118**:1323–1329.

93. Poissonnier MH, Picone O, Brossard Y, Lepercq J. Intravenous fetal exchange transfusion before 22 weeks of gestation in early and severe red-cell fetomaternal alloimmunization. *Fetal Diagn Ther.* 2003;**18**:467–471.

94. Lindenburg IT, van Kamp IL, van Zwet EW, et al. Increased perinatal loss after intrauterine transfusion for alloimmune anaemia before 20 weeks of gestation. *BJOG.* 2013;**120**:847–852.

95. Ruma MS, Moise KJ, Kim E, et al. Combined plasmapheresis and intravenous immune globulin for the treatment of severe maternal red cell alloimmunization. *Am J Obstet Gynecol.* 2007;**196**:138.e1-6.

96. Lindenburg IT, Wolterbeek R, Oepkes D, et al. Quality control for intravascular intrauterine transfusion using cumulative sum (CUSUM) analysis for the monitoring of individual performance. *Fetal Diagn Ther.* 2011;**29**:307–314.

97. Watts DH, Luthy DA, Benedetti TJ, et al. Intraperitoneal fetal transfusion under direct ultrasound guidance. *Obstet Gynecol.* 1988;**71**:84–88.

98. De Boer IP, Zeestraten EC, Lopriore E, et al. Pediatric outcome in Rhesus hemolytic disease treated with and without intrauterine transfusion. *Am J Obstet Gynecol.* 2008;**198**(54).e1-4.

99. Rath ME, Smits-Wintjens VE, Oepkes D, et al. Iron status in infants with alloimmune haemolytic disease in the first three months of life. *Vox Sang.* 2013;**105**:328–333.

100. Watson WJ, Wax JR, Miller RC, Brost BC. Prevalence of new maternal alloantibodies after intrauterine transfusion for severe Rhesus disease. *Am J Perinatol.* 2006;**23**:189–192.

101. Lindenburg IT, Smits-Wintjens VE, van Klink JM, et al. Long-term neurodevelopmental outcome after intrauterine transfusion for hemolytic disease of the fetus/newborn: the LOTUS study. *Am J Obstet Gynecol.* 2012;**206**:141. e1-8.

Twin-Twin Transfusion Syndrome

6

Rupi Mavi Parikh and Jose L. Peiro

Monochorionic pregnancies comprise 40% of twin gestations and in 99% of these cases, each twin has its own amniotic sac. These monochorionic and diamniotic (MCDA) twin pregnancies are subject to a high risk of complications including severe selective growth restriction, twin-to-twin transfusion syndrome (TTTS), twin retrograde arterial perfusion syndrome (TRAP), and discordant malformations.

Twin-to-twin transfusion syndrome is a common complication in monochorionic twin pregnancies because of the shared placental circulation. The incidence of TTTS is approximately 1:40 to 1:60 of twin pregnancies, 9–15% of monochorionic diamniotic pregnancies, and 6% of monoamniotic pregnancies.[1] The exact incidence may vary, however, as some fetal losses in monochorionic multiple gestations in the first half of pregnancy may be related to undiagnosed TTTS. This condition is associated with a high risk of fetal/neonatal mortality, and fetuses that survive are at risk of severe cardiac, neurologic, and developmental disorders. Severe TTTS may result in cardiovascular, central nervous system (CNS) and other end organ sequelae because of vascular compromise in one or both twins. Up to 8% of TTTS cases have evidence of CNS injury on fetal MRI. These CNS findings range from ischemic insult or hemorrhage, to dilation of cerebral venous sinuses.[1]

Inter-twin vascular connections within the placenta are critical for the development of TTTS. There are three main types of anastomoses in monochorionic placenta, that is venovenous (VV), arterioarterial (AA), and arteriovenous (AV). The imbalance of blood flow through these placental anastomoses leads to volume depletion in the donor twin resulting in oliguria and oligohydramnios, and volume overload in the recipient twin causing polyuria and polyhydramnios. Both AA and VV anastomoses are direct superficial connections on the placental surface with the potential for bidirectional flow. Arteriovenous vessels are also present on the placental surface, but the area of anastomoses is in the cotyledon, located deep within the placenta. Arteriovenous connections are linked through large capillary beds and are usually overall balanced in both directions so TTTS does not occur. These AV anastomoses can, however, result in unidirectional blood flow from one twin to the other and if uncompensated can lead to circulatory imbalance between the twins. The size of the AV anastomoses in addition to placental vascular resistance influences the volume of inter-twin transfusion more than the number of anastomoses (Figure 6.1). Mortality from TTTS is highest in the absence of AA and lowest when AA anastomoses are present (42% vs. 15%) as these anastomoses allow for bidirectional flow, which may compensate for the unidirectional flow through AV anastomoses.[3]

Both unbalanced vascular anastomoses and the cardiovascular response to circulatory imbalance play a role in the pathophysiology of TTTS. The precipitating event for the development of TTTS is likely to be a relative hypovolemia in one twin (donor twin) in

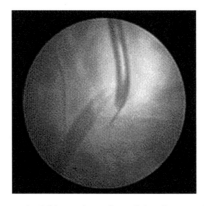

Figure 6.1 Arteriovenous anastomosis visible on the surface of the placenta, darker donor artery (at 12 o'clock) feeding into the lighter recipient vein at 7 o'clock.
With permission from Bamberg and Hecher.[2]

response to the imbalance in placental vascular anastomoses. In an attempt to restore intravascular volume, several vasoactive mediators are released. The donor twin's renin-angiotensin system is upregulated, and vasopressin levels are elevated. The recipient twin experiences hypervolemia, which causes atrial enlargement and release of both atrial and brain natriuretic peptide. The release of these hormones contributes to fetal polyuria and eventual polyhydramnios in the recipient sac. Hypervolemia and increased levels of vaso-active mediators also result in cardiac hypertrophy, cardiomegaly, and cardiac dysfunction in the recipient twin.[1,4]

Screening and Staging of Twin-Twin Transfusion

Prenatal diagnosis is by conventional ultrasound and Doppler. Two criteria are used for the diagnosis: the presence of a monochorionic diamniotic pregnancy and the presence of oligohydramnios in one sac and polyhydramnios in the other. The degree of polyhydramnios in the recipient twin dictates the diagnosis and staging of TTTS. Polyhydramnios is assessed by measuring the deepest vertical pocket on ultrasound. A vertical deep pocket measurement of 8 cm or greater < 20 weeks' gestation and > 10 cm at > 20 weeks' gestation in the amniotic sac of the recipient is in alignment with a diagnosis of TTTS.[5] Because of the oligohydramnios in the donor twin, the deepest vertical pocket measures < 2 cm; it is not uncommon for the donor to be stuck within its membranes, against the wall of the uterus or the placenta as a result of the accompanying polyhydramnios in the recipient twin. Measurement of the deepest vertical pocket is typically performed at 20 weeks; however, signs of TTTS may be detectable even at 18 weeks. In this scenario, a maximum vertical pocket measurement of 6 cm is believed to be a more sensitive and suggestive sign of TTTS.

The most commonly used staging system for TTTS was developed by Quintero et al. in 1999 and includes five stages.[6] The proposed five stages of disease are based on findings from two-dimensional ultrasound and Doppler velocimetry in the umbilical artery, umbilical vein, and ductus venosus. These stages range from mild disease with isolated discordant amniotic fluid volume to severe disease with demise of one or both twins.

Stage I   – oligohydramnios and polyhydramnios sequence, and the bladder of the donor twin is visible. Normal Doppler in both twins.

Stage II – oligohydramnios and polyhydramnios sequence, but bladder of donor twin not visualized. Normal Doppler in both twins.

Stage III – oligohydramnios and polyhydramnios sequence, nonvisualized bladder, abnormal dopplers. Absent/reversed end-diastolic velocity in the umbilical artery, reversed flow in the a-wave of ductus venosus, pulsatile flow in the umbilical vein in either fetus.

Stage IV – one or both fetuses show signs of hydrops.

Stage V – one or both fetuses have died.

See Table 6.1.[6]

Quintero's method of classification for TTTS considers a sequence of progressive ultrasonographic features. This may be better suited for monitoring disease progression as it has potential limitations in guiding therapy. Atypical presentations can occur which do not fall under the precise definitions for the Quintero stages. For example, some Stage I TTTS fetuses show signs of heart failure and cases of intrauterine fetal demise have occurred even with a diagnosis of Stage I TTTS.

The Cincinnati modification of the Quintero staging system is a cardiovascular scoring system based on progressively worsening fetal echocardiographic findings in the recipient fetus.[4] Echocardiographic features include the presence and severity of atrioventricular valve incompetence, ventricular wall thickening, and diminished ventricular function. These abnormalities often represent a more concrete indication for intervention. Table 6.2 highlights the components of Quintero staging and Cincinnati modification.

Twin-to-twin transfusion syndrome usually presents in the second trimester and can either remain stable or rapidly progress to affect fetal well-being. In terms of surveillance, women with a twin pregnancy should be evaluated with ultrasonography at 10–13 weeks' gestation to assess fetal viability, chorionicity, nuchal translucency, and crown-rump length. Particular guidelines have been set for the monitoring of twin pregnancies by the International Society of Ultrasound in Obstetrics and Gynecology and others.[7] After the

Table 6.1 Quintero staging

Stage	Poly/oligohydramnios	Absent bladder in donor	Critically abnormal Dopplers	Ascites, pericardial, or pleural effusion, scalp edema, or overt hydrops present	Demise of one or both twins
I	+	−	−	−	−
II	+	+	−	−	−
III	+	+	+	−	−
IV	+	+	+	+	−
V	+	+	+	+	+

-Polyhydramnios represents maximum vertical pocket of >8 cm.
-Oligohydramnios is a maximum vertical pocket of <2 cm.
-Critically abnormal Dopplers is characterized by at least one of the following: a) absent or reverse end-diastolic velocity in the umbilical artery b) reverse flow in the ductus venosus, or c) pulsatile umbilical venous flow.[6]

Table 6.2 Quintero and Cincinnati staging for TTTS

TTTS Staging System

Quintero staging   Cincinnati staging

		Observations			
Stages	Donor Bladder	Amniotic Fluid: Donor/Recipient	Doppler Wave Forms	Other	
I	Visible	Oligohydramnios/ polyhydramnios	Normal		
II	Not visible	Oligohydramnios/ polyhydramnios	Normal		Cardiomyopathy
III	Visible or not visible	Oligohydramnios/ polyhydramnios	Abnormal		IIIa mild IIIb moderate IIIc severe
IV				Fetal hydrops or abdominal ascites	
V				Demise of either fetus	

first trimester scan, uncomplicated dichorionic twin pregnancies should be scanned every four weeks. For screening for the development of twin-twin syndrome or twin reverse arterial perfusion sequence in monochorionic twin pregnancies, bi-weekly ultrasound surveillance is recommended from 16 weeks onward.[3,7,8]

This level of close monitoring of twin pregnancies is necessary because while the clinical picture of Stage I TTTS may remain stable, if progression does occur it will happen quickly. Sonographic surveillance occurring less frequently than every two weeks, from 16 weeks onward, has been associated with a higher incidence of late stage diagnosis of TTTS. This emphasizes the importance of establishing chorionicity in twin pregnancies as early as possible. Besides monitoring MCDA pregnancies for the development of amniotic fluid abnormalities, other findings have been associated with TTTS. Inter-twin nuchal transparency (NT) > 50%, inter-twin crown-rump length discrepancy and reversed ductus venosus flow within the first trimester are suggestive of TTTS.[9]

Inter-twin membrane folding has also been associated with development of TTTS in more than one-third of cases. If these findings are established it may be a good idea to undergo more frequent ultrasound surveillance, at least every one to two weeks, for TTTS. Doppler evaluation is not typically performed in uncomplicated MCDA gestations, and while it may improve TTTS detection, it is not specifically recommended as part of routine surveillance.[3]

Severe discordance of amniotic fluid in both twins is usually the main prenatal finding. However, fetal echocardiography is also warranted in all monochorionic twins as the risk of cardiac anomalies is increased nine-fold in MCDA twins and 14-fold when TTTS is present. Screening for congenital heart disease in twins with TTTS is therefore essential.[3] Most of the cardiac conditions detected are atrial or ventricular septal defects and pulmonary stenosis has also been reported with some frequency. Cases of right ventricular outflow tract obstruction have also been reported secondary to the existing increased preload, afterload, and activation of the renin-angiotensin system. The functional abnormalities that complicate TTTS occur primarily in the recipient twin as volume overload causes cardiomegaly, increased aortic and pulmonary velocities, and atrioventricular valve regurgitation. Over time, the recipient twin develops progressive biventricular hypertrophy and diastolic dysfunction. Recipient twins in TTTS who show evidence of cardiac involvement have poor outcomes while those with normal cardiac function have improved survival. Although fetal cardiac findings are not officially part of the TTTS staging system, many centers routinely perform fetal echocardiography in cases of TTTS. It is possible that early diagnosis of recipient twin cardiomyopathy may identify those MCDA gestations that would benefit from early intervention.[3]

Growth discordance and intrauterine growth restriction (IUGR) often can overlap and complicate TTTS.[3] Unequal placental sharing occurs in approximately 20% of MCDA gestations and can coexist with TTTS, therefore complicating the diagnosis and management. Distinguishing TTTS complicated by growth restriction from selective IUGR can be difficult as the IUGR fetus in both circumstances may have oligohydramnios. The amniotic fluid volume is the distinguishing factor between these entities. In TTTS, the normally grown fetus is usually the recipient and often has excess amniotic fluid. Determining the true diagnosis of TTTS versus selective IUGR is important in deciding on therapeutic options. Laser photocoagulation of abnormal placental anastomoses is the treatment of choice for TTTS while the treatment of IUGR is variable and depends on gestational age.[1]

Mothers with TTTS often remain asymptomatic but symptoms related to excessive uterine distension (polyhydramnios) may occur such as inability to lay flat, insomnia, lower abdominal pain, worsening gastroesophageal reflux symptoms, and pelvic pressure.

Management

There are numerous treatment options for TTTS, which include selective fetocide, cord coagulation, placental blood-letting, maternal medical therapy with digoxin or indomethacin, serial amnioreduction, microseptostomy of the inner-twin membrane, and nonselective or selective fetoscopic laser photocoagulation.

Amnioreduction was initially used for the management of maternal discomfort in the presence of polyhydramnios. Survival following aggressive amnioreduction under ultrasound guidance is only 50%, with the possibility of approximately 30% of babies suffering severe neurological sequelae after birth.[10] In addition, as the underlying cause of hemodynamic imbalance is not addressed by this mode of therapy, recurrence frequently occurs, necessitating the need to repeat the procedure.

Nonselective laser photocoagulation of all vessels crossing the inter-twin membrane is problematic, as it may sacrifice vessels not responsible for the TTTS resulting in a higher death rate of the donor twin from acute placental insufficiency.

Selective fetoscopic laser photocoagulation has become widely accepted as the treatment of choice for TTTS. A multicenter randomized trial by Senat et al.[10] found that selective fetoscopic laser photocoagulation (SFLP) was associated with a higher incidence of survival of at least one twin, higher gestational age at delivery and better neurological outcomes compared to amnioreductions.[10,11] Fetoscopic laser photocoagulation not only arrests shunting of blood from the donor to recipient, but also halts the transfer of potentially harmful vasoactive mediators. Ville and associates[12] reported 53% survival with a fetoscopic laser technique, which was better than the survival observed with serial amnioreduction (37%). The goal of SFLP is to ablate all abnormal communicating placental anastomoses. However, after standard therapy, some communications may still remain. This resulted in the development of a new laser technique, the "Solomon method,"[13] in which a thin line is drawn with the laser from one edge of the placenta to the other thereby ablating the entire vascular equator and minimizing the risk of residual placental communications which are not visible to the naked eye. The goal is to functionally separate the placenta into two regions through the vascular equator with each one supplying a twin.

A randomized study comparing the Solomon technique with standard SFLP revealed that the Solomon technique was associated with decreased incidence of recurrent TTTS and post-laser twin anemia polycythemia sequence (TAPS).[13]

Patients with Stage I TTTS are often managed expectantly as over 75% of cases remain stable or spontaneously regress. In a literature review of Stage I TTTS, the overall survival rates were 86% after expectant management, 77% after amnioreduction, and 86% after laser therapy.[3] Contraindications for the use of ablative laser therapy include associated major fetal malformations, fetal demise, rupture of membranes, and a maternal condition that requires termination of pregnancy.

Extensive counseling should be provided to patients with pregnancies complicated by TTTS, including natural history of the disease, management options, as well as detailed risks and benefits. Currently, SFLP of placental anastomoses is considered by most experts to be the best available approach and superior to serial amnioreduction for the management of Stage II, III, and IV TTTS in pregnancies < 26 weeks' gestation. In high-volume fetal treatment centers, double survival is 70% and single survival is 90% with a 10% incidence of long-term neurologic sequalae in survivors following SFLP therapy.[2]

Laser photocoagulation is performed under ultrasound guidance. An initial mapping of the placental vasculature is performed followed by placement of a sheath into the recipient amniotic cavity, and insertion of an endoscope.[3] Prior to laser photocoagulation of vascular anastomoses, extensive mapping of the anastomoses at the inter-twin amniotic membrane level is performed to identify vessels that communicate with both fetuses and to exclude the nutritional vessels of each fetus and the placenta (Figure 6.2). In a sequential manner, and guided by the previous mapping, the arteriovenous anastomoses that run from the donor to the recipient and then those from the recipient to the donor are coagulated first, thereby decreasing the possibility of hemodynamic disturbances between the fetuses during the procedure. Minimizing the duration of laser treatment after detailed mapping has occurred can avoid hemodynamic disturbances between the fetuses.

The Solomon technique involves delineation of the placental equator and obliteration of vascular anastomoses even when they are small. The intensity of the laser is usually 25–40 W for the Nd-YAG or diode laser (Figure 6.3). At the end of the procedure, amnioreduction is performed on the amniotic cavity of the recipient to restore a normal volume of amniotic fluid.

Selective coagulation of all vessel types (AA, AV, and VV) is routinely performed over nonselective ablation as this is thought to lead to a lower rate of postoperative fetal mortality.[14] In general, overall survival rates of 50–70% can be expected after SFLP treatment of TTTS. In experienced centers, the risk of this procedure may be as low as 10% however, there does remain a 10–30% risk of fetal loss with laser photocoagulation. In

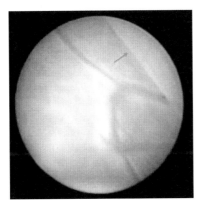

Figure 6.2 Visualization of the inter-twin membrane. Fetoscopic visualization (arrow) is useful to identify crossing vessels and to map the inter-twin connections.
Photo courtesy of Jose Piero MD.

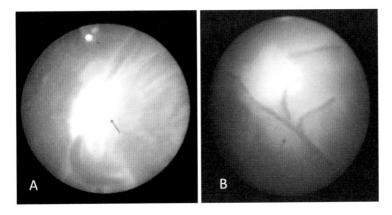

Figure 6.3 Laser photocoagulated vascular connection on the surface of the placenta. (A) Nd-YAG laser, and (B) diode laser.
Photo courtesy of Jose Piero MD.

scenarios where the recipient twin demonstrates signs of cardiomyopathy, improved survival of the recipient twin has been reported with maternal administration of nifedipine up to 24–48 hours before SFLP is performed. While perioperative maternal treatment with nifedipine may require intraoperative support of the maternal blood pressure with vasoactive agents, no statistically significant difference in five-day fetal survival was noted following delivery.[15] After SFLP, the recipient twin's cardiac function tends to normalize within four weeks, and pulmonic valve defects also appear to stabilize. Overall, 87% of post-laser recipient twins who survive are reported to have normal echocardiograms by about two years of age.[16]

Twin Anemia Polycythemia Sequence

This condition, characterized by anemia in the donor twin, and polycythemia in the recipient twin without accompanying oligohydramnios or polyhydramnios[17] can occur spontaneously or post-laser therapy for TTTS in 1–5% or 16% of patients, respectively.[17–20] The pathophysiology includes chronic feto-fetal transfusion in monochorionic twins in the presence of minimal abnormal placenta vascular connections. Diagnosis is made in-utero by prenatal Doppler findings of middle cerebral artery peak systolic velocity (MCA-PSV) of ≥ 1.5 MoM (multiples of the median) in the donor, which is suggestive of anemia. In the recipient fetus, the MoM is ≤ 1.0, suggestive of polycythemia. Postnatal diagnosis is by an inter-twin hemoglobin difference of ≥ 8 g/dL and one of either small residual placental anastomoses or a reticulocyte count ratio (reticulocyte count donor/reticulocyte count recipient ≥ 1.7). The optimal management of TAPS is not known but treatment options include fetoscopic laser therapy, intrauterine blood transfusion to the donor with or without combination of partial exchange blood transfusion in the recipient, expectant management, or fetocide.[21]

Anesthetic Management

Preoperative Considerations

The preoperative preparation is the same as for other fetoscopic procedures and includes a complete maternal history and physical examination. This involves assessment of the airway as well as landmarks for regional anesthesia when applicable. Full disclosure of the anesthetic options, associated risks of local, neuraxial, and general anesthesia, and the benefits of each should be discussed with the patient. Mothers should be informed that medicines to induce light sedation will be administered in conjunction with local anesthetic infiltration for the procedure. In addition, their cooperation may be required during the procedure in terms of regulating their respiratory pattern. It is important to enquire about previous procedures that may have been performed such as amnioreduction, or placement of fetal thoracoabdominal or pleural shunts, as these may increase the mother's anxiety level. Risks of intravenous sedation such as vomiting, or pruritus and that of regional anesthesia including hypotension, bleeding, infection, nerve damage, post dural puncture headache, failed regional anesthetic, sedation, and need for general anesthesia with risks of intubation should also be discussed.

Apart from when indicated, general anesthesia should also be mentioned as a possible backup in situations of failed regional anesthesia, heightened maternal anxiety, inability to lay flat, or persistent vomiting during the procedure, and/or difficult surgical exposure. For pregnant women, general anesthesia is associated with increased morbidity and mortality particularly because of airway-related complications and the increased risk of hemorrhage from uterine atony. Adequate preparations should be made to manage these situations.

Risks of the procedure including preterm labor, chorioamniotic separation, infection, hemorrhage, blood transfusion, pulmonary edema, fetal demise, and postoperative bed rest should be discussed with the mother by the procedural physician.

Laboratory studies are ordered by the fetal surgeons or maternal-fetal medicine (MFM) team, and include CBC (complete blood count), electrolyte panel, and a type and cross for two units packed red blood cells (PRBCs) in case of unexpected maternal bleeding or an emergent cesarean section becomes necessary (when the fetuses are viable). Additional laboratory studies to consider include coagulation studies, maternal echocardiogram, ECG (electrocardiogram), chest X-ray, and maternal pulmonary function tests as the medical history indicates.

Preoperative orders which should be in place prior to taking the patient to the operating room include intravenous antibiotics for the mother, and magnesium sulfate infusion for postoperative tocolysis (or intraoperative administration as indicated), and local anesthetics for regional anesthesia.

Assessment of the fetus includes determination of estimated gestational age (usually 18–24 weeks) and estimated fetal weight. Fetal echocardiogram findings, fetal karyotype, significant ultrasound and fetal ultrafast MRI findings should also be noted.

Medications including oral citric acid and sodium citrate (Bicitra®), as well as intravenous H-2 antagonists and prokinetic agents for gastrointestinal reflux prophylaxis, should be administered preoperatively. Depending on the patient's anxiety level, intravenous midazolam may be required for anxiolysis.

When sedation is employed, the mothers remain spontaneously ventilating with a nasal cannula in place. A nasal cannula with a CO_2 sampling port allows for proper monitoring of ventilation. In addition, the required resources for administration of general anesthesia should be readily available such as airway equipment for mother (adult laryngoscope, styletted smaller sized endotracheal tube), and difficult airway equipment. Rapid sequence induction medications for the mother, propofol and succinylcholine (if not contraindicated), should also be readily accessible.

In terms of anesthetic choice for SFLP and treatment of TTTS in general, a variety of modalities have been employed. These include maternal intravenous sedation, and/or neuraxial techniques such as spinal, epidural or combined spinal/epidural anesthesia. The position of the placenta may influence the surgical approach as well as the mode of anesthesia. In the case of a posterior placenta, the access to the fetus is straightforward and typically is amenable to intravenous sedation with local anesthesia. Maternal sedation with remifentanil 0.08–0.1 mcg/kg/min or a propofol infusion (25–50 mcg/kg/min), in addition to local infiltration of the skin and subcutaneous tissues with local anesthetics is a common anesthetic modality for these patients. A remifentanil infusion is often used as it is easy to titrate, readily crosses the placenta causing fetal immobility, and reliably provides maternal sedation.[22] Ephedrine and phenylephrine are often required intraoperatively to maintain hemodynamics as anesthetic medications commonly result in a decrease in systemic vascular resistance and subsequent hypotension. Regardless of the medication administered for sedation, bolus administration of additional sedative, midazolam or analgesics such as fentanyl may be necessary depending on the patient's level of anxiety during the procedure. A low-dose propofol infusion for sedation, in addition to fentanyl and midazolam, may also be included as part of the anesthetic plan. The use of dexmedetomidine bolus and infusion may also be considered for intravenous sedation of the obese pregnant patient.

When the placenta is located anteriorly, the surgical approach may depend on the presence or absence of a surgical window. If an access window is detected on ultrasound examination that will facilitate placement of a fetoscope, either intravenous sedation or neuraxial anesthesia may be administered for the procedure. In the absence of a surgical access window, laparoscopic assisted SFLP may be indicated.[23–25] Laparoscopic assisted SFLP warrants general anesthesia as the placement of a scope in the lower epigastric region and the patient's flank is best tolerated under general anesthesia.

Rossi et al.[19] compared local anesthesia with intravenous sedation to general anesthesia to determine the optimal anesthetic technique for SFLP. Their analysis of 266 patients revealed that patients undergoing general anesthesia for SFLP were likely to have more fluctuations in maternal blood pressure and maternal heart rate before, during, and after surgery compared to those who received local anesthesia. There was also a trend toward more maternal complications with the use of general anesthesia. General anesthesia was also associated with an increased risk for intra-amniotic bleeding; likely a result of refractory uterine myometrial relaxation from halogenated inhalation anesthetics. In contrast, local anesthesia was associated with similar pregnancy outcomes to general anesthesia but fewer maternal complications. The authors of this study also concluded that local anesthesia was associated with perioperative hemodynamic stability, which optimizes oxygenation and perfusion to the mother and fetus.[19]

The operative site in SFLP is specifically the placenta, therefore, fetal anesthesia and analgesia are not indicated. Nevertheless, minimization of fetal movement via maternal sedation with remifentanil helps facilitate the procedure.

Intraoperative Management

The patient is positioned supine with a left lateral tilt by placing a wedge underneath the right flank. Standard ASA monitors are placed, as well as a nasal cannula for oxygen if applicable.

If epidural catheter placement is warranted, the patient will be placed in the sitting position for catheter insertion typically in the lumbar region (commonly at the L2–3 level). Prior to the start of the procedure, a T6 sensory level of anesthesia is confirmed and the patient is placed in a supine position with left uterine displacement. Foley catheter placement will be necessary if the patient receives a neuraxial block. Following adequate sterile preparation and draping of the patient, an ultrasound is performed by the MFM team to identify placental location and surgical window for intervention.

For the patient receiving intravenous sedation, the process is commenced as the monitors are being placed to ensure adequate sedation by the time the procedure begins. Maternal comfort during the procedure is further accomplished with verbal reassurance and additional sedation as necessary.

Maternal mean arterial pressure (MAP) should be maintained within 10–20% of baseline to preserve uteroplacental perfusion. The blood pressure can be maintained in this range with the administration of ephedrine and phenylephrine boluses. If the patient is already on magnesium sulfate for preterm contractions, intravenous fluid should be administered judiciously to prevent pulmonary edema.

Continuous uterus irrigation is performed with warmed normal saline through a hotline if necessary. An ongoing tally of the fluid volume in and out of the patient must be kept to prevent excess fluid absorption that could lead to pulmonary edema. Fetal surgeons and the operating room nursing team carefully monitor the input of fluid from the rapid transfuser and the amount of fluid taken off at the end of the case. Depending on how sick the fetuses are, persistent fetal bradycardia or fetal compromise may occur during the procedure requiring administration of emergency fetal resuscitation drugs or an emergency cesarean section for viable fetuses. When the fetuses are viable, it is imperative to know the estimated fetal weight to prepare resuscitation drugs for the fetus such as atropine and epinephrine if this becomes necessary. Epinephrine should be available in low (1 mcg/kg) or high (10 mcg/kg) doses. The anesthesiologist should also have required drugs for an emergency cesarean section readily available during the procedure in case an emergency delivery of viable fetuses becomes necessary. Otherwise, the fetus typically does not require any medication during SFLP and the focus of anesthetic management rests on the mother.

Postoperative tocolysis is an essential consideration as preterm labor is common following fetal interventions. Impaired uterine blood flow or partial placental separation can also occur postoperatively because of uterine manipulation or incisions. If indicated, a magnesium sulfate infusion may be started perioperatively, as requested by the MFM team, with a bolus of 4–6 gm over 20-30 minutes followed by an infusion of 2–3 gm/Hr based on MFM preference. On completion of the procedure, the incision is closed and the sedation medications are discontinued. If an epidural catheter has been placed and used for the procedure, it should be removed on completion of the procedure with confirmation and documentation of an intact catheter tip. The patient is then transported to the recovery room where a tocodynamometer is reapplied and fetal heart rates are documented.

While SFLP has become mainstream therapy for TTTS, a common complication of this procedure remains preterm premature rupture of membranes. Consequently, patients are closely monitored postoperatively for this complication. Studies are ongoing to investigate how this complication can best be prevented.

References

1. Faye-Peterson O, Crombleholme T. Twin-twin transfusion: part 2: infant anomalies, clinical intervention and placental examination. *Neoreviews.* 2008;**9**(9):e380.

2. Bamberg C, Hecher K. Update on twin-to-twin transfusion syndrome. *Best Pract Res Clin Obstet Gynaecol.* 2019;**58**:55–65.

3. Society for Maternal-Fetal Medicine, Simpson LL. Twin-twin transfusion syndrome. *Am J Obstet Gynecol.* 2013;**208**(1):3–18.

4. Michelfelder E, Gottliebson W, Border W, et al. Early manifestations and spectrum of recipient twin cardiomyopathy in twin-twin transfusion syndrome: relation to Quintero stage. *Ultrasound Obstet Gynecol.* 2007;**30**(7):965–971.

5. Johnson A. Diagnosis and management of twin-twin transfusion syndrome. *Clin Obstet Gynecol.* 2015;**58**(3):611–631.

6. Quintero RA, Morales WJ, Allen MH, et al. Staging of twin-twin transfusion syndrome. *J Perinatol.* 1999; **19**(8 Pt 1):550–555.

7. Khalil A, Rodgers M, Baschat A, et al. ISUOG Practice Guidelines: role of ultrasound in twin pregnancy. *Ultrasound Obstet Gynecol.* 2016;**47**(2):247–263.

8. Oepkes D, Sueters M. Antenatal fetal surveillance in multiple pregnancies. *Best Pract Res Clin Obstet Gynaecol.* 2017;**38**:59–70.

9. Stagnati V, Zanardini C, Fichera A, et al. Early prediction of twin-to-twin transfusion syndrome: systematic review and meta-analysis. *Ultrasound Obstet Gynecol.* 2017;**49**(5):573–582.

10. Senat MV, Deprest J, Boulvain M, et al. Endoscopic laser surgery versus serial amnioreduction for severe twin-to-twin transfusion syndrome. *N Engl J Med.* 2004;**351**(2):136–144.

11. Salomon LJ, Ortqvist L, Aegerter P, et al. Long-term developmental follow-up of infants who participated in a randomized clinical trial of amniocentesis vs laser photocoagulation for the treatment of twin-to-twin transfusion syndrome. *Am J Obstet Gynecol.* 2010;**203**(5):444.e1–444.e7.

12. Ville Y, Hyett J, Hecher K, Nicolaides K. Preliminary experience with endoscopic laser surgery for severe twin-twin transfusion syndrome. *N Engl J Med.* 1995;**332**(4):224–227.

13. Slaghekke F, Oepkes D. Solomon technique versus selective coagulation for twin-twin

transfusion. *Twin Research Hum Genet.* 2016;**19**(3):217–221.

14. Quintero RA, Comas C, Bornick PW, et al. Selective versus non-selective laser photocoagulation of placental vessels in twin-to-twin transfusion syndrome. *Ultrasound Obstet Gynecol.* 2000;**16** (3):230–236.

15. Ngamprasertwong P, Habli M, Boat A, et al. Maternal hypotension during fetoscopic surgery: incidence and its impact on fetal survival outcomes. *ScientificWorldJournal.* 2013;2013:709059.

16. Van Mieghem T, Klaritsch P, Done E, et al. Assessment of fetal cardiac function before and after therapy for twin-to-twin transfusion syndrome. *Am J Obstet Gynecol.* 2009;**200**(4):400.e1–400.e7.

17. Lopriore E, Middeldorp JM, Oepkes D, Klumper FJ, Walther FJ, Vandenbussche FP. Residual anastomoses after fetoscopic laser surgery in twin-to-twin transfusion syndrome: frequency, associated risks and outcome. *Placenta.* 2007; **28**(2-3):204–208.

18. Gupta R, Kilby M, Cooper G. Fetal surgery and anaesthetic implications. *BJA Educ.* 2008;**8**(2):71–75.

19. Rossi AC, Kaufman MA, Bornick PW, Quintero RA. General vs local anesthesia for the percutaneous laser treatment of twin-twin transfusion syndrome. *Am J Obstet Gynecol.* 2008;**199**(2):137.e1–137.e7.

20. Lewi L, Jani J, Blickstein I, et al. The outcome of monochorionic diamniotic twin gestations in the era of invasive fetal therapy: a prospective cohort study. *Am J Obstet Gynecol.* 2008;**199**(5):514.e1–514.e8.

21. Slaghekke F, Zhao DP, Middeldorp JM, et al. Antenatal management of twin-twin transfusion syndrome and twin anemia-polycythemia sequence. *Expert Rev Hematol.* 2016;**9**(8):815–820.

22. Van de Velde M, Van Schoubroeck D, Lewi LE, et al. Remifentanil for fetal immobilization and maternal sedation during fetoscopic surgery: a randomized, double-blind comparison with diazepam. *Anesth Analg.* 2005;**101**(1):251–258.

23. Middeldorp JM, Lopriore E, Sueters M, et al. Laparoscopically guided uterine entry for fetoscopy in twin-to-twin transfusion syndrome with completely anterior placenta: a novel technique. *Fetal Diagn Ther.* 2007;**22**(6):409–415.

24. Papanna R, Johnson A, Ivey RT, et al. Laparoscopy-assisted fetoscopy for laser surgery in twin-twin transfusion syndrome with anterior placentation. *Ultrasound Obstet Gynecol.* 2010;**35**:65–70.

25. Shamshirsaz AA, Javadian P, Ruano R, et al. Comparison between laparoscopically assisted and standard fetoscopic laser ablation in patients with anterior and posterior placentation in twin-twin transfusion syndrome: a single center study. *Prenat Diagn.* 2015;**35**(4):376–381.

Fetal Endoscopic Tracheal Occlusion (FETO)

Mariatu Verla, Candace C. Style, Olutoyin A. Olutoye, and Oluyinka O. Olutoye

Indications for FETO

Congenital Diaphragmatic Hernia

Congenital diaphragmatic hernia (CDH) is the partial or complete loss of the diaphragm which results in herniation of the abdominal contents into the chest. It occurs in approximately 1 in 2,500–4,000 live births and the mortality ranges between 15% and 50%.[1] A failure in the formation of the pleuroperitoneal fold plays a role in development of this congenital anomaly; however, a clear understanding of the pathogenesis is still unknown.[2–5] This defect most commonly occurs on the left side of the diaphragm (85–90%), but can also occur on the right (10–15%) or bilaterally (< 1%). The factors that resulted in the improper development of diaphragm as well as the intrathoracic herniation of the abdominal viscera probably also contribute to impairment of the fetus' lung development, which leads to pulmonary hypoplasia and pulmonary hypertension. There is a direct correlation between the severity of pulmonary hypoplasia and pulmonary hypertension to the morbidity and mortality of CDH.

Congenital diaphragmatic hernia is typically detected prenatally by ultrasound. Increasingly, magnetic resonance imaging (MRI) is being used as an adjunct to better characterize the hernia and the severity of the defect (Figure 7.1).[6,7] Measurement indices such as the percent liver herniation, lung-to-head ratio (LHR), and lung volumes are strong prenatal predictors of postnatal survival.[8–10] The severe form of CDH can be defined as an observed-to-expected lung-to-head ratio (O/E-LHR) < 0.25 on ultrasound, or observed-to-expected total fetal lung volume (O/E TFLV) < 0.35 and percentage of liver herniation > 21% by MRI.[11]

The current standard of care for CDH patients primarily focuses on postnatal management. This regimen includes conventional mechanical ventilation and/or high-frequency oscillation ventilation (HFOV) with non-emergent surgical CDH repair. Though somewhat controversial, the use of inhaled nitric oxide (iNO), other pulmonary vasodilators, and extracorporeal membrane oxygenation (ECMO) has been incorporated into the algorithm of standard of care treatment for CDH at some institutions. However, patients with the most severe forms of CDH continue to have high morbidity and mortality rates.

Fetal endoscopic tracheal occlusion is not widely accepted as standard of care in the management of CDH. It is still an experimental procedure, reserved for isolated, severe diaphragmatic hernia cases.[11–13] Recent trials performed in Europe, and North and South America have been promising. Fetuses treated with FETO had increased lung volumes,

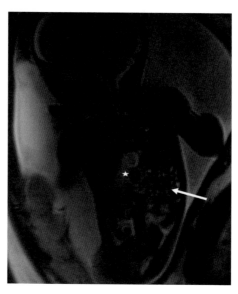

Figure 7.1 Large left diaphragmatic hernia with significant amount of bowel and liver herniated into the left hemithorax (arrow). Stomach (*) is also herniated across midline posterior to the heart into the right hemithorax.

higher survival rates and reduced need for ECMO compared to fetuses who only received postnatal therapy.[13–15]

Severe Pulmonary Hypoplasia from ePPROM

Similar to the pulmonary hypoplasia seen in CDH, fetuses with early preterm premature rupture of membranes (ePPROM) before 22 weeks' gestation can also develop severe pulmonary hypoplasia.[11] It is hypothesized that the significant amniotic fluid loss from the ruptured membranes leads to anhydramnios. This puts the fetus at risk for chronic external chest compression from the uterine wall which results in restriction of lung growth and development. Animal studies where fetal tracheostomy resulted in pulmonary hypoplasia suggest that an imbalance in the intra-amniotic and airway pressure may be a more plausible explanation. Based on the same physiologic principle and benefit that we have seen with tracheal occlusion in CDH, experimental studies using FETO in ePPROM cases have been described in the literature.[11,16,17]

Brief History of FETO and CDH

Prior to the 1990s, emergent surgical repair after birth was considered the standard of care.[18] Nevertheless, the outcomes of severe CDH remained poor. During this same time period, Harrison et al. studied the possibility of in-utero CDH repair to improve outcomes. Their early attempts at in-utero CDH repair did not offer a survival advantage and in those with the "liver up" position, the repair was technically challenging, resulted in kinking of the ductus venosus as the liver was reduced from the chest and was associated with a high risk of fetal death.[19–24] However, the observation that fetuses with tracheal obstruction had remarkable lung growth and successes in experimental animal studies paved the way for the development of the FETO procedure. In-utero tracheal ligation studies performed in the fetal rabbit and lamb model demonstrated accelerated lung growth.[25–32] After the trachea was ligated, there was an accumulation of pulmonary fluid which led to a significant increase in hydrostatic pressure. This pressure was thought to stimulate alveolar cell proliferation and lung growth and in turn improve respiratory function.[25,26,28] After numerous experimental studies, the first tracheal occlusion study in human fetuses was performed in the 1990s by Harrison and colleagues.[33]

Since its inception, various techniques and devices have been tested to identify the best temporary tracheal occlusion mechanism that is both reversible and least injurious to the airway.[30,33] One such device was the internal foam plug. It was easily inserted via a translaryngeal approach to occlude the trachea; but was abandoned because it caused tracheomalacia.[30,33] Next, tracheal metal clips were introduced that caused minimal tracheal damage. To remove the clips, the ex-utero intrapartum treatment (EXIT) procedure was performed at the time of delivery. The EXIT procedure provided a controlled environment to secure the neonate's airway and remove the clips prior to dividing the umbilical cord.[33,34] Although the clips were not directly damaging to the trachea, the actual in-utero placement required a neck dissection which posed significant risk of injury to the recurrent laryngeal nerve and trachea.[1,35,36]

Despite the initial disappointments with in-utero temporary endotracheal occlusion, the concept was revisited. A detachable, inflatable, silicone balloon was successfully developed that could be inserted using endoscopic techniques (Fetendo).[36,37] This new technique eliminated the need for the hazardous neck dissection required for the tracheal clip placement. The Fetendo balloon technique has been further refined over the years. A laparotomy or hysterotomy is no longer indicated for fetal exposure during tracheal balloon placement. Today, FETO is performed completely via a percutaneous endoscopic approach; this change has dramatically reduced postoperative preterm labor and thus the associated maternal and fetal morbidity and mortality.[14,24,38–41]

The FETO Procedure

Preoperative Considerations

Patients whose fetuses will undergo FETO are typically prehydrated with lactated Ringer's solution, receive a prophylactic 2 g dose of IV cefazolin (first generation cephalosporin) and an antacid such as oral citrate, metoclopramide, or ranitidine.[12,39,42–44] Based on the institution's tocolysis protocol, the patient may also receive tocolytic agents such as nifedipine, magnesium sulfate, terbutaline, or atosiban pre-, intra- and postoperatively.[12,42,44] The breech presentation is the desired position to perform the FETO procedure. Ideally the fetus' back should be directed toward the posterolateral wall of the uterus and the face directed to the opposite uterine wall.[45] Gentle external manipulation can be performed to achieve the optimal fetal position.[15,45]

Maternal and Fetal Anesthesia

Fetal endoscopic tracheal occlusion is generally performed between 26 and 30 weeks' gestation under maternal continuous epidural, combined spinal-epidural anesthesia (through the L3–L4 or L4–L5 intervertebral spaces), local anesthesia with intravenous sedation, or general anesthesia.[12,13,39,42–45] General anesthesia is rarely performed for this indication today. The choice of anesthetic is based on institutional preference, the expected duration of the procedure, and the perceived need for fetal manipulation and positioning. Obtaining the optimum fetal position for placement of the tracheal balloon can be a limiting factor for this procedure.

Once the desired fetal position is achieved under ultrasound guidance, a 20- or 22-gauge needle is used to administer an intramuscular injection into the fetal arm or leg to provide fetal analgesia and immobilization. Typical anesthetic agents administered to the fetus include a combination of fentanyl 15 mcg/kg and pancuronium 0.2–2 mg/kg or vecuronium 0.2 mg/kg. Atropine 20 mcg/kg can also be administered to prevent fetal bradycardia.[12,13,39,42–44] Maternal anxiolytic, if indicated, is usually withheld until after the baby has been positioned and fetal medications administered. Administration of midazolam to the mother prior to verification of adequate fetal position may make version of the baby difficult.

Continuous fetal monitoring with ultrasonography is performed throughout the procedure to monitor the fetus' status. In the case of polyhydramnios, drainage of some of the excessive amniotic fluid may be necessary to ease fetal access.[15]

Insertion of Tracheal Occlusion Balloon

Under ultrasound guidance, uterine access can be either with a metallic sheath and trocar or a disposable 10 or 12 Fr sheath using the Seldinger technique. The sheath is inserted percutaneously through the abdominal and uterine walls into the amniotic cavity. A judicious attempt should be made to ensure that no placenta is present between the desired fetoscopic entry site on the maternal skin and the fetal mouth. Once within the amniotic cavity, the trocar is removed and replaced by a 1.0–1.3 mm cannula with a fetoscope. The sheath also allows concurrent insertion of the balloon occlusion system (a microcatheter loaded with a detachable latex balloon) with the fetoscope. Using a combination of ultrasound guidance and direct fetoscopic visualization, the fetoscope is directed toward the fetus' mouth and into the pharynx and larynx, under the epiglottis, through the vocal cords and into the trachea. Once the carina is identified, the balloon is positioned proximal to the carina and about midway between the carina and the vocal cords (Figure 7.2). The balloon is then filled with about 0.8 mL saline solution or an isotonic contrast agent, and detached from the catheter to rest within the preselected trachea position. (Centers that favor decompression of the balloon by needle guided puncture favor placing the balloon higher up in the neck for ease of access at the time of desufflation.) The balloon position can be confirmed by ultrasound and/or the fetoscope. Once the balloon position has been confirmed and the mother and fetus are stable, all the instruments are removed, and the procedure is ended. Operative time can range from 3 to 90 minutes.[15] Factors that can prolong the operative time include undesired fetal positions and polyhydramnios. There is a higher risk of rupture of membranes with long operative times.[15]

Postoperative Considerations

Upon completion of the FETO procedure, patients are generally placed on bedrest and monitored for uterine contractions. The duration of monitoring varies between groups but can be up to 24–48 hours in the hospital with continuous fetal monitoring.[42,44,45] In the first 24 postoperative hours, the patients may receive nifedipine as a prophylactic tocolytic, low molecular weight heparin, and analgesics as needed.[39,43,45] Ultrasounds are performed biweekly to evaluate the structural integrity and position of the tracheal occlusion balloon, fetal pulmonary response, amniotic fluid volume, and fetal growth.[12,42,44] In the event of

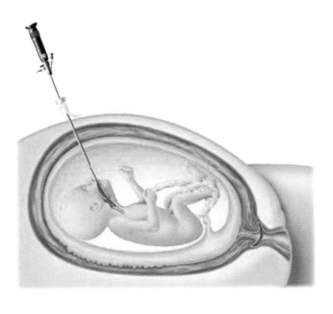

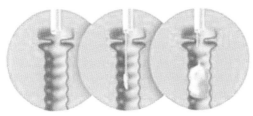

Figure 7.2 Percutaneous, transuterine insertion of endoscope into fetal trachea for placement of endoluminal balloon. Inset shows mid-tracheal placement of a detachable balloon for tracheal occlusion.
With permission from Deprest J, et al. *Ultrasound Obstet Gynecol.* 2004;24(2):121–126, First published: 27 July 2004, DOI: (10.1002/uog.1711).

a preterm delivery, corticosteroids are typically administered.[39,43,44] If the hospital course is uneventful, the patient can be discharged home. At our institution, during the FETO period, we require all our patients to stay in the same city as our fetal center in the event of preterm delivery or the need for emergent balloon extraction. Some centers obtain an MRI after about four weeks of tracheal occlusion to assess fetal lung growth and help with prognostication.

Reversal of Tracheal Occlusion

Balloon removal is typically performed between 32 and 34 weeks' gestation.[15,44,45] Reversal of tracheal occlusion permits lung maturation. Most of the lung growth from the tracheal occlusion peaks by the second or third week following balloon occlusion. Thereafter, as the fetus grows, the increase in the size of the trachea renders the balloon less occlusive. We had performed some mathematical modeling taking into account the rate of lung fluid production and the pressure generated within the airways with tracheal occlusion and theorized that a mere 0.1 mm gap between the balloon and fetal trachea will result in effective loss of occlusion. Other situations that may necessitate balloon reversal outside of this time frame include rupture of membrane with or without labor and infection.[15] The tracheal balloon can be removed in-utero via fetoscopy, by ultrasound-guided puncture, or at the time of delivery by EXIT.[12,13,39,42–46] The EXIT procedure allows the fetus to remain attached to the placental circulation until the tracheal balloon is retrieved and an endotracheal tube is inserted.[42] Nowadays, tracheal occlusion reversal is preferably performed fetoscopically.[13] If performed fetoscopically, the balloon is punctured with a sharp stylet with care not to advance the stylet beyond the carina or to cause damage to surrounding structures.[15] Ultrasound-guided puncture of the balloon is accomplished by inserting a 20- or 22-gauge needle through the maternal abdomen and the fetal thorax while directed at the trachea.[15,39,43] The fluid produced by the lungs then washes out the balloon.[15] If a patient presents in advanced labor or is very preterm with balloon in-situ, vaginal delivery may be performed. The balloon may be removed using a tracheoscope or it can be punctured using a 20- or 22-gauge needle which is inserted through the neck and under the cricoid cartilage.[39,43] In a controlled setting with a well-prepared team, the reversal should only take a few seconds.[15] The EXIT procedure is another option for tracheal occlusion reversal if these emergent cases arise.

Complications

In the hands of a well-trained surgeon and experienced fetal team, FETO can be performed quickly and safely. However, certain complications such as premature rupture of membranes (PROM) or preterm delivery may be inevitable.[13] This is the most common complication of FETO and the risk is especially heightened at the time of the balloon insertion and at the reversal procedure. Thus, these patients should always be monitored after the procedure and should stay close by and/or have easy access to a FETO center during this time period. Some centers have delayed the second intervention for balloon deflation until about 36 weeks to further delay the onset of PROM. This approach should only be entertained in centers that are set up for ready access and emergent balloon removal should the patient present in labor with a balloon in-situ.

References

1. Verla MA, Style CC, Olutoye OO. Prenatal intervention for the management of congenital diaphragmatic hernia. *Pediatr Surg Int.* 2018;**34**(6):579–587.

2. Allan DW, Greer JJ. Pathogenesis of nitrofen-induced congenital diaphragmatic hernia in fetal rats. *J Appl Physiol.* 1997;**83**(2):338–347.

3. Butler N, Claireaux AE. Congenital diaphragmatic hernia as a cause of perinatal mortality. *Lancet.* 1962;**1**(7231):659–663.

4. Harrison MR, Adzick NS, Estes JM, Howell LJ. A prospective study of the outcome for fetuses with diaphragmatic hernia. *JAMA.* 1994;**271**(5):382–384.

5. Mah VK, Zamakhshary M, Mah DY, et al. Absolute vs relative improvements in congenital diaphragmatic hernia survival: what happened to "hidden mortality." *J Pediatr Surg.* 2009;**44**(5):877–882.

6. Mehollin-Ray AR, Cassady CI, Cass DL, Olutoye OO. Fetal MR imaging of congenital diaphragmatic hernia. *Radiographics.* 2012;**32**(4):1067–1084.

7. Mesas Burgos C, Hammarqvist-Vejde J, Frenckner B, Conner P. Differences in outcomes in prenatally diagnosed congenital diaphragmatic hernia compared to postnatal detection: a single-center experience. *Fetal Diagn Ther.* 2016;**39**(4):241–247.

8. Akinkuotu AC, Cruz SM, Abbas PI, et al. Risk-stratification of severity for infants

with CDH: Prenatal versus postnatal predictors of outcome. *J Pediatr Surg.* 2016;**51**(1):44–48.

9. Jani J, Nicolaides KH, Keller RL, et al. Observed to expected lung area to head circumference ratio in the prediction of survival in fetuses with isolated diaphragmatic hernia. *Ultrasound Obstet Gynecol.* 2007;**30**(1):67–71.

10. Zamora IJ, Olutoye OO, Cass DL, et al. Prenatal MRI fetal lung volumes and percent liver herniation predict pulmonary morbidity in congenital diaphragmatic hernia (CDH). *J Pediatr Surg.* 2014;**49**(5):688–693.

11. Kohl T. Minimally invasive fetoscopic interventions: an overview in 2010. *Surg Endosc.* 2010;**24**(8):2056–2067.

12. Ruano R, Ali RA, Patel P, et al. Fetal endoscopic tracheal occlusion for congenital diaphragmatic hernia: indications, outcomes, and future directions. *Obstet Gynecol Surv.* 2014;**69**(3):147–158.

13. Peiro JL, Carreras E, Guillen G, et al. Therapeutic indications of fetoscopy: a 5-year institutional experience. *J Laparoendosc Adv Surg Tech A.* 2009;**19**(2):229–236.

14. Belfort MA, Olutoye OO, Cass DL, et al. Feasibility and outcomes of fetoscopic tracheal occlusion for severe left diaphragmatic hernia. *Obstet Gynecol.* 2017;**129**(1):20–29.

15. Deprest J, Nicolaides K, Done E, et al. Technical aspects of fetal endoscopic tracheal occlusion for congenital diaphragmatic hernia. *J Pediatr Surg.* 2011;**46**(1):22–32.

16. Kohl T, Muller A, Franz A, et al. Temporary fetoscopic tracheal balloon occlusion enhanced by hyperoncotic lung distension: is there a role in the treatment of fetal pulmonary hypoplasia from early preterm premature rupture of membranes? *Fetal Diagn Ther.* 2007;**22**(6):462–465.

17. Kohl T, Geipel A, Tchatcheva K, et al. Life-saving effects of fetal tracheal occlusion on pulmonary hypoplasia from preterm premature rupture of membranes. *Obstet Gynecol.* 2009;**113** (2 Pt 2):480–483.

18. Lally KP. Congenital diaphragmatic hernia – the past 25 (or so) years. *J Pediatr Surg.* 2016;**51**(5):695–698.

19. Harrison MR, Adzick NS, Bullard KM, et al. Correction of congenital diaphragmatic hernia in utero VII: a prospective trial. *J Pediatr Surg.* 1997;**32**(11):1637–1642.

20. Harrison MR, Adzick NS, Longaker MT, et al. Successful repair in utero of a fetal diaphragmatic hernia after removal of herniated viscera from the left thorax. *N Engl J Med.* 1990;**322**(22):1582–1584.

21. Harrison MR, Adzick NS, Flake AW, Jennings RW. The CDH two-step: a dance of necessity. *J Pediatr Surg.* 1993;**28**(6):813–816.

22. Harrison MR, Adzick NS, Flake AW, et al. Correction of congenital diaphragmatic hernia in utero: VI. Hard-earned lessons. *J Pediatr Surg.* 1993;**28**(10):1411–1417.

23. MacGillivray TE, Jennings RW, Rudolph AM, et al. Vascular changes with in utero correction of diaphragmatic hernia. *J Pediatr Surg.* 1994;**29**(8):992–996.

24. Skarsgard ED, Meuli M, VanderWall KJ, et al. Fetal endoscopic tracheal occlusion ('Fetendo-PLUG') for congenital diaphragmatic hernia. *J Pediatr Surg.* 1996;**31**(10):1335–1338.

25. Alcorn D, Adamson TM, Lambert TF, et al. Morphological effects of chronic tracheal ligation and drainage in the fetal lamb lung. *J Anat.* 1977;**123**(Pt 3):649–660.

26. Carmel JA, Friedman F, Adams FH. Fetal tracheal ligation and lung development. *Am J Dis Child.* 1965;**109**(5):452–456.

27. Lanman JT, Schaffer A, Herod L, et al. Distensibility of the fetal lung with fluid in sheep. *Pediatr Res.* 1971;5:586.

28. Wilson JM, DiFiore JW, Peters CA. Experimental fetal tracheal ligation prevents the pulmonary hypoplasia associated with fetal nephrectomy: possible application for congenital diaphragmatic hernia. *J Pediatr Surg.* 1993;**28**(11):1433–1439.

29. Beierle EA, Langham MR, Jr., Cassin S. In utero lung growth of fetal sheep with diaphragmatic hernia and tracheal stenosis. *J Pediatr Surg.* 1996;**31**(1):141–146.

30. Bealer JF, Skarsgard ED, Hedrick MH, et al. The 'PLUG' odyssey: adventures in experimental fetal tracheal occlusion. *J Pediatr Surg.* 1995;**30**(2):361–364.

31. DiFiore JW, Fauza DO, Slavin R, et al. Experimental fetal tracheal ligation reverses the structural and physiological effects of pulmonary hypoplasia in congenital diaphragmatic hernia. *J Pediatr Surg.* 1994;**29**(2):248–256.

32. Hedrick MH, Estes JM, Sullivan KM, et al. Plug the lung until it grows (PLUG): a new method to treat congenital diaphragmatic hernia in utero. *J Pediatr Surg.* 1994;**29**(5):612–617.

33. Harrison MR, Adzick NS, Flake AW, et al. Correction of congenital diaphragmatic hernia in utero VIII: Response of the hypoplastic lung to tracheal occlusion. *J Pediatr Surg.* 1996;**31**(10):1339–1348.

34. Mychaliska GB, Bealer JF, Graf JL, et al. Operating on placental support: the ex utero intrapartum treatment procedure. *J Pediatr Surg.* 1997;**32**(2):227–230.

35. Harrison MR, Albanese CT, Hawgood SB, et al. Fetoscopic temporary tracheal occlusion by means of detachable balloon for congenital diaphragmatic hernia. *Am J Obstet Gynecol.* 2001;**185**(3):730–733.

36. Harrison MR, Sydorak RM, Farrell JA, et al. Fetoscopic temporary tracheal occlusion for congenital diaphragmatic hernia: prelude to a randomized, controlled trial. *J Pediatr Surg.* 2003;**38**(7):1012–1020.

37. Chiba T, Albanese CT, Farmer DL, et al. Balloon tracheal occlusion for congenital diaphragmatic hernia: experimental studies. *J Pediatr Surg.* 2000;**35**(11):1566–1570.

38. Longaker MT, Golbus MS, Filly RA, et al. Maternal outcome after open fetal surgery. A review of the first 17 human cases. *JAMA.* 1991;**265**(6):737–741.

39. Deprest J, Gratacos E, Nicolaides KH. Fetoscopic tracheal occlusion (FETO) for severe congenital diaphragmatic hernia: evolution of a technique and preliminary results. *Ultrasound Obstet Gynecol.* 2004;**24**(2):121–126.

40. Luks FI, Gilchrist BF, Jackson BT, Piasecki GJ. Endoscopic tracheal obstruction with an expanding device in a fetal lamb model: preliminary considerations. *Fetal Diagn Ther.* 1996;**11**(1):67–71.

41. Kohl T. Fetoscopic surgery: where are we today? *Curr Opin Anaesthesiol.* 2004;**17**(4):315–321.

42. Ruano R, Yoshisaki CT, da Silva MM, et al. A randomized controlled trial of fetal endoscopic tracheal occlusion versus postnatal management of severe isolated congenital diaphragmatic hernia. *Ultrasound Obstet Gynecol.* 2012;**39**(1):20–27.

43. Deprest J, Jani J, Gratacos E, et al. Fetal intervention for congenital diaphragmatic hernia: the European experience. *Semin Perinatol.* 2005;**29**(2):94–103.

44. Jani J, Gratacos E, Greenough A, et al. Percutaneous fetal endoscopic tracheal occlusion (FETO) for severe left-sided congenital diaphragmatic hernia. *Clin Obstet Gynecol.* 2005;**48**(4):910–922.

45. Peralta CF, Sbragia L, Bennini JR, et al. Fetoscopic endotracheal occlusion for severe isolated diaphragmatic hernia: initial experience from a single clinic in Brazil. *Fetal Diagn Ther.* 2011;**29**(1):71–77.

46. Jani JC, Nicolaides KH, Gratacos E, et al. Severe diaphragmatic hernia treated by fetal endoscopic tracheal occlusion. *Ultrasound Obstet Gynecol.* 2009;**34**(3):304–310.

Fetal Cardiac Intervention

Olutoyin A. Olutoye and Shaine Morris

Over the past 20 years, fetal cardiac intervention has expanded from a few centers to many centers across the world.[1,2] During this time, indications have expanded, selection criteria have been refined, and procedural mortality has declined.[2–8]

Prevalence of Fetal Cardiac Disease

While there is an appreciable increase in fetal cardiac intervention procedures, the actual incidence of fetal congenital heart disease (CHD) is difficult to assess as a certain percentage of affected fetuses die in-utero prior to a prenatal diagnosis. The most important conditions to diagnose in the prenatal period are those with critical congenital heart disease (CCHD), which includes conditions requiring intervention within the first year of life, and particularly within the first few days of life. International estimates of the birth prevalence of CCHD are between 10 and 30 pregnancies with CHD per 10,000 pregnancies.[9] Although some studies suggest a decreasing birth prevalence of CCHD, detailed studies suggest that the actual fetal prevalence of CCHD may be stable. The observed declining birth prevalence may be secondary to increasing prenatal diagnosis rates and subsequent increasing termination of pregnancies for fetuses with CCHD.[10–12]

All fetal screening evaluations include screening for cardiac conditions, as most fetal heart disease occurs in low-risk populations. The mid-gestation obstetric ultrasound can detect > 50% of severe cardiac malformations when it includes the four-chamber view.[13] When evaluation of the three vessels, outflow tracts, and trachea are added to the study, the sensitivity to detect cardiac anomalies increases to 90%.[14,15] Detection of any abnormality on an obstetric scan warrants a more in-depth study via fetal echocardiography. The risk of CHD is greater than that of the general population in the presence of certain maternal conditions such as a maternal history of cardiac disease, diabetes mellitus, autoimmune disease, or drug exposure. In these situations, fetal echocardiography is also recommended in addition to the assessments previously mentioned.[13] Isolated fetal conditions that trigger dedicated cardiac imaging include monochorionic twinning (associated with a 2–9% incidence of cardiac malformations),[16,17] heart rate abnormalities (brady- or tachyarrhythmias), or noncardiac anomalies such as chromosomal abnormalities, abnormalities of the umbilical cord or venous system, nonimmune hydrops and increased nuchal translucency (subcutaneous swelling on back of the fetus neck), on first trimester screening.

Fetal Echocardiography

Fetal echocardiography can detect many cardiac conditions in-utero provided the fetus has an optimal lie and the image resolution is adequate. In experienced hands, fetal echocardiography detects approximately 90–98% of serious congenital heart disease in low-risk patient populations.[18–22] Some cardiac conditions may remain undetected in-utero such as atrial septal defects (because of the obligate patency of the foramen ovale in-utero), and small ventricular septal defects (because of the equal ventricular pressures), but these tend to be minor lesions which do not pose a threat to life. A fetal echocardiogram is preferentially performed between 18 and 22 weeks' gestation and is most performed after the mid-trimester obstetric ultrasound screening. The timing of the fetal echocardiogram may, however, be influenced by the timing of the patient referral from the outside institution, or the time at which the patient commences her prenatal visits. First trimester fetal echocardiography is possible in some institutions and has a reasonable detection rate for major anomalies.[23] Because of the suboptimal negative predictive value of the study at this stage of gestation, at-risk pregnant mothers undergoing first trimester fetal echocardiography should undergo a repeat examination in the second trimester.[24] A repeat second or possibly third trimester fetal echocardiogram may be necessary after the first cardiac evaluation depending on the timing of the first screen, course of identified lesion, or nature of progression of the identified disease.[13]

The initial assessment in the fetal echocardiogram involves evaluation of the four-chamber view which allows assessment of cardiac size, angulation of the apex, and determination of size and situs of the atria and ventricles. Additional views to evaluate the outflow tracts, three-vessel and trachea view, are also obtained (Figure 8.1).[25] Fetal echocardiography also includes a detailed 2D/gray-scale imaging of the cardiovascular structures including color Doppler interrogation of all the valves, veins, arteries, atrial and ventricular septae; pulsed Doppler of the valves and ductus venosus, as well as assessment of cardiac rhythm and function using 2D, M-mode, and pulsed Doppler imaging (Figure 8.2).[26] Additional information that can be obtained which is useful to the fetal specialist, includes cardiac biometry, additional Doppler measures and quantitative evaluation of cardiac function. These additional measurements can facilitate the diagnosis of other subtle cardiac conditions. Color Doppler enhances assessment of the fetal heart as it provides detailed information on the patency of the ventricular inflow and outflow tracts, anatomy and flow through the arches and competency of atrioventricular and semilunar valves.[27–29] The use of color Doppler is particularly helpful at earlier gestational ages.[30,31] The heart rate, as well as the relationship between the atrial and ventricular contractions can also be assessed. The latter is particularly important in assessment of arrhythmias. Differentiation between specific types of arrhythmias is important as this helps guide treatment options.[32,33]

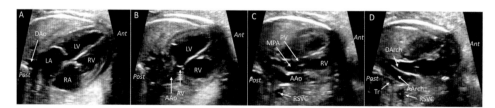

Figure 8.1 Basic cardiac evaluation in the fetus first involves evaluation of the heart sweeping from the four-chamber view (A), to the left ventricular outflow tract (B), to the right ventricular outflow tract (C), to the three-vessel and trachea view (D). AAo: Ascending aorta, AArch: Aortic arch, Ant: Anterior, AV: Aortic valve, DAo: Descending aorta, DArch: Ductal arch, LA: Left atrium, LV: Left ventricle, MPA: Main pulmonary artery, Post: Posterior, PV: Pulmonary valve, RA: Right atrium, RSVC: Right superior vena cava, RV: Right ventricle, Tr: Trachea.

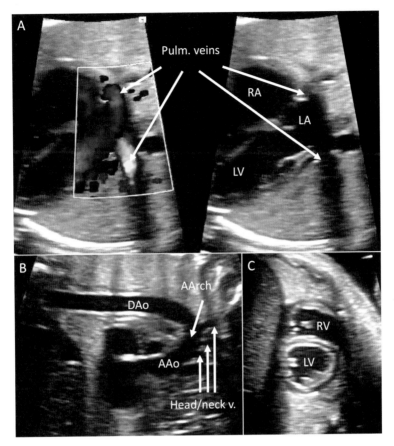

Figure 8.2 A sample of additional images collected during fetal echocardiography. (A) Color Doppler interrogation from the four-chamber view demonstrated normal return of at least two pulmonary veins. (B) The aortic arch in long axis. (C) Short-axis view of the right and left ventricles. AAo: Ascending aorta, AArch: Aortic arch, DAo: Descending aorta, Head/neck v.: head and neck vessels, LA: Left atrium, LV: Left ventricle, Pulm. veins: Pulmonary veins, RA: Right atrium, RV: Right ventricle.

Extracardiac Anomalies and Genetic Conditions

Following a diagnosis of a fetal cardiac condition which may likely benefit from intervention, it is important to rule out any extracardiac anomalies as the presence of one anomaly in the fetus commonly signifies the presence of another congenital malformation.[34] Associated anomalies may be detected via prenatal radiologic evaluation including ultrasound and fetal magnetic resonance imaging (MRI). Genetic testing for aneuploidy and for copy number variation (typically using microarray technology), should also be strongly considered via chorionic villus sampling or amniocentesis, as up to 21% of fetuses with congenital heart disease will have a pathogenic variant detected by one of these methods.[35] Whole exome sequencing is not universally available prenatally, but can have significant additional diagnostic yield; a study limited to fetuses with left-sided lesions showed 18% had aneuploidy or copy number variation, and an additional 16% had evidence of single gene defects detected by whole exome sequencing, for a total of 34% with a clear genetic abnormality.[36]

Trisomy 21, 13 and 18 are among the most common chromosomal anomalies. Other microduplications and microdeletions including 22q11.21 deletion are also common. Single genes for which variants cause CHD include *PTPN11, KMT2D, NOTCH1, CHD7*, among many others.[37] For conditions compatible with life where postnatal management is considered, genetic testing allows for proper management of the parents' expectations as some conditions are amenable to successful postnatal intervention while others are not and are associated with a tenuous course postdelivery.

Genetic testing is highly important in the face of an existing diagnosis of fetal congenital heart disease for many reasons; it allows for investigation of additional anomalies, may provide information on the recurrence risk for the parents of the fetus, or for the child when he/she reaches reproductive age. Most importantly, it guides parental decision on pregnancy termination (depending on the gestational age at diagnosis and the country in which the patient resides). It also informs whether aggressive postnatal management should be considered. Lastly, information obtained from genetic testing may preclude a discussion on possible in-utero cardiac intervention because of the high mortality of the detected cardiac lesion.

Cardiac Interventions

In-utero cardiac intervention is available for multiple fetal cardiac conditions, and reduces the morbidity or mortality associated with certain lesions. Cardiac interventions can usually be grouped into: pharmacologic intervention, in which the fetus receives medical therapy, typically transplacental via maternal administration; catheter-based intervention, in which techniques using needle insertion followed by catheter introduction to the fetal heart are employed; and open fetal surgery, in which the fetus' heart is directly exposed for a surgical procedure. Examples of each of these interventions are listed in Table 8.1.

Open fetal surgery as well as ex-utero intrapartum therapy with resection of intracardiac tumor on placental support, have both been described for the management of intrapericardial tumors.[42,51] Intrapericardial tumors are rare and lethal tumors, consisting of all three germ layers.[52] They can be challenging to manage as the prognosis typically depends on the time of diagnosis, rate of growth, as well as the presence of pericardial tamponade and/or hydrops fetalis. Indications for treatment include increase in tumor size and a decrease in cardiac output. In the absence of hydrops, mid-gestation in-utero resection as well as resection on uteroplacental support, via the EXIT procedure have been successful.[42]

General anesthesia, required for open fetal surgery and the EXIT procedure (exit-to-resection, in this case), is the same regardless of the indication, and is discussed in later chapters.

The mode of anesthesia required for catheter-based procedures, which comprise most fetal cardiac interventions, will be discussed in this chapter following the description of the individual conditions.

Catheter-Based Fetal Cardiac Intervention

Three main fetal cardiac conditions may be subject to catheter-based intervention: Severe aortic stenosis with evolving hypoplastic left heart syndrome (eHLHS), hypoplastic left heart syndrome (HLHS) with intact or severely restrictive atrial septum, and pulmonary stenosis/atresia with intact ventricular septum (PA/IVS). Atrial septoplasty and atrial

Table 8.1 Categories of fetal cardiac intervention[2,6,7,13,38–50]

Group	Condition	Intervention
Pharmacologic	Tachyarrhythmia	Transplacental antiarrhythmic medication (e.g. digoxin, flecainide, sotalol, amiodarone)
	Heart block	Steroids
	Myocarditis	Steroids, intravenous immunoglobulin
	Left heart hypoplasia	Chronic maternal hyperoxygenation
	Ebstein anomaly and tricuspid valve dysplasia	Transplacental nonsteroidal anti-inflammatory medication to induce ductal restriction Chronic maternal hyperoxygenation
Catheter-based	Severe aortic stenosis	Aortic valvuloplasty
	Hypoplastic left heart syndrome with intact or restrictive atrial septum	Atrial septal septoplasty and/or stenting
	Severe pulmonary valve stenosis	Pulmonary valvuloplasty
Open surgery	Pericardial teratoma	Open tumor resection
Other	Pericardial effusion	Pericardiocentesis
	Heart block	Fetal pacemaker implantation

stenting of a restrictive atrial foramen may preserve the pulmonary function and improve stability in cases of HLHS with a restrictive atrial septum, thereby increasing the chances of successful postnatal surgery. In cases of semilunar valve stenosis, or atresia, however, fetal valvuloplasty aims to achieve a biventricular, rather than univentricular, circulation.[53]

Aortic Stenosis with Evolving HLHS

Fetal aortic valvuloplasty for aortic stenosis with eHLHS is the most performed fetal cardiac catheter-based intervention.[54] Severe aortic stenosis in this condition results in a dilated and severely dysfunctional left ventricle (Figure 8.3). If left untreated, left ventricle growth gradually slows down, is eventually halted, and hypoplastic left heart develops as the rest of the heart grows around the arrested left ventricle. Prenatal intervention via balloon valvuloplasty, if successful, improves antegrade flow, diastolic function, and ventricular filling, thereby increasing the chances of bidirectional circulation at the time of delivery.[53] While some data suggest that chances of a biventricular circulation are higher following fetal aortic valvuloplasty, compared to no intervention, mortality benefit has not been clearly demonstrated.[2,55,56]

The success of fetal aortic valvuloplasty depends on careful patient selection. Criteria must first select those most fated to develop HLHS. Once this is established, criteria are used to determine fetuses who are most likely to benefit from the intervention. The features most strongly associated with progression of fetal aortic stenosis to HLHS include retrograde flow in the transverse aortic arch, left to right blood flow across the foramen ovale, moderate to severe left ventricular dysfunction, and monophasic mitral valve inflow.[57] Physiologic criteria that suggest a favorable response to aortic valvuloplasty include higher left ventricular (LV) pressure, larger ascending aorta, improved LV diastolic function, and higher LV

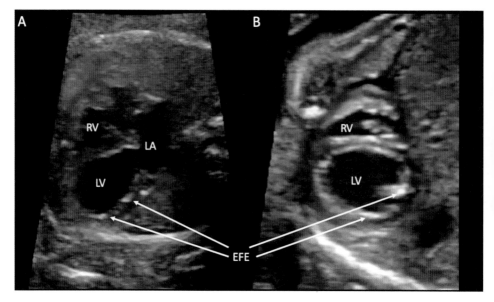

Figure 8.3 Fetal echocardiogram of a fetus with severe aortic stenosis. (A) 2D four-chamber view demonstrating a dilated and globular left ventricle with some endocardial fibroelastosis. (B) Short axis view of the ventricles showing the same. EFE: endocardial fibroelastosis, LA: left atrium, LV: left ventricle, RV: right ventricle.

long-axis z-scores.[7] The gestational age at which diagnosis is made is also important, as this is a progressive fetal condition. When severe aortic stenosis is noted in the second trimester, HLHS will likely evolve, although when detected in the third trimester this progression is much less likely. Of note, aortic stenosis early in gestation is very subtle and often missed on obstetric ultrasonography.[56]

Approach to Intervention

Figure 8.4 shows an example of an operating room setup for fetal cardiac catheter-based intervention. Under ultrasound guidance, typically a styletted 18- or 19-gauge needle is inserted through the maternal abdomen, uterine wall, fetal chest, and into the apex of the left ventricle. A wire and small coronary angioplasty balloon are then placed through the needle and positioned across the aortic valve. The balloon is then inflated across the valve and withdrawn (Figure 8.5). Success is determined following color Doppler evidence of anterograde flow across the aorta.[58]

HLHS or Other Critical Left Heart Obstruction With Intact or Restrictive Atrial Septum

A restrictive septum is present in about 22% of all HLHS patients and 6% have an intact atrial septum.[59] A severely restrictive or intact atrial septum poses severe danger to the fetus in-utero as the impaired egress of blood from the left atrium results in overburdening of the pulmonary venous system with progressive damage to the pulmonary vasculature, resulting in pulmonary hypertension and eventual damage to the lung parenchyma.[59–61] Neonatal intervention includes rapid left atrial decompression by performing an atrial septal

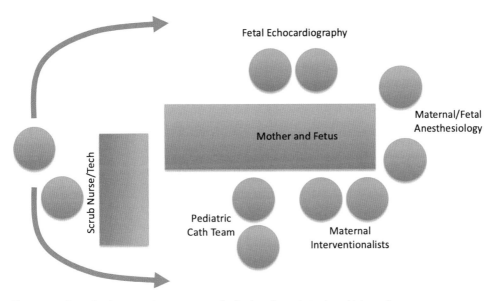

Figure 8.4 Example of an operating room setup for fetal cardiac catheter-based intervention.

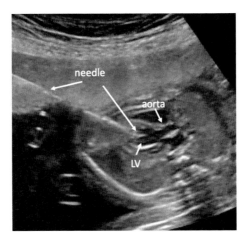

Figure 8.5 Fetal echocardiogram during fetal aortic valvuloplasty. In this image, the needle has been advanced into the left ventricular cavity.

intervention either in the catheterization lab or via surgery, in the operating room. Nevertheless, this scenario is associated with a poor prognosis. HLHS with a severely restrictive or intact atrial septum is associated with high mortality, reported as ~50% before Stage II palliation, ~70% at 1 year and up to 100% shortly after the Fontan procedure.[59,62–66] Given the severity of this condition, fetal atrial septal intervention has been employed to slow or halt the progression of pulmonary vascular disease. As with aortic valvuloplasty, selection criteria are important to determine fetuses who have the highest risk of neonatal instability following delivery. One of the best predictors of severe postnatal atrial septal restriction and neonatal instability in the fetus is the ratio of the pulmonary venous Doppler velocity time integral measures of prograde to retrograde flow < 2.7–3.[67,68] Atrial septal intervention in critical left heart obstruction has been associated with a lower cesarean section rate and a more stable neonate, but a mortality benefit has not been definitely demonstrated.[6,69,70] The limitations of studies of fetal atrial septal intervention to date include small sample sizes, inconsistent candidacy criteria across institutions, and heterogeneous severity of obstruction.

At times, severe aortic stenosis is associated with severe mitral valve regurgitation and left atrial dilation. In this circumstance, a restrictive atrial septum is often present and hydrops occurs.[4,71,72] Fetal cardiac intervention, consisting of aortic valvuloplasty and/or atrial septal intervention may be employed in this condition for the typical reasons, and also in an attempt to prolong gestation by reversing hydrops which may be present because of the high venous pressures.[73]

Approach to Intervention

Both balloon septoplasty and stent placement have been used as modes of intervention. Stent placement is advantageous in fetuses with thick atrial septae and provides a persistently patent communication compared to balloon septoplasty.[70] An 18- or 19-gauge needle is inserted into either the right or left atrium and a 22-gauge needle or stylette is often used to puncture and cross the atrium. A balloon or balloon-mounted stent is then inflated across the septum. This procedure has been shown to be more technically challenging than valvuloplasty procedures.[70] One challenge is that a fair amount of manual force is needed to perforate the typically thick atrial septum, but there is a risk of atrial wall tearing or injury to the pulmonary veins. Recently, a laser technique has been utilized to more smoothly cross the atrial septum.[74] Current estimates suggest a technical success rate of ~77% and a fetal mortality rate as a result of the procedure of ~13% (Figure 8.6).

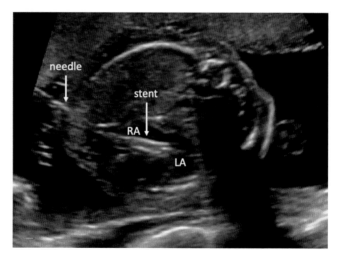

Figure 8.6 Fetal echocardiogram during atrial septal stent placement. The stent has been inflated, causing the "railroad track" look with parallel white lines on echocardiography. LA: left atrium, RA: right atrium.

Pulmonary Atresia With Intact Intraventricular Septum (PA/IVS)

There is much more experience with valvuloplasty for stenosis of the aortic valve compared to that of the pulmonary valve, but there have been significant reports of the latter.[2,75–77] The concern with pulmonary stenosis/atresia in the presence of an intact ventricular septum is that, similar to what occurs with critical left heart obstruction, the right ventricle may experience growth arrest, and become too hypoplastic at birth to support a complete cardiac output. A severely hypoplastic right ventricle necessitates a single ventricle palliation. Potentially in-utero pulmonary valvuloplasty may allow egress from the right ventricle and support continued right ventricular growth, thereby allowing for a postnatal biventricular repair. The ultimate goal in treatment is to restore right ventricular function and promote biventricular function.[54] To date, the evidence to support this intervention has been suboptimal.[2] Candidacy would ideally be limited to fetuses at risk of progressing to single ventricle circulation, who also have a patent infundibulum and an identifiable pulmonary valve.[78] Several centers have addressed this question, and predictors usually involve fetal tricuspid valve z-score, tricuspid regurgitation, and/or ratios of right to left sided structures.[76,79–81] Although some centers have reported a high rate of ultimate biventricular repair, many of the fetuses undergoing intervention would not have been predicted to have single ventricle circulation.[5]

Approach to Intervention

Technically, the approach to pulmonary valvuloplasty is similar to that of aortic valvuloplasty, the only difference being the approach to the right ventricular outflow tract which lies behind the sternum and may be difficult to access. Access is best obtained via the subcostal or intercostal approach. Once an 18- or 19-gauge needle is inserted into the right ventricle, the stylette is removed and wire with a coronary balloon is inserted across the valve and inflated. Like the treatment of aortic stenosis, success is confirmed with color Doppler evidence of anterograde flow across the valve.

Complications

Maternal morbidity following these procedures are minimal and reports suggesting some morbidity are limited to the beginning phases of commencing these interventions where the mothers were undergoing general anesthesia, for abdominal laparotomy and some experienced fluid overload and wound hematomas.[2,58] The majority of complications following these procedures have been observed in fetuses of earlier gestational ages in whom the procedures can be technically challenging. The risk of technical challenge must always be balanced with the chance of disease progression if intervention is performed later in gestation.

Both aortic and pulmonary valvuloplasty may be complicated by bradycardia, ventricular dysfunction, hemopericardium, or fetal demise. Balloon septoplasty or stent placement for HLHS can have all these same complications in addition to stent dislodgement or embolization.[6,70,82,83]

Anesthesia for Fetal Cardiac Intervention

Like the considerations for fetal cardiac intervention, the mode of anesthesia for fetal cardiac intervention has evolved over the years. The proper maternal candidate must be selected to undergo anesthesia for this procedure as the mother's safety comes first and must be prioritized over the health or safety of the fetus when any fetal cardiac intervention is considered. This holds true also for any fetal intervention. Mothers with American Society of Anesthesiology (ASA) Class 1 or 2 classification are typically considered for these procedures.

A thorough preoperative history and physical examination is performed with necessary consultations obtained. Recommendations made by consultants should be strictly followed to optimize the mother's general health condition prior to surgery.

General anesthesia was initially described for patients undergoing fetal cardiac intervention[58] and is still required in rare instances where a maternal hysterotomy will be necessary to accomplish the procedure. Inhalational anesthetics utilized for general anesthesia provide the added benefit of uterine relaxation. In most cases nowadays, however, this form of anesthesia has not been required. Neuraxial anesthesia via epidural, combined spinal-epidural, or spinal routes are more commonly employed for fetal cardiac interventions.

When the plan includes an epidural catheter, this is placed prior to the patient arriving in the operating room. A test dose must be administered in addition to a small dose of bupivacaine to ensure the expected response can be elicited, that is some paresthesia (confirmation that the catheter is working), prior to wheeling the patient into the operating room. Full dosing of the catheter should not occur before the patient arrives in the operating room as an adequate fetal lie (imperative to success of the procedure), must be confirmed by the maternal-fetal medicine physicians before the required T6 sensory level of anesthesia is obtained.

On arrival in the operating room, the patient is positioned on the operating bed in a left lateral position and ASA monitors are placed. The maternal-fetal medicine and fetal cardiac interventionist teams perform an ultrasound to determine the lie of the baby and presence of adequate surgical access to perform the procedure. It is important not to administer any sedative to the mother prior to confirmation of an adequate fetal lie, because transplacental passage of sedatives to the fetus may sedate the fetus and make it challenging for a successful version if this is necessary for the procedure to be performed. Once the fetus' position has been confirmed to be adequate for precise catheter placement and fetal medication has been administered for analgesia and relaxation, the mother may receive some sedation depending on her anxiety level. The fetus typically receives an intramuscular injection of a combination medication into the gluteal muscle, thigh, or shoulder depending on position. This combination usually includes fentanyl for pain (5-10 mcg/kg) or higher, atropine (20 mcg/kg) and vecuronium (0.4 mg/kg). Small volumes of medication are preferred so the medications should not be overdiluted. Vecuronium, for example, should be diluted to 2 mg/mL prior to dispensing the weight-based dose for the fetus. After the fetus receives the medication and while the surgeons are scrubbing for surgery, dosing of the mother's epidural catheter with 0.25% bupivacaine or 0.2% ropivicaine should occur with the goal of achieving a T6 sensory level. Prior to commencing surgery, an adequate sensory level of anesthesia should be confirmed using a skin pinch to ensure the epidural is working adequately. As the duration of the procedure varies greatly, approximately half of the required volume to achieve the T6 level should be administered via the epidural catheter every 60–90 minutes to maintain the sensory level.

Combined spinal epidural anesthesia may be considered; however, there can be a lot of down time before the procedure finally starts with requirements for positioning of the fetus as well as preparation of equipment for the procedure. In addition, intrathecal administration of medication may accentuate maternal hypotension, which is unfavorable for a fetus who already has a baseline marginal cardiac status. Either of these modes of anesthesia provides the necessary relaxation required for version of the fetus if this is required, to facilitate the procedure.

Confirmation of adequate fetal lie is the main prerequisite for success of fetal cardiac interventions and procedures may occasionally be rescheduled because of an inability to get the fetus in the right position. Version of the fetus can be uncomfortable but a neuraxial block with either an epidural or combined-spinal anesthesia allows the mother to tolerate this uncomfortable preparatory phase of the procedure. Spinal anesthesia may be considered as a mode of anesthesia; however, the side effect of hypotension which is not desirable especially for fetal cardiac conditions plus the limited duration of this block make it a less desirable option. General and spinal anesthesia are both associated with maternal hypotension and increased use of vasopressors. While the intraoperative use of vasopressors helps maintain maternal blood pressure within 20% of baseline during obstetric surgery, vasopressors can also alter normal placental perfusion and fetal blood flow.[84]

Once the procedure is under way, maternal sedation may be required to allay any anxiety the mother may have. This can be accomplished by intermittent boluses or infusions of sedatives such as remifentanil or dexmedetomidine. These procedures usually involve a lot of ongoing discussion among the MFM physicians, interventional cardiologists, and cardiologists so maternal sedation is usually helpful.

The fetus is continuously monitored during these procedures by a cardiologist using ultrasound to guide the intervention and assess the fetal heart rate, cardiac volume status, and myocardial contractility. Fetal brady- or tachyarrhythmias commonly occur during fetal cardiac interventions. As such, additional fetal resuscitative medications and measures may be required to treat the fetus. These include atropine, epinephrine, calcium gluconate, lactated Ringer's fluid boluses (10cc aliquots), and occasionally direct administration of blood to the fetus. It is not uncommon for these to be administered via the intracardiac route during fetal resuscitation. Fetal bradycardia, cardiac tamponade, and cerebral hemorrhage are all described complications of fetal cardiac intervention. Valvular regurgitation commonly occurs, particularly when an aortic valvuloplasty is performed and this is better tolerated in-utero than in the postnatal period.[85,86]

Despite the documented intraprocedure complications, mortality from these procedures has improved in centers where they are performed regularly. Fetal demise in these centers is down to 5–10% but still ranges from 32% in centers that do not see these cases on a regular basis.[2,87] This emphasizes the need for these cases to be performed at centers where personnel with experienced hands abound. Overall, when contemplating candidacy for a procedure, the care teams must balance potential risks, benefits, and goals of the parents.

References

1. Gardiner HM, Kovacevic A, Tulzer G, et al. Natural history of 107 cases of fetal aortic stenosis from a European multicenter retrospective study. *Ultrasound Obstet Gynecol.* 2016;48(3):373–381. doi: 10.1002/uog.15876 [doi].

2. Moon-Grady AJ, Morris SA, Belfort M, et al. International fetal cardiac intervention registry: A worldwide collaborative description and preliminary outcomes. *J Am Coll Cardiol.* 2015;66(4):388–399. doi: 10.1016/j.jacc.2015.05.037 [doi].

3. Freud LR, McElhinney DB, Marshall AC, et al. Fetal aortic valvuloplasty for evolving hypoplastic left heart syndrome: Postnatal outcomes of the first 100 patients. *Circulation.* 2014;130(8):638–645. doi: 10.1161/CIRCULATIONAHA.114.009032 [doi].

4. Mallmann MR, Herberg U, Gottschalk I, et al. Fetal cardiac intervention in critical aortic stenosis with severe mitral regurgitation, severe left atrial enlargement, and restrictive foramen ovale. *Fetal Diagn Ther.* 2020;**47** (5):440–447. doi: 10.1159/000502840 [doi].

5. Tulzer A, Arzt W, Gitter R, et al. Immediate effects and outcome of in-utero pulmonary valvuloplasty in fetuses with pulmonary atresia with intact ventricular septum or critical pulmonary stenosis. *Ultrasound Obstet Gynecol.* 2018;**52** (2):230–237. doi: 10.1002/uog.19047 [doi].

6. Jantzen DW, Moon-Grady AJ, Morris SA, et al. Hypoplastic left heart syndrome with intact or restrictive atrial septum: A report from the international fetal cardiac intervention registry. *Circulation.* 2017;**136** (14):1346–1349. doi: 10.1161/ CIRCULATIONAHA.116.025873 [doi].

7. Friedman KG, Sleeper LA, Freud LR, et al. Improved technical success, postnatal outcome and refined predictors of outcome for fetal aortic valvuloplasty. *Ultrasound Obstet Gynecol.* 2018;**52** (2):212–220. doi: 10.1002/uog.17530 [doi].

8. Nugent AW, Kowal RC, Juraszek AL, Ikemba C, Magee K. Model of magnetically guided fetal cardiac intervention: Potential to avoid direct cardiac puncture. *J Matern Fetal Neonatal Med.* 2013;**26** (18):1778–1781. doi: 10.3109/ 14767058.2013.818116 [doi].

9. Bakker MK, Bergman JEH, Krikov S, et al. Prenatal diagnosis and prevalence of critical congenital heart defects: An international retrospective cohort study. *BMJ Open.* 2019;**9**(7):e028139-2018– 028139. doi: 10.1136/bmjopen-2018- 028139 [doi].

10. Lytzen R, Vejlstrup N, Bjerre J, et al. Live-born major congenital heart disease in Denmark: Incidence, detection rate, and termination of pregnancy rate from 1996 to 2013. *JAMA Cardiol.* 2018;**3**(9):829–837. doi: 10.1001/jamacardio.2018.2009 [doi].

11. Idorn L, Olsen M, Jensen AS, et al. Univentricular hearts in Denmark 1977 to 2009: Incidence and survival. *Int J Cardiol.* 2013;**167**(4):1311–1316. doi: 10.1016/j. ijcard.2012.03.182 [doi].

12. Egbe A, Uppu S, Lee S, Ho D, Srivastava S. Changing prevalence of severe congenital heart disease: A population-based study. *Pediatr Cardiol.* 2014;**35**(7):1232–1238. doi: 10.1007/s00246-014-0921-7 [doi].

13. Donofrio MT, Moon-Grady AJ, Hornberger LK, et al. Diagnosis and treatment of fetal cardiac disease: A scientific statement from the American Heart Association. *Circulation.* 2014;**129** (21):2183–2242. doi: 10.1161/01. cir.0000437597.44550.5d [doi].

14. Kirk JS, Riggs TW, Comstock CH, Lee W, Yang SS, Weinhouse E. Prenatal screening for cardiac anomalies: The value of routine addition of the aortic root to the four-chamber view. *Obstet Gynecol.* 1994;**84**(3):427–431.

15. Del Bianco A, Russo S, Lacerenza N, et al. Four chamber view plus three-vessel and trachea view for a complete evaluation of the fetal heart during the second trimester. *J Perinat Med.* 2006;**34**(4):309–312. doi: 10.1515/JPM.2006.059 [doi].

16. Bahtiyar MO, Dulay AT, Weeks BP, et al. Prevalence of congenital heart defects in monochorionic/diamniotic twin gestations: A systematic literature review. *J Ultrasound Med.* 2007;**26**(11):1491–1498. doi: 26/11/1491 [pii].

17. Lopriore E, Bokenkamp R, Rijlaarsdam M, et al. Congenital heart disease in twin-to-twin transfusion syndrome treated with fetoscopic laser surgery. *Congenit Heart Dis.* 2007;**2**(1):38–43. doi: 10.1111/j.1747- 0803.2007.00070.x [doi].

18. Stumpflen I, Stumpflen A, Wimmer M, Bernaschek G. Effect of detailed fetal echocardiography as part of routine prenatal ultrasonographic screening on detection of congenital heart disease. *Lancet.* 1996;**348**(9031):854–857. doi: S0140-6736(96)04069-X [pii].

19. Yagel S, Weissman A, Rotstein Z, et al. Congenital heart defects: Natural course and in utero development. *Circulation.* 1997;**96**(2):550–555. doi: 10.1161/01. cir.96.2.550 [doi].

20. Rakha S, El Marsafawy H. Sensitivity, specificity, and accuracy of fetal echocardiography for high-risk pregnancies in a tertiary center in Egypt. *Arch Pediatr.* 2019;**26**(6):337–341. doi: S0929-693X(19)30117-4 [pii].

21. Pinheiro DO, Varisco BB, Silva MBD, et al. Accuracy of prenatal diagnosis of congenital cardiac MalformationsAcuracia do diagnostico pre-natal de cardiopatias congenitas. *Rev Bras Ginecol Obstet.* 2019;**41**(1):11–16. doi: 10.1055/s-0038-1676058 [doi].

22. Pasierb MM, Penalver JM, Vernon MM, Arya B. The role of regional prenatal cardiac screening for congenital heart disease: A single center experience. *Congenit Heart Dis.* 2018;**13**(4):571–577. doi: 10.1111/chd.12611 [doi].

23. Yu D, Sui L, Zhang N. Performance of first-trimester fetal echocardiography in diagnosing fetal heart defects: Meta-analysis and systematic review. *J Ultrasound Med.* 2020;**39**(3):471–480. doi: 10.1002/jum.15123 [doi].

24. McBrien A, Hornberger LK. Early fetal echocardiography. *Birth Defects Res.* 2019;**111**(8):370–379. doi: 10.1002/bdr2.1414 [doi].

25. Rychik J, Ayres N, Cuneo B, et al. American Society of Echocardiography guidelines and standards for performance of the fetal echocardiogram. *J Am Soc Echocardiogr.* 2004;**17**(7):803–810. doi: 10.1016/j.echo.2004.04.011 [doi].

26. Hornberger LK, Sahn DJ. Rhythm abnormalities of the fetus. *Heart.* 2007;**93**(10):1294–1300. doi: 93/10/1294 [pii].

27. Stewart PA, Wladimiroff JW. Fetal echocardiography and color doppler flow imaging: The Rotterdam experience. *Ultrasound Obstet Gynecol.* 1993;**3**(3):168–175. doi: 10.1046/j.1469-0705.1993.03030168.x [doi].

28. Copel JA, Morotti R, Hobbins JC, Kleinman CS. The antenatal diagnosis of congenital heart disease using fetal echocardiography: Is color flow mapping necessary? *Obstet Gynecol.* 1991;**78**(1):1–8.

29. Gembruch U, Chatterjee MS, Bald R, et al. Color doppler flow mapping of fetal heart. *J Perinat Med.* 1991;**19**(1–2):27–32.

30. Moon-Grady A, Shahanavaz S, Brook M, et al. Can a complete fetal echocardiogram be performed at 12 to 16 weeks' gestation? *J Am Soc Echocardiogr.* 2012;**25**(12):1342–1352. doi: 10.1016/j.echo.2012.09.003 [doi].

31. Comas Gabriel C, Galindo A, Martinez JM, et al. Early prenatal diagnosis of major cardiac anomalies in a high-risk population. *Prenat Diagn.* 2002;**22**(7):586–593. doi: 10.1002/pd.372 [doi].

32. Fouron JC, Fournier A, Proulx F, et al. Management of fetal tachyarrhythmia based on superior vena cava/aorta doppler flow recordings. *Heart.* 2003;**89**(10):1211–1216. doi: 10.1136/heart.89.10.1211 [doi].

33. Carvalho JS, Prefumo F, Ciardelli V, et al. Evaluation of fetal arrhythmias from simultaneous pulsed wave doppler in pulmonary artery and vein. *Heart.* 2007;**93**(11):1448–1453. doi: hrt.2006.101659 [pii].

34. Copel JA, Pilu G, Kleinman CS. Congenital heart disease and extracardiac anomalies: Associations and indications for fetal echocardiography. *Am J Obstet Gynecol.* 1986;**154**(5):1121–1132. doi: 0002-9378(86)90773-8 [pii].

35. Cai M, Huang H, Su L, et al. Fetal congenital heart disease: Associated anomalies, identification of genetic anomalies by single-nucleotide polymorphism array analysis, and postnatal outcome. *Medicine (Baltimore).* 2018;**97**(50):e13617. doi: 10.1097/MD.0000000000013617 [doi].

36. Sun H, Yi T, Hao X, et al. Contribution of single-gene defects to congenital cardiac left-sided lesions in the prenatal setting. *Ultrasound Obstet Gynecol.* 2020;**56**(2):225–232. doi: 10.1002/uog.21883 [doi].

37. Lord J, McMullan DJ, Eberhardt RY, et al. Prenatal exome sequencing analysis in fetal structural anomalies detected by ultrasonography (PAGE): A cohort study. *Lancet.* 2019;**393**(10173):747–757. doi: S0140-6736(18)31940-8 [pii].

38. Schidlow DN, Freud L, Friedman K, Tworetzky W. Fetal interventions for structural heart disease. *Echocardiography.* 2017;**34**(12):1834–1841. doi: 10.1111/echo.13667 [doi].

39. Krishnan A, Arya B, Moak JP, Donofrio MT. Outcomes of fetal echocardiographic surveillance in anti-SSA exposed fetuses at a large fetal cardiology center. *Prenat Diagn.* 2014;**34**(12):1207–1212. doi: 10.1002/pd.4454 [doi].

40. Co-Vu J, Lopez-Colon D, Vyas HV, et al. Maternal hyperoxygenation: A potential therapy for congenital heart disease in the fetuses? A systematic review of the current literature. *Echocardiography.* 2017;**34**(12):1822–1833. doi: 10.1111/echo.13722 [doi].

41. Cuneo BF, Moon-Grady AJ, Sonesson SE, et al. Heart sounds at home: Feasibility of an ambulatory fetal heart rhythm surveillance program for anti-SSA-positive pregnancies. *J Perinatol.* 2017;**37**(3):226–230. doi: 10.1038/jp.2016.220 [doi].

42. Rychik J, Khalek N, Gaynor JW, et al. Fetal intrapericardial teratoma: Natural history and management including successful in utero surgery. *Am J Obstet Gynecol.* 2016;**215**(6):780.e1-780.e7. doi: S0002-9378(16)30575-0 [pii].

43. Riskin-Mashiah S, Moise KJ, Jr., Wilkins I, et al. In utero diagnosis of intrapericardial teratoma: A case for in utero open fetal surgery. *Prenat Diagn.* 1998;**18**(12):1328–1330. doi: 10.1002/(SICI)1097-0223(199812)18:123.0.CO;2-7 [pii].

44. Edwards LA, Lara DA, Sanz Cortes M, et al. Chronic maternal hyperoxygenation and effect on cerebral and placental vasoregulation and neurodevelopment in fetuses with left heart hypoplasia. *Fetal Diagn Ther.* 2019;**46**(1):45–57. doi: 10.1159/000489123 [doi].

45. Arunamata A, Axelrod DM, Bianco K, et al. Chronic antepartum maternal hyperoxygenation in a case of severe fetal Ebstein's anomaly with circular shunt physiology. *Ann Pediatr Cardiol.* 2017;**10**(3):284–287. doi: 10.4103/apc.APC_20_17 [doi].

46. Lara DA, Morris SA, Maskatia SA, et al. Pilot study of chronic maternal hyperoxygenation and effect on aortic and mitral valve annular dimensions in fetuses with left heart hypoplasia. *Ultrasound Obstet Gynecol.* 2016;**48**(3):365–372. doi: 10.1002/uog.15846 [doi].

47. Zeng S, Zhou Q, Zhang M, et al. Features and outcome of fetal cardiac aneurysms and diverticula: A single center experience in China. *Prenat Diagn.* 2016;**36**(1):68–73. doi: 10.1002/pd.4714 [doi].

48. Garcia Rodriguez R, Rodriguez Guedes A, Garcia Delgado R, et al. Prenatal diagnosis of cardiac diverticulum with pericardial effusion in the first trimester of pregnancy with resolution after early pericardiocentesis. *Case Rep Obstet Gynecol.* 2015;2015:154690. doi: 10.1155/2015/154690 [doi].

49. Carpenter RJ, Jr., Strasburger JF, Garson A, Jr., et al. Fetal ventricular pacing for hydrops secondary to complete atrioventricular block. *J Am Coll Cardiol.* 1986;**8**(6):1434–1436. doi: S0735-1097(86)80319-9 [pii].

50. Zhou L, Vest AN, Chmait RH, et al. A percutaneously implantable fetal pacemaker. *Conf Proc IEEE Eng Med Biol Soc.* 2014;2014:4459–4463. doi: 10.1109/EMBC.2014.6944614 [doi].

51. Nassr AA, Shazly SA, Morris SA, et al. Prenatal management of fetal intrapericardial teratoma: A systematic review. *Prenat Diagn.* 2017;**37**(9):849–863. doi: 10.1002/pd.5113 [doi].

52. Heerema-McKenney A, Harrison MR, Bratton B, et al. Congenital teratoma: A clinicopathologic study of 22 fetal and neonatal tumors. *Am J Surg Pathol.* 2005;**29**(1):29–38. doi: 00000478-200501000-00004 [pii].

53. Gardiner HM. In utero intervention for severe congenital heart disease. *Best Pract Res Clin Obstet Gynaecol.* 2019;58:42–54. doi: S1521-6934(19)30003-3 [pii].

54. Gellis L, Tworetzky W. The boundaries of fetal cardiac intervention: Expand or tighten? *Semin Fetal Neonatal Med.*

2017;**22**(6):399–403. doi: S1744-165X(17)30095-1 [pii].

55. Kovacevic A, Ohman A, Tulzer G, et al. Fetal hemodynamic response to aortic valvuloplasty and postnatal outcome: A European multicenter study. *Ultrasound Obstet Gynecol.* 2018;**52**(2):221–229. doi: 10.1002/uog.18913 [doi].

56. Freud LR, Moon-Grady A, Escobar-Diaz MC, et al. Low rate of prenatal diagnosis among neonates with critical aortic stenosis: Insight into the natural history in utero. *Ultrasound Obstet Gynecol.* 2015;**45**(3):326–332. doi: 10.1002/uog.14667 [doi].

57. Makikallio K, McElhinney DB, Levine JC, et al. Fetal aortic valve stenosis and the evolution of hypoplastic left heart syndrome: Patient selection for fetal intervention. *Circulation.* 2006;**113**(11):1401–1405. doi: CIRCULATIONAHA.105.588194 [pii].

58. Tworetzky W, Wilkins-Haug L, Jennings RW, et al. Balloon dilation of severe aortic stenosis in the fetus: Potential for prevention of hypoplastic left heart syndrome: Candidate selection, technique, and results of successful intervention. *Circulation.* 2004;**110**(15):2125–2131. doi: 01.CIR.0000144357.29279.54 [pii].

59. Rychik J, Rome JJ, Collins MH, et al. The hypoplastic left heart syndrome with intact atrial septum: Atrial morphology, pulmonary vascular histopathology and outcome. *J Am Coll Cardiol.* 1999;**34**(2):554–560. doi: S0735-1097(99)00225-9 [pii].

60. Vlahos AP, Lock JE, McElhinney DB, van der Velde ME. Hypoplastic left heart syndrome with intact or highly restrictive atrial septum: Outcome after neonatal transcatheter atrial septostomy. *Circulation.* 2004;**109**(19):2326–2330. doi: 10.1161/01.CIR.0000128690.35860.C5 [doi].

61. Goltz D, Lunkenheimer JM, Abedini M, et al. Left ventricular obstruction with restrictive inter-atrial communication leads to retardation in fetal lung maturation. *Prenat Diagn.* 2015;**35**(5):463–470. doi: 10.1002/pd.4559 [doi].

62. Arai S, Fujii Y, Kotani Y, et al. Surgical outcome of hypoplastic left heart syndrome with intact atrial septum. *Asian Cardiovasc Thorac Ann.* 2015;**23**(9):1034–1038. doi: 10.1177/0218492315606581 [doi].

63. Bichell D. Invited commentary. *Ann Thorac Surg.* 2020;**109**(3):833–834. doi: S0003-4975(19)31550-4 [pii].

64. Salve GG, Datar GM, Perumal G, et al. Impact of high-risk characteristics in hypoplastic left heart syndrome. *World J Pediatr Congenit Heart Surg.* 2019;**10**(4):475–484. doi: 10.1177/2150135119852319 [doi].

65. Vida VL, Bacha EA, Larrazabal A, et al. Hypoplastic left heart syndrome with intact or highly restrictive atrial septum: Surgical experience from a single center. *Ann Thorac Surg.* 2007;**84**(2):581–585; discussion 586. doi: S0003-4975(07)00729-1 [pii].

66. Glatz JA, Tabbutt S, Gaynor JW, et al. Hypoplastic left heart syndrome with atrial level restriction in the era of prenatal diagnosis. *Ann Thorac Surg.* 2007;**84**(5):1633–1638. doi: S0003-4975(07)01367-7 [pii].

67. Gellis L, Drogosz M, Lu M, et al. Echocardiographic predictors of neonatal illness severity in fetuses with critical left heart obstruction with intact or restrictive atrial septum. *Prenat Diagn.* 2018;**38**(10):788–794. doi: 10.1002/pd.5322 [doi].

68. Divanovic A, Hor K, Cnota J, et al. Prediction and perinatal management of severely restrictive atrial septum in fetuses with critical left heart obstruction: Clinical experience using pulmonary venous doppler analysis. *J Thorac Cardiovasc Surg.* 2011;**141**(4):988–994. doi: 10.1016/j.jtcvs.2010.09.043 [doi].

69. Chaturvedi RR, Ryan G, Seed M, et al. Fetal stenting of the atrial septum: Technique and initial results in cardiac lesions with left atrial hypertension. *Int J Cardiol.* 2013;**168**(3):2029–2036. doi: 10.1016/j.ijcard.2013.01.173 [doi].

70. Kalish BT, Tworetzky W, Benson CB, et al. Technical challenges of atrial septal stent placement in fetuses with hypoplastic left heart syndrome and intact atrial septum. *Catheter Cardiovasc Interv.* 2014;**84**(1):77–85. doi: 10.1002/ccd.25098 [doi].

71. Rogers LS, Peterson AL, Gaynor JW, et al. Mitral valve dysplasia syndrome: A unique form of left-sided heart disease. *J Thorac Cardiovasc Surg.* 2011;**142**(6):1381–1387. doi: 10.1016/j.jtcvs.2011.06.002 [doi].

72. Vogel M, McElhinney DB, Wilkins-Haug LE, et al. Aortic stenosis and severe mitral regurgitation in the fetus resulting in giant left atrium and hydrops: Pathophysiology, outcomes, and preliminary experience with pre-natal cardiac intervention. *J Am Coll Cardiol.* 2011;**57**(3):348–355. doi: 10.1016/j.jacc.2010.08.636 [doi].

73. Ide T, Miyoshi T, Kitano M, et al. Fetal critical aortic stenosis with natural improvement of hydrops fetalis due to spontaneous relief of severe restrictive atrial communication. *J Obstet Gynaecol Res.* 2015;**41**(7):1137–1140. doi: 10.1111/jog.12681 [doi].

74. Belfort MA, Morris SA, Espinoza J, et al. Thulium laser-assisted atrial septal stent placement: First use in fetal hypoplastic left heart syndrome and intact atrial septum. *Ultrasound Obstet Gynecol.* 2019;**53** (3):417–418. doi: 10.1002/uog.20161 [doi].

75. Tulzer G, Arzt W, Franklin RC, et al. Fetal pulmonary valvuloplasty for critical pulmonary stenosis or atresia with intact septum. *Lancet.* 2002;**360**(9345):1567–1568. doi: S0140-6736(02)11531-5 [pii].

76. Gomez Montes E, Herraiz I, Mendoza A, Galindo A. Fetal intervention in right outflow tract obstructive disease: Selection of candidates and results. *Cardiol Res Pract.* 2012;2012:592403. doi: 10.1155/2012/592403 [doi].

77. Polat T, Danisman N. Pulmonary valvulotomy in a fetus with pulmonary atresia with intact ventricular septum: First experience in Turkey. *Images Paediatr Cardiol.* 2012;**14**(3):6–11.

78. Tworetzky W, McElhinney DB, Marx GR, et al. In utero valvuloplasty for pulmonary atresia with hypoplastic right ventricle: Techniques and outcomes. *Pediatrics.* 2009;**124**(3):e510-8. doi: 10.1542/peds.2008-2014 [doi].

79. Roman KS, Fouron JC, Nii M, et al. Determinants of outcome in fetal pulmonary valve stenosis or atresia with intact ventricular septum. *Am J Cardiol.* 2007;**99**(5):699–703. doi: S0002-9149(06)02277-6 [pii].

80. Gardiner HM. In-utero intervention for severe congenital heart disease. *Best Pract Res Clin Obstet Gynaecol.* 2008;**22** (1):49–61. doi: 10.1016/j.bpobgyn.2007.06.003.

81. Gottschalk I, Strizek B, Menzel T, et al. Severe pulmonary stenosis or atresia with intact ventricular septum in the fetus: The natural history. *Fetal Diagn Ther.* 2020;**47** (5):420–428. doi: 10.1159/000502178 [doi].

82. Marshall AC, Levine J, Morash D, et al. Results of in utero atrial septoplasty in fetuses with hypoplastic left heart syndrome. *Prenat Diagn.* 2008;**28**(11):1023–1028. doi: 10.1002/pd.2114 [doi].

83. Jaeggi E, Renaud C, Ryan G, Chaturvedi R. Intrauterine therapy for structural congenital heart disease: Contemporary results and Canadian experience. *Trends Cardiovasc Med.* 2016;**26**(7):639–646. doi: 10.1016/j.tcm.2016.04.006 [doi].

84. Ferschl MB, Feiner J, Vu L, et al. A comparison of spinal anesthesia versus monitored anesthesia care with local anesthesia in minimally invasive fetal surgery. *Anesth Analg.* 2020;**130** (2):409–415. doi: 10.1213/ANE.0000000000003947 [doi].

85. McElhinney DB, Marshall AC, Wilkins-Haug LE, et al. Predictors of technical success and postnatal biventricular outcome after in utero aortic valvuloplasty for aortic stenosis with evolving hypoplastic left heart syndrome. *Circulation.* 2009;**120** (15):1482–1490. doi: 10.1161/CIRCULATIONAHA.109.848994 [doi].

86. Arzt W, Wertaschnigg D, Veit I, et al. Intrauterine aortic valvuloplasty in fetuses with critical aortic stenosis: Experience and results of 24 procedures. *Ultrasound Obstet Gynecol.* 2011;**37**(6):689–695. doi: 10.1002/uog.8927 [doi].

87. Galindo A, Gomez-Montes E, Gomez O, et al. Fetal aortic valvuloplasty: Experience and results of two tertiary centers in Spain. *Fetal Diagn Ther.* 2017;**42**(4):262–270. doi: 10.1159/000460247 [doi].

Antepartum Fetal Monitoring

Jimmy Espinoza

The conventional view is that fetal hypoxia and acidosis leads to multi-systemic fetal injury and death. The objective of antenatal fetal surveillance (AFS) is to identify the compromised fetus with the intention of providing an opportunity to intervene before permanent damage or death occurs.[1] Antenatal fetal surveillance relies on the premise that the fetus whose well-being is challenged, will respond with a series of adaptive or maladaptive responses, which can be detected by the methods used in AFS. In humans and pregnant animals, the fetal heart rate pattern, fetal movements, and fetal muscular tone are sensitive to hypoxemia and acidemia.[2–5] AFS techniques use some of these metrics to evaluate fetal wellbeing including the nonstress test (NST), biophysical profile (BPP), modified BPP, contraction stress test (CST), and umbilical artery Doppler velocimetry. Maternal-fetal movement assessment, also known as "fetal kick counts," is frequently used as an AFS technique as well. It is important to keep in mind that although abnormal AFS results may be associated with acidemia and hypoxemia, these results do not reflect the severity nor the duration of acid-base disturbance.[1] The gestational age upon initiation of AFS testing and frequency of testing may vary by hospital and by institution. Institutions are encouraged to standardize their AFS according to the recommendations from regulatory bodies including The American College of Obstetricians and Gynecologists.

In humans, the reference range of normal umbilical blood gas parameters has been established by fetal blood sampling (FBS) and can vary by gestational age.[6] The degree of hypoxemia and acidemia at which various indices of fetal well-being become abnormal is not completely known; however, some reports have provided important insight in this regard. For example, in one study, fetal surveillance was performed immediately before FBS in fetuses with growth restriction and in those affected by maternal alloimmunization.[7] The authors reported that poor biophysical profile scores were associated with a pH < 7.20, whereas the pH was > 7.20 when the biophysical profile score was normal.[7]

Antenatal fetal surveillance is generally used to assess the risk of fetal death in pregnancies at increased risk for fetal demise because of maternal medical conditions or conditions associated with abnormal fetal or placental development (see Table 9.1). Beginning at 32–34 weeks' gestation until delivery, AFS is typically performed once or twice weekly. However, in very high-risk pregnancies AFS can be started as early as 28 weeks. A normal AFS test result is considered reassuring; however, this test result can also be false negative. A false negative AFS result is defined as an incidence of stillbirth occurring within one week of a normal test result. The incidence of a false negative NST once a week is approximately 3.2 stillbirths/1,000 pregnancies;[8] and twice a week is 1.9 stillbirths/1,000 pregnancies.[9] For BPP and modified BPP, the incidence of a false negative test is 0.8 stillbirths/1,000 pregnancies;[10,11] and in CST is 0.4 stillbirths/1,000 pregnancies.[8]

Table 9.1 Indications for antepartum fetal surveillance

Maternal conditions	Pregnancy-related conditions
• Pregestational diabetes mellitus	• Gestational hypertension
• Hypertension	• Preeclampsia
• Systemic lupus erythematosus	• Decreased fetal movement
• Chronic renal disease	• Gestational diabetes mellitus (poorly controlled or
• Antiphospholipid syndrome	medically treated)
• Hyperthyroidism (poorly controlled)	• Oligohydramnios
• Hemoglobinopathies	• Fetal growth restriction
• Cyanotic heart disease	• Post-term pregnancy
• Malignancies	• Isoimmunization
	• Previous fetal demise
	• Multiple gestation with significant fetal growth discordance

The high false positive rate (an abnormal test resulting in an uncompromised fetus) of various testing protocols (up to 50% with the NST), limits the utility of interpreting a test in isolation.[8]

It is important to note that there is little evidence from randomized controlled trials that AFS decreases the risk of fetal death, and some reports suggest that it may actually be detrimental as AFS may increase the rate of iatrogenic prematurity.[12] Nevertheless, AFS remains one of the cornerstones of assessing fetal well-being during prenatal care.

Maternal-Fetal Movement Assessment

A decrease in fetal movement may precede fetal death in some cases by several days.[13] This is the basis for the evaluation of the maternal perception of fetal movements as a means of AFS in high-risk populations. In the low-risk pregnancy, this technique is frequently the only form of fetal surveillance that is performed. Fetal movement is perceptible to the mother by 19–20 weeks.[14] Other factors can also affect maternal perceptions of movement, including gestational age, placental location, medications, maternal activity, position, and obesity.[15,16] Periods of active fetal movements generally last 40 minutes whereas quiet periods last about 20 minutes.[15,17]

Women are advised to do "kick counts" by lying on their side and counting the number of fetal movements. The perception of 10 distinct movements in two hours is commonly regarded as reassuring.[1,18] In the absence of a reassuring count, further fetal assessment is recommended.

One report indicated that evaluation of fetal movements has important limitations as a means of AFS. In a randomized controlled trial which involved over 68,000 low-risk women, women were allocated to either fetal movement evaluation (intervention group) or routine care (control group). The fetal death rate was similar in both groups, that is 2.9/1,000 in the intervention group versus 2.7/1,000 in the control group.[19] An important limitation of this study was that only 46% of women in the intervention group were compliant in reporting decreased fetal movement. Of note, a systematic review published in the Cochrane Database concluded that there is insufficient evidence to recommend routine counting of fetal movement to prevent stillbirth.[20]

Nonstress Test

Nonstress test is the most common screening test used in antepartum fetal surveillance, consisting of a recording of the fetal heart rate (FHR) with simultaneous documentation of uterine activity using an external fetal monitor. Interpretation of the NST is based on the premise that the heart rate of the fetus that is not acidotic or neurologically depressed, will temporarily accelerate with fetal movements.[1]

Nonstress test results are categorized as being either reactive (normal) or nonreactive. Reactivity is defined by two or more accelerations observed within a 20 minute period.[21] If reactivity has not occurred during the first 20 minutes, FHR and contraction monitoring may be continued for an additional 20 minutes. A nonreactive NST is one that lacks sufficient FHR accelerations over a 40 minute period[1] but does not demonstrate absence of variability or decelerations.

Fetal heart rate is evaluated for a period of up to 20 minutes, although it may be extended for up to 40 minutes to allow for variations in the fetal sleep-wake cycle. The FHR pattern, including baseline heart rate, variability, and the presence or absence of accelerations and decelerations are evaluated in NST interpretation (Figure 9.1).

The FHR baseline is thought to be regulated by the autonomic nervous system, which is also modulated by an interplay of sympathetic and parasympathetic signals.[22] The FHR baseline is the average number of beats per minute (rounded to zero or five) over a 10-minute period. Periods of marked variability (amplitude of the FHR greater than 25 beats per minute above the baseline) should not be used to determine the baseline. Additionally the baseline should be recognizable for at least two minutes during the NST, although the two minutes may not be contiguous.[23]

If the NST is not reactive, an alternative approach of assessment is the use of vibroacoustic stimulation. A 2014 systematic review found that the use of vibroacoustic stimulation shortened the mean overall testing time by almost seven minutes and reduced the frequency of nonreactive NSTs by 40% (OR 0.62, 95% CI 0.48–0.81).[24] To perform vibroacoustic stimulation, the device is positioned on the maternal abdomen and a stimulus is applied for one to two seconds. If vibroacoustic stimulation fails to elicit a response, it may be repeated up to three times for longer durations of up to three seconds.

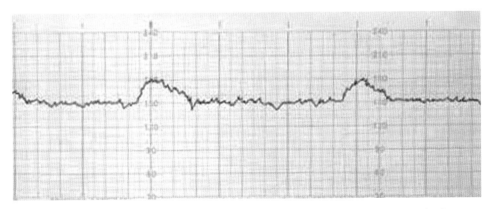

Figure 9.1 Reassuring nonstress test tracing showing moderate fetal heart rate variability with amplitude ranging from six to 25 beats.

Most healthcare providers use a subjective approach to determine the FHR baseline by "eyeballing" the tracing as opposed to using computerized techniques. The normal baseline FHR ranges from 110 to 160 beats per minute; the baseline tends to be in the higher end of the normal range early in gestation and decreases as gestation advances.[25] Maturation of the fetal nervous system occurs throughout gestation and affects NST interpretation. Between 24 and 28 weeks, up to 50% of NSTs will not be reactive because of immaturity of the fetal nervous system, which limits the utility of the test in the midtrimester.[26] The number of nonreactive tests decreases to 15% between the gestational ages of 28 and 32 weeks.[27,28]

Variability refers to the fluctuations in the baseline FHR that are quantified in beats per minute.[23] Variability can be absent, minimal (Figure 9.2), moderate (Figure 9.1), or marked. Moderate variability, in which the amplitude ranges between six and 25 beats per minute, is considered reassuring.[22] Fetal heart rate variability is rare before 24 weeks but should be present after 28 weeks. Absence of variability in the third trimester should be considered abnormal until further evaluation. Tracings demonstrating minimal variability (amplitude less than six beats per minute) or absent variability (amplitude range is undetectable) warrant further investigation, especially when the gestational age is in the mid- to late third trimester.[22]

Accelerations are defined as a rapid increase in FHR with onset to peak less than 30 seconds. The frequency and amplitude of FHR accelerations increase with advancing gestational age, which contributes to the decrease in nonreactive NSTs as gestational age increases.[29,30] In a fetus that is 32 weeks' gestation or greater, the acceleration should peak at

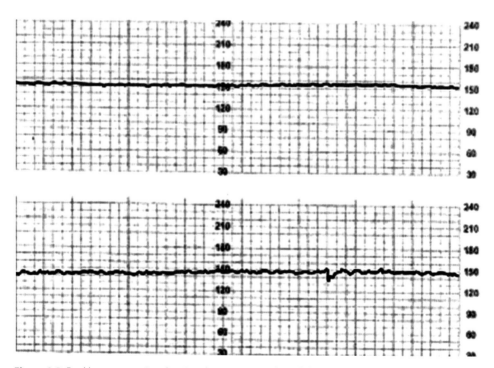

Figure 9.2 Fetal heart rate tracing showing absent, or minimal variability.

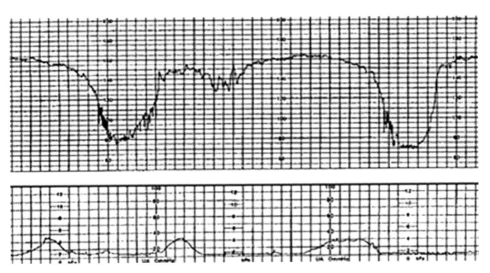

Figure 9.3 Fetal heart rate tracing depicting late decelerations; there is a gradual decrease in fetal heart rate with a time frame of 30 seconds from onset to nadir.

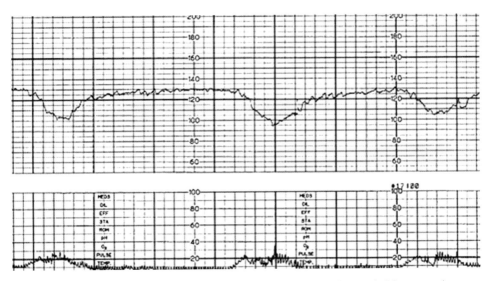

Figure 9.4 Fetal heart rate tracing depicting early decelerations, characterized by a gradual decrease and return to baseline with time from onset of the deceleration to the lowest point of the deceleration (nadir) > 30 seconds. The nadir of the early deceleration occurs with the peak of a contraction.

at least 15 beats per minute above the baseline and persist for at least 15 seconds (Figure 9.1). In a fetus less than 32 weeks, the peak of the acceleration should be at least 10 beats per minute above baseline and persist for at least 10 seconds.

Decelerations are classified as late (Figure 9.3), early (Figure 9.4), or variable (Figure 9.5) and differ in their onset, nadir, and recovery in relation to uterine contractions. Late

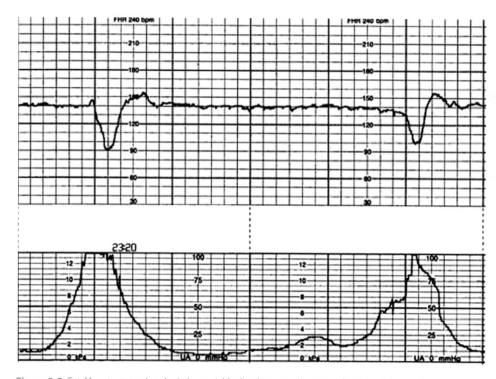

Figure 9.5 Fetal heart rate tracing depicting variable decelerations; decrease of ≥ 15 beats lasting for ≥15 seconds. Time to onset and resolution (return to baseline) is typically two minutes.

decelerations represent fetal hypoxia, early decelerations represent head compression particularly in the second stage of labor, and variable decelerations represent transient cord compression. The correct identification of the type of deceleration impacts FHR interpretation and management.

A sinusoidal FHR pattern is relatively rare and is defined as a sine wave-like undulating pattern in the FHR baseline with a cycle frequency of three to five/minute that persists for over 20 minutes (Figure 9.6). It is considered abnormal and requires prompt attention, in particular because of its association with fetal anemia. However, sinusoidal FHR patterns have been described in 75% of patients receiving butorphanol during labor without an association with adverse outcomes.[31]

Intrapartum Fetal Monitoring

In 2009, a Practice Bulletin published by the American College of Obstetricians and Gynecologists and supported by other regulatory bodies, recommended the use of a new three-tiered system to interpret FHR tracings.[22,23] Although the emphasis in this report is on intrapartum FHR patterns, the delineated classification of tracings may also be extrapolated to the antepartum setting. The new three-tiered system is as follows:

1) Category I FHR tracings: Normal tracings which are strongly predictive of normal fetal acid–base status at the time of observation. In Category I FHR tracings, no specific action is required. These tracings may include any of the following:

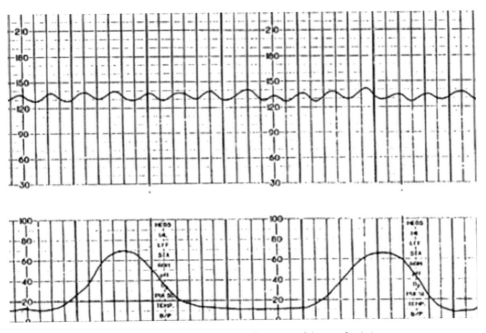

Figure 9.6 Sinusoidal fetal heart rate pattern with a cycle frequency of three to five/minute.

   a. Baseline rate: 110–160 beats/per minute

   b. Moderate baseline FHR variability

   c. Absent late or variable decelerations

   d. Early decelerations could be present or absent

   e. Accelerations could be present or absent.

2) Category II FHR tracings: These are not predictive of abnormal fetal acid–base status, yet presently there is inadequate evidence to classify these as Category I or Category III. Category II FHR tracings require evaluation, continued surveillance and reevaluation. In some circumstances, ancillary tests to ensure fetal well-being or intrauterine resuscitative measures may be required with Category II tracings. See Table 9.2 [22] for the description of Category II FHR.

3) Category III tracings: These are associated with abnormal fetal acid–base status at the time of observation. Category III FHR tracings require prompt evaluation. Efforts to expeditiously resolve the abnormal FHR pattern may include provision of maternal oxygen, change in maternal position, discontinuation of labor stimulation, treatment of maternal hypotension, and treatment of tachysystole with FHR changes. If a Category III tracing does not resolve with these measures, delivery should be performed. The following FHR rate patterns are considered Category III:

   a. Absent baseline FHR variability and any of the following:

      i. Recurrent late decelerations

      ii. Recurrent variable decelerations

      iii. Bradycardia

   b. Sinusoidal pattern.

Table 9.2 Examples of Category II tracings

Baseline rate	Baseline FHR variability	Accelerations	Periodic or episodic decelerations
• Bradycardia not accompanied by absent baseline variability • Tachycardia	• Minimal baseline variability • Absent baseline variability without recurrent decelerations • Marked baseline variability	• Absence of induced accelerations after fetal stimulation	• Recurrent variable decelerations with minimal or moderate variability • Prolonged decelerations more than two minutes but less than 10 minutes • Recurrent late decelerations with moderate baseline variability • Variable decelerations with slow return to baseline, overshoots or shoulders

Source: ACOG Practice Bulletin Number 106, July 2009.[22]

Despite widespread use of the NST, there are limited data to support its efficacy in the prevention of stillbirth. A Cochrane review reported that performing a NST had no significant effect on the rate of stillbirth or any measure of perinatal morbidity.[32] However, the trials included in this meta-analysis were conducted in the early 1980s, when testing was first being introduced and may not reflect how these tests are utilized and interpreted today. Traditionally, the NST was performed on a weekly basis. However, increasing NST to twice a week in women with at-risk pregnancies was found to reduce the rate of stillbirth after a reactive NST to 1.9/1,000 compared to a previously published rate of 6.1/1,000.[9] Twice weekly testing remains the most common recommendation in most clinical circumstances.

Contraction Stress Test

Contraction stress test evaluates the FHR using external monitoring during uterine contractions, which are associated with transient decreased oxygenation.[1] Contractions can occur spontaneously or can be induced via nipple stimulation or intravenous oxytocin administration. The goal of a CST is to identify the fetus at risk for compromise by observing the fetus during transient "stress." Once three contractions in a 10-minute period are achieved, the CST is characterized as negative if no late or significant variable decelerations are observed following ≥ 50% of the contractions.[33] Contraction stress test results can also be categorized as equivocal, suspicious, or unsatisfactory. Suspicious is considered in the presence of intermittent late decelerations or significant variable decelerations; equivocal is when decelerations occur in the presence of contractions more frequent than every two minutes or lasting longer than 90 seconds; and unsatisfactory CST is when fewer than three contractions in 10 minutes are achieved or when the tracing is uninterpretable.[1]

Contraindications to CST include conditions that prohibit a vaginal delivery or increase the risk of preterm delivery, uterine rupture, or bleeding. These conditions include preterm labor, preterm premature rupture of membranes (PPROM), and history of extensive uterine surgery, classical cesarean delivery, or known placenta previa. Contraction stress test could be used to evaluate the placental and fetal reserve in complicated pregnancies that are suggestive of placental insufficiency such as fetal growth restriction, to evaluate if the fetus could tolerate labor.

Biophysical Profile

The BPP is an AFS method that utilizes several metrics that can be independently affected by fetal hypoxemia. The BPP consists of an NST combined with four observations made by ultrasonography. These four components include an assessment of fetal movements, fetal breathing, fetal tone, and amniotic fluid volume (AFV). The presence of normal biophysical activity is indirect evidence that the central nervous system which controls activity is intact and functioning and there is most likely no hypoxia. The absence of a biophysical parameter is more difficult to interpret, as it may reflect either pathologic depression or periodic physiological changes.

The biophysical activities that first become active in fetal development are the last to disappear when asphyxia affects the biophysical activities.[34] The fetal tone center is the earliest to function in-utero, at 7.5–8.5 weeks' gestation. The fetal movement center starts functioning at approximately nine weeks' gestation. Regular fetal breathing does not occur until 20–21 weeks' gestation. The last of the biophysical activities to appear is FHR reactivity, which is not consistently present until the late second trimester or early third trimester.[34] The FHR reactivity center is the most sensitive to hypoxia, whereas the fetal tone is the last to disappear during asphyxia.[34] The fetus with suboptimal oxygenation will usually present with nonreactive NST and absence of fetal breathing at the initial stages of hypoxia. If hypoxia becomes worse, the fetal body movements and fetal tone will be abolished. Amniotic fluid volume is not acutely influenced by alterations in fetal central nervous system function.[34] Oligohydramnios is typically the result of a chronic process thought to be secondary to redistribution of fetal blood flow to prioritize critical organs including the fetal brain, heart, and adrenals.

In a study that looked at the relationship between fetal biophysical scores, cord blood gases, and acid-base measurements in nonlabored fetuses within three hours of a cesarean delivery, the first manifestations of fetal hypoxemia and acidemia were loss of FHR reactivity and breathing movements. Fetal movements and tone were subsequently compromised with increasing degrees of hypoxemia, acidemia, and hypercapnia.[34] Some studies have demonstrated a relationship between lower BPP scores and increased perinatal morbidity and mortality rates, as well as increased risk for cerebral palsy.[35]

Each of the five components of the BPP is assigned a score of either two (normal or present) or zero (abnormal, absent, or insufficient).[1] A composite score of eight (with normal amniotic fluid) or 10 is normal, indicating the absence of a fetal indication for intervention. A score of six is considered equivocal, posing a possible risk of fetal asphyxia, and generally prompts delivery in the term fetus. In a preterm fetus, a repeat BPP may be considered in 24 hours. A score of four or less is abnormal,[1] suggesting probable fetal asphyxia, and generally warrants delivery.

Points are awarded for fetal movement if two or more discrete body or limb movements are observed within 30 minutes. Fetal tone is defined as one or more episodes of extension with return to flexion in a limb or opening and closing of the hand. Fetal breathing is defined as a sustained episode of chest wall movements > 20 seconds.[1] Points are also awarded for a reactive NST and a deepest vertical pocket (DVP) of at least 2 cm.[36,37] The more components of the BPP that are absent, the higher the incidence of acidemia.[34,38–41]

A normal BPP score (8/10 or 10/10) is reassuring and makes it highly unlikely that the fetus is hypoxemic. However, an abnormal score does not necessarily prove that hypoxemia is present. The fetus has adaptive responses to states of low oxygen, which include reduced fetal activity, increased oxygen extraction, increased fetal hemoglobin, and redistribution of blood flow to increase perfusion to the fetal brain, heart, and adrenals.[41] In some cases of chronic fetal disease, such as growth restriction, biophysical variables may initially be absent but can subsequently reappear. As such, the presence of certain components of the BPP does not guarantee that the fetus is not hypoxic and may explain why stillbirths still occur following a "normal" BPP.[42] The false negative rate, or risk of fetal death within a week of a normal test result, ranges between 0.4 and 0.6/1,000 live births, a rate that is about 10% of the observed perinatal mortality rate in any high-risk study population.[10,43] These deaths may also be caused by acute events that cannot be anticipated such as a cord prolapse, abruption, or accidental cord compression.

It has been proposed that the presence or absence of normal amniotic fluid volume can have different effects on the interpretation of BPP. For example, with a BPP of 8/10 or 10/10 (including two points for amniotic fluid), the risk of developing fetal asphyxia within one week in the absence of any intervention is low (about 1/1,000). When the BPP is 6/10 or 8/10 (with no points awarded for amniotic fluid) the risk of developing fetal asphyxia within one week without intervention is increased, from 20/1,000 to 30/1,000 to more than 50/1,000.[44] A 6/10 score, which includes two points for amniotic fluid, is considered equivocal, and management depends on gestational age and the indication for testing. The possibility of developing fetal asphyxia cannot be excluded with an equivocal test result, and the test should be repeated within 24 hours in the setting of prematurity; if the fetus is at or near term, delivery may be recommended. A score of 0/10 to 4/10 is ominous and is associated with a 115/1,000 to 550/1,000 risk of fetal asphyxia within one week if no intervention occurs.[44]

Management must be individualized. A low biophysical score warrants immediate investigation for factors other than hypoxia that may be present, such as prolonged fetal sleep cycles, maternal sedative medications, fetal anomalies, and maternal disease. In the absence of any confounding factors, a low score increases the risk for fetal acidemia and the likelihood of fetal compromise and death.

Modified Biophysical Profile

The modified BPP combines the NST with the evaluation of amniotic fluid volume. An amniotic fluid volume index (AFI) > 5 cm represents an adequate volume of amniotic fluid. Thus, the modified BPP is considered normal if the NST is reactive and the AFI is > 5, and abnormal if either the NST is nonreactive or the AFI is ≤ 5.

Performing a full BPP can take up to 50 minutes, including 30 minutes for the ultrasound examination and 20 minutes for the NST. In 1989 Clark et al.[45] first introduced the modified BPP, which combines the NST and the AFI. The original study used vibroacoustic stimulation after five minutes of the NST if spontaneous accelerations were absent. A second stimulus was administered if no accelerations were noted in 10 minutes. Once two accelerations were noted, the NST was discontinued. The AFI was measured using the four-quadrant technique. The NST, using vibroacoustic stimulation if needed, served as an indicator of short-term fetal oxygenation status, whereas the AFI served as an indicator of uteroplacental function.[46] Today the modified BPP is often performed using a traditional NST along with an amniotic fluid assessment via formal AFI or DVP. The modified BPP is considered normal if the DVP is > 2 cm or AFI is at least 5 cm and the NST is reactive. If either of these parameters is not met, further investigation including a full BPP is indicated. In a review that included 12,620 high-risk patients, the predictive value of the four ultrasound components of the BPP (when normal) was found to be equivalent to that of the full BPP (including the NST).[47] This observation was demonstrated in a subsequent prospective study evaluating the use of NST only when values for one or more of the ultrasound components was abnormal and was found to reduce the need for NSTs in 95% of cases.[48] An NST should always be performed if any of the ultrasound components is abnormal. However, a BPP score of 8/10 is as accurate as a score of 10/10 for the prediction of fetal well-being, as long as points are not deducted for fluid.[49] There is limited information comparing the full BPP to the modified BPP. In one trial comparing the two, no difference was noted in neonatal outcomes between the groups.[11] Comparing the modified BPP as the primary testing method and the complete BPP as the backup test, antepartum fetal death was 6.75 times less common in high-risk women who were tested than in their nontested counterparts. However, the modified BPP is associated with a high rate of false positive results (60%), which led to iatrogenic prematurity in 1.5% of women tested before term.[11] Despite the limited data, the modified BPP is frequently utilized for fetal surveillance because it is less time consuming than a full BPP.

Doppler Evaluation of the Umbilical Artery

Doppler assessment of the fetal circulation is an important adjunct for assessing the likelihood of adverse outcomes with fetal growth retardation (FGR). In this context, one should be aware of the early and late forms of FGR with an arbitrary cutoff that is typically set at 32 weeks.[50] Early onset FGR is more likely associated with vascular abnormalities of the maternal-fetal placental circulation. Ultrasound findings include abnormal Doppler waveforms that suggest high vascular impedance of the uterine and umbilical arteries. This could signify a 40–70% risk of associated preeclampsia and potential problems of prematurity. Late onset FGR is more likely to involve placental villous diffusion and perfusion defects that cause cerebral or umbilical artery Doppler abnormalities. Antenatal surveillance for late FGR revolves around identifying fetuses at risk for stillbirth.

Clinical management, based on Doppler evaluation of the umbilical artery in fetuses with FGR, is associated with fewer perinatal deaths, inductions of labor, and cesarean deliveries.[51] The Society for Maternal Fetal Medicine (SMFM) guidelines recommended that umbilical artery Doppler velocimetry can be performed at the level of the abdominal cord insertion, in the absence of maternal respiration, and when the waveforms are uniform[52] (Figure 9.7). The preference at our institution is to choose a free umbilical cord loop with a minimal angle of insonation. Measurement of umbilical artery systolic to diastolic ratio (S/D ratio) or pulsatility index (PI) should be documented. The latter is useful when the end diastolic velocity is absent or reversed.

The SMFM currently does not recommend Doppler assessment of other maternal or fetal vascular territories including uterine arteries, middle cerebral artery, ductus venosus, umbilical vein, and aortic isthmus to guide clinical management in FGR.[53] A more recent literature review,

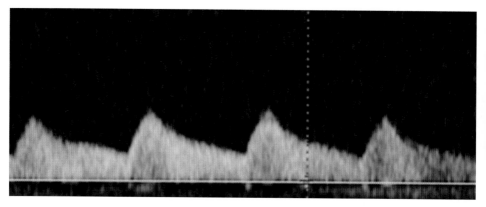

Figure 9.7 Umbilical artery Doppler velocimetry showing uniform high-velocity systolic and diastolic flow waveforms within the umbilical artery.

however, describes the potential utility of calculating cerebroplacental ratio (CPR) as the ratio of the PI from MCA and umbilical artery (UA) Doppler waveforms.[54] This ratio reflects the degree of fetal cerebrovascular dilatation resulting from hypoxia and increased placental vascular impedance that leads to decreased UA diastolic flow. Despite mounting evidence of the association between CPR and adverse outcomes including stillbirth, most healthcare providers are awaiting the results of randomized controlled trials to provide guidance on how to best interpret these results for patient care.[55,56]

Other Doppler parameters such as the ductus venosus and umbilical venous flow have also been reported for growth restricted fetuses. The ductus venosus waveform reflects pressure-volume changes in the heart. When an absence or reversal of the a-wave is noted (Figure 9.8), fetal survival of greater than one week is unlikely.[57] Umbilical vein pulsations (Figure 9.9) are also an ominous pattern.[58–60] The evaluation of umbilical vein pulsations is best performed via an intra-abdominal portion of the umbilical vein. This approach is more reliable than insonating a free loop of cord because pulsations from the umbilical artery can sometimes be transmitted to the umbilical vein.

Doppler ultrasonography can be used to observe flow velocity waveforms in the fetal umbilical arteries. In the normal fetus, high-velocity systolic and diastolic flow is noted within the umbilical artery (Figure 9.7). Increased resistance in placental vasculature may increase the impedance to flow resulting in diminished diastolic flow such that the ratio of systolic to diastolic flow is high.[61–63] In the setting of growth restriction, studies have shown that a systolic/diastolic ratio two standard deviations above the mean for a given gestational age is abnormal, warrants close surveillance, and consideration of antenatal steroids or delivery depending on gestational age.[64] As flow resistance increases, absent or reversed diastolic flow can be observed (Figure 9.8). Both of these findings are ominous and increase the risk for perinatal fatality. The use of Doppler evaluation in the setting of fetal growth restriction is associated with a reduction in the rate of perinatal death by as much as 29%.[51,64]

Fetal Monitoring During Fetal Surgery

Acute cardiovascular changes can take place during fetal surgery. These are probably secondary to the effects of cardiac dysfunction associated with the specific anomaly, transient umbilical

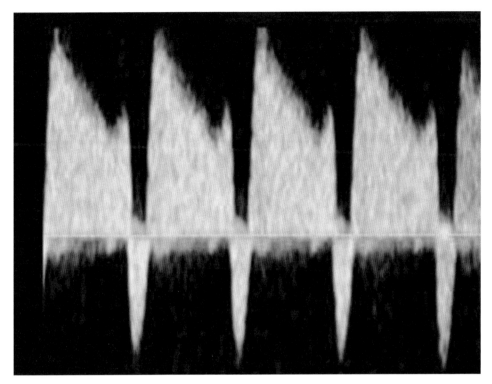

Figure 9.8 The ductus venosus waveform reflecting pressure-volume changes in the heart; reversed diastolic flow is observed.

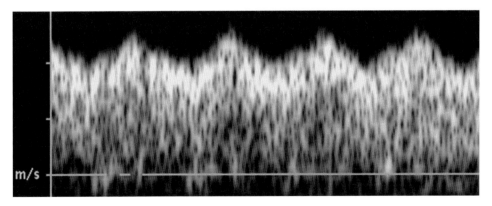

Figure 9.9 Umbilical vein pulsations detected by Doppler ultrasound.

cord compression, surgical stress, tocolytic agents, and anesthesia or a combination of the above. Doppler interrogation of the umbilical artery, ductus venosus and MCA as well as fetal echocardiography during open or fetoscopic intrauterine surgery, is challenging because of the significant oligohydramnios that is present as a result of the intentional or unintentional removal of the amniotic fluid and frequent fetal manipulation required to accomplish the surgery. Echocardiographic monitoring during fetal surgery is an important adjunct in the management of these patients. In a study that included cases of fetal surgery for myelomeningocele (MMC) repair, resection of intrathoracic masses, tracheal occlusion for congenital diaphragmatic hernia, and resection of sacrococcygeal teratoma, the authors performed fetal echocardiography before, during, and early after surgery.[65] The authors reported that during fetal surgery, heart rate increased acutely, and combined cardiac output diminished at the time of fetal incision for all groups including those with myelomeningocele, which suggested diminished stroke volume. Ventricular and valvular dysfunction were identified in all groups, as was acute constriction of the ductus arteriosus. Tricuspid regurgitation (TR) was present in all groups preoperatively, and the frequency and severity of TR increased for all groups intraoperatively. Although TR diminished 24 hours after surgery, grade 2 TR persisted beyond 24 hours in 4% of myelomeningocele cases (2/51) and 25% of fetuses with sacrococcygeal teratoma. Mitral regurgitation was not observed preoperatively in any fetuses with myelomeningocele or congenital diaphragmatic hernia but was present as grade 1 in 20% of intrathoracic masses and 25% of sacrococcygeal teratoma patients. The frequency and severity of mitral regurgitation increased for all groups intraoperatively. Mitral regurgitation was not detected in any group 24 hours after surgery.[65] The authors also reported that no cardiac dysfunction was observed late after surgery in fetuses with myelomeningocele repair, resection of intrathoracic masses, or tracheal occlusion for congenital diaphragmatic hernia, but cardiac dysfunction was present in 50% of fetuses who underwent sacrococcygeal teratoma resection. The authors concluded that echocardiographic monitoring of the heart during fetal surgery reveals that important hemodynamic derangements commonly occur but tend to be transient.[65]

In another study, researchers performed a longitudinal evaluation of blood flow patterns in the ductus arteriosus (DA) during the perioperative period in 10 fetal myelomeningocele cases, the authors reported that in all fetuses, both the DA times for average mean, and end diastolic velocity, increased significantly between baseline and the time of inhaled anesthesia exposure; and decreased significantly between inhaled anesthesia exposure and postoperative day two.[66] Thus abnormal DA flow patterns culminating in significant DA constriction occurred during fetal MMC repair and the authors proposed that limiting maternal exposure to indomethacin, supplemental oxygen, and inhaled anesthesia may reduce the incidence and severity of DA constriction during open fetal surgery.[66]

Conclusions

Antenatal fetal surveillance is considered standard of care in the management of high-risk pregnancies. However, there is limited scientific evidence supporting the use of AFS to decrease fetal death. Thus, clinical recommendations on the use of AFS are based largely on consensus and expert opinions. An important benefit of AFS is that it provides an opportunity to evaluate the health of both the mother and the fetus on a more frequent basis. Because of the high rate of false positive findings with each of the AFS testing methods, providers are encouraged to interpret the AFS according to the indication for AFS, gestational age, and intrinsic limitations of each test. AFS testing should not be performed in pregnancies that are provable or complicated by lethal fetal abnormalities unless other circumstances apply. Frequency and duration of surveillance should be based on the indication and chronicity of the maternal and fetal condition.

References

1. Practice bulletin no. 145: antepartum fetal surveillance. *Obstet Gynecol.* 2014;**124**:182–192.

2. Manning FA, Platt LD. Maternal hypoxemia and fetal breathing movements. *Obstet Gynecol.* 1979;**53**:758–760.

3. Boddy K, Dawes GS, Fisher R, et al. Foetal respiratory movements, electrocortical and cardiovascular responses to hypoxaemia and hypercapnia in sheep. *J Physiol.* 1974;**243**:599–618.

4. Natale R, Clewlow F, Dawes GS. Measurement of fetal forelimb movements in the lamb in utero. *Am J Obstet Gynecol.* 1981;**140**:545–551.

5. Murata Y, Martin CB, Jr., Ikenoue T, et al. Fetal heart rate accelerations and late decelerations during the course of intrauterine death in chronically catheterized rhesus monkeys. *Am J Obstet Gynecol.* 1982;**144**:218–223.

6. Weiner CP, Sipes SL, Wenstrom K. The effect of fetal age upon normal fetal laboratory values and venous pressure. *Obstet Gynecol.* 1992;**79**:713–718.

7. Manning FA, Snijders R, Harman CR, et al. Fetal biophysical profile score. VI. Correlation with antepartum umbilical venous fetal pH. *Am J Obstet Gynecol.* 1993;**169**:755–763.

8. Freeman RK, Anderson G, Dorchester W. A prospective multi-institutional study of antepartum fetal heart rate monitoring. II. Contraction stress test versus nonstress test for primary surveillance. *Am J Obstet Gynecol.* 1982;**143**:778–781.

9. Boehm FH, Salyer S, Shah DM, Vaughn WK. Improved outcome of twice weekly nonstress testing. *Obstet Gynecol.* 1986;**67**:566–568.

10. Manning FA, Morrison I, Harman CR, et al. Fetal assessment based on fetal biophysical profile scoring: experience in 19,221 referred high-risk pregnancies. II. An analysis of false-negative fetal deaths. *Am J Obstet Gynecol.* 1987;**157**:880–884.

11. Miller DA, Rabello YA, Paul RH. The modified biophysical profile: antepartum testing in the 1990s. *Am J Obstet Gynecol.* 1996;**174**:812–817.

12. Thacker SB, Berkelman RL. Assessing the diagnostic accuracy and efficacy of selected antepartum fetal surveillance techniques. *Obstet Gynecol Surv.* 1986;**41**:121–141.

13. Pearson JF, Weaver JB. Fetal activity and fetal wellbeing: an evaluation. *Br Med J.* 1976;**1**:1305–1307.

14. Andersen HF, Johnson TR, Jr., Flora JD, Jr., Barclay ML. Gestational age assessment. II. Prediction from combined clinical observations. *Am J Obstet Gynecol.* 1981;**140**:770–774.

15. Neldam S. Fetal movements as an indicator of fetal well-being. *Dan Med Bull.* 1983;**30**:274–278.

16. O'Neill E, Thorp J. Antepartum evaluation of the fetus and fetal well being. *Clin Obstet Gynecol.* 2012;**55**:722–730.

17. Patrick J, Campbell K, Carmichael L, et al. Patterns of gross fetal body movements over 24-hour observation intervals during the last 10 weeks of pregnancy. *Am J Obstet Gynecol.* 1982;**142**:363–371.

18. Moore TR, Piacquadio K. A prospective evaluation of fetal movement screening to reduce the incidence of antepartum fetal death. *Am J Obstet Gynecol.* 1989;**160**:1075–1080.

19. Grant A, Elbourne D, Valentin L, Alexander S. Routine formal fetal movement counting and risk of antepartum late death in normally formed singletons. *Lancet.* 1989;**2**:345–349.

20. Mangesi L, Hofmeyr GJ, Smith V, Smyth RM. Fetal movement counting for assessment of fetal wellbeing. *Cochrane Database Syst Rev.* 2015;CD004909.

21. Evertson LR, Gauthier RJ, Schifrin BS, Paul RH. Antepartum fetal heart rate testing. I. Evolution of the nonstress test. *Am J Obstet Gynecol.* 1979;**133**:29–33.

22. ACOG Practice Bulletin No. 106: Intrapartum fetal heart rate monitoring: nomenclature, interpretation, and general management principles. *Obstet Gynecol.* 2009;**114**:192–202.

23. Macones GA, Hankins GD, Spong CY, et al. The 2008 National Institute of Child Health

and Human Development workshop report on electronic fetal monitoring: update on definitions, interpretation, and research guidelines. *J Obstet Gynecol Neonatal Nurs.* 2008;37:510–515.

24. Tan KH, Smyth RM, Wei X. Fetal vibroacoustic stimulation for facilitation of tests of fetal wellbeing. *Cochrane Database Syst Rev.* 2013;CD002963.

25. Wheeler T, Murrills A. Patterns of fetal heart rate during normal pregnancy. *Br J Obstet Gynaecol.* 1978;85:18–27.

26. Bishop EH. Fetal acceleration test. *Am J Obstet Gynecol.* 1981;141:905–909.

27. Druzin ML, Gratacos J, Keegan KA, Paul RH. Antepartum fetal heart rate testing. VII. The significance of fetal bradycardia. *Am J Obstet Gynecol.* 1981;139:194–198.

28. Lavin JP, Jr., Miodovnik M, Barden TP. Relationship of nonstress test reactivity and gestational age. *Obstet Gynecol.* 1984;63:338–344.

29. Park MI, Hwang JH, Cha KJ, et al. Computerized analysis of fetal heart rate parameters by gestational age. *Int J Gynaecol Obstet.* 2001;74:157–164.

30. Sadovsky G, Nicolaides KH. Reference ranges for fetal heart rate patterns in normoxaemic nonanaemic fetuses. *Fetal Ther.* 1989;4:61–68.

31. Hatjis CG, Meis PJ. Sinusoidal fetal heart rate pattern associated with butorphanol administration. *Obstet Gynecol.* 1986;67:377–380.

32. Grivell RM, Alfirevic Z, Gyte GM, Devane D. Antenatal cardiotocography for fetal assessment. *Cochrane Database Syst Rev.* 2012;12:CD007863.

33. ACOG practice bulletin. Antepartum fetal surveillance. Number 9, October 1999 (replaces Technical Bulletin Number 188, January 1994). Clinical management guidelines for obstetrician-gynecologists. *Int J Gynaecol Obstet.* 2000;68:175–185.

34. Vintzileos AM, Gaffney SE, Salinger LM, et al. The relationship between fetal biophysical profile and cord pH in patients undergoing cesarean section before the onset of labor. *Obstet Gynecol.* 1987;70:196–201.

35. Manning FA, Bondaji N, Harman CR, et al. Fetal assessment based on fetal biophysical profile scoring. VIII. The incidence of cerebral palsy in tested and untested perinates. *Am J Obstet Gynecol.* 1998;178:696–706.

36. Chamberlain PF, Manning FA, Morrison I, et al. Ultrasound evaluation of amniotic fluid volume. I. The relationship of marginal and decreased amniotic fluid volumes to perinatal outcome. *Am J Obstet Gynecol.* 1984;150:245–249.

37. Manning FA, Harman CR, Morrison I, et al. Fetal assessment based on fetal biophysical profile scoring. IV. An analysis of perinatal morbidity and mortality. *Am J Obstet Gynecol.* 1990;162:703–709.

38. Nabhan AF, Abdelmoula YA. Amniotic fluid index versus single deepest vertical pocket as a screening test for preventing adverse pregnancy outcome. *Cochrane Database Syst Rev.* 2008;CD006593.

39. Vintzileos AM, Gaffney SE, Salinger LM, et al. The relationships among the fetal biophysical profile, umbilical cord pH, and Apgar scores. *Am J Obstet Gynecol.* 1987;157:627–31.

40. Vintzileos AM, Campbell WA, Nochimson DJ, Weinbaum PJ. The use and misuse of the fetal biophysical profile. *Am J Obstet Gynecol.* 1987;156:527–533.

41. Vintzileos AM, Fleming AD, Scorza WE, et al. Relationship between fetal biophysical activities and umbilical cord blood gas values. *Am J Obstet Gynecol.* 1991;165:707–713.

42. Martin CB, Jr. Normal fetal physiology and behavior, and adaptive responses with hypoxemia. *Semin Perinatol.* 2008;32:239–242.

43. Dayal AK, Manning FA, Berck DJ, et al. Fetal death after normal biophysical profile score: An eighteen-year experience. *Am J Obstet Gynecol.* 1999;181:1231–1236.

44. Manning FA. Fetal biophysical profile. *Obstet Gynecol Clin North Am.* 1999;26:557–577,v.

45. Clark SL, Sabey P, Jolley K. Nonstress testing with acoustic stimulation and amniotic fluid volume assessment: 5973 tests without unexpected fetal death. *Am J Obstet Gynecol.* 1989;**160**:694–697.

46. Rutherford SE, Phelan JP, Smith CV, Jacobs N. The four-quadrant assessment of amniotic fluid volume: an adjunct to antepartum fetal heart rate testing. *Obstet Gynecol.* 1987;**70**:353–356.

47. Manning FA, Morrison I, Lange IR, et al. Fetal assessment based on fetal biophysical profile scoring: experience in 12,620 referred high-risk pregnancies. I. Perinatal mortality by frequency and etiology. *Am J Obstet Gynecol.* 1985;**151**:343–350.

48. Manning FA, Menticoglou S, Harman CR, et al. Antepartum fetal risk assessment: the role of the fetal biophysical profile score. *Baillieres Clin Obstet Gynaecol.* 1987;**1**:55–72.

49. Manning FA. Antepartum fetal surveillance. *Curr Opin Obstet Gynecol.* 1995;7:146–149.

50. Seravalli V, Baschat AA. A uniform management approach to optimize outcome in fetal growth restriction. *Obstet Gynecol Clin North Am.* 2015;**42**:275–288.

51. Alfirevic Z, Stampalija T, Gyte GM. Fetal and umbilical Doppler ultrasound in high-risk pregnancies. *Cochrane Database Syst Rev.* 2010;CD007529.

52. Berkley E, Chauhan SP, Abuhamad A. Doppler assessment of the fetus with intrauterine growth restriction. *Am J Obstet Gynecol.* 2012;**206**:300–308.

53. DeVore GR. The importance of the cerebroplacental ratio in the evaluation of fetal well-being in SGA and AGA fetuses. *Am J Obstet Gynecol.* 2015;**213**:5–15.

54. Dunn L, Sherrell H, Kumar S. Review: Systematic review of the utility of the fetal cerebroplacental ratio measured at term for the prediction of adverse perinatal outcome. *Placenta.* 2017;**54**:68–75.

55. Khalil A, Morales-Rosello J, Townsend R, et al. Value of third-trimester cerebroplacental ratio and uterine artery Doppler indices as predictors of stillbirth and perinatal loss. *Ultrasound Obstet Gynecol.* 2016;**47**:74–80.

56. Seravalli V, Miller JL, Block-Abraham D, Baschat AA. Ductus venosus Doppler in the assessment of fetal cardiovascular health: an updated practical approach. *Acta Obstet Gynecol Scand.* 2016;**95**:635–644.

57. Baschat AA, Harman CR. Antenatal assessment of the growth restricted fetus. *Curr Opin Obstet Gynecol.* 2001;**13**:161–168.

58. Gudmundsson S, Tulzer G, Huhta JC, Marsal K. Venous Doppler in the fetus with absent end-diastolic flow in the umbilical artery. *Ultrasound Obstet Gynecol.* 1996;7:262–267.

59. Hofstaetter C, Dubiel M, Gudmundsson S. Two types of umbilical venous pulsations and outcome of high-risk pregnancy. *Early Hum Dev.* 2001;**61**:111–117.

60. Erskine RL, Ritchie JW. Umbilical artery blood flow characteristics in normal and growth-retarded fetuses. *Br J Obstet Gynaecol.* 1985;**92**:605–610.

61. Giles WB, Trudinger BJ, Baird PJ. Fetal umbilical artery flow velocity waveforms and placental resistance: pathological correlation. *Br J Obstet Gynaecol.* 1985;**92**:31–38.

62. Reuwer PJ, Bruinse HW, Stoutenbeek P, Haspels AA. Doppler assessment of the fetoplacental circulation in normal and growth-retarded fetuses. *Eur J Obstet Gynecol Reprod Biol.* 1984;**18**:199–205.

63. Devoe LD, Gardner P, Dear C, Faircloth D. The significance of increasing umbilical artery systolic-diastolic ratios in third-trimester pregnancy. *Obstet Gynecol.* 1992;**80**:684–687.

64. Giles W, Bisits A. Clinical use of Doppler ultrasound in pregnancy: information from six randomised trials. *Fetal Diagn Ther.* 1993;**8**:247–255.

65. Rychik J, Tian Z, Cohen MS, et al. Acute cardiovascular effects of fetal surgery in the human. *Circulation.* 2004;**110**:1549–1556.

66. Howley L, Wood C, Patel SS, et al. Flow patterns in the ductus arteriosus during open fetal myelomeningocele repair. *Prenat Diagn.* 2015;**35**:564–570.

Myelomeningocele Repair

Chapter

10

William Whitehead and Titilopemi Aina

Introduction

Myelomeningocele (MMC) is an open neural tube defect (NTD) involving the spinal cord. In MMC, both cerebrospinal fluid (CSF) and spinal tissue are exposed through a skin defect (Figure 10.1). Neural tube defects occur as a result of a failure of fusion of the neural tube in the third week of development around the twentieth day. This failure affects development of the brain, spinal cord, meninges, and vertebral body.[1] MMC occurs in ~1 in 1,500 live births per year in the United States. Outcomes vary, but the majority of patients are afflicted with one or more long-term morbidities including hydrocephalus, neurogenic bladder, bowel incontinence, and lower extremity paraparesis.

Traditionally, MMCs are repaired postnatally within the first two to three days of life. The goal of surgery is to untether the spinal cord from the surrounding skin and close the tissue defect in multiple layers with the final layer being skin closure. Surgical repair of MMC stops the egress of CSF, prevents meningitis, and protects functioning nerves; however, it does not restore or improve neurologic function.

The idea for in-utero repair of MMC originates from the observation that neurologic function deteriorates during gestation. This is supported by animal experiments in the mid-1980s and 1990s with sheep and primates. The surgical creation of a NTD in-utero followed by repair several weeks later led to preserved neurologic function in the animals, whereas no repair resulted in paraparesis and neurogenic bladder as seen in patients with spina bifida.[2–5] In the mid-1990s, in-utero repair for MMC was introduced by Bruner et al. using a multiport, percutaneous fetoscopic approach.[6] A second group at University of California at San

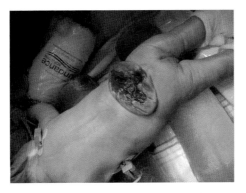

Figure 10.1 Exposed neural placode in a newborn with myelomeningocele. Photo courtesy of Dr. William Whitehead.

Francisco also attempted fetoscopic repair, but the results from both groups were dismal. They reported a 50% fetal mortality rate, a 100% need for postnatal MMC wound revision, and 75% rate of shunt dependence in surviving patients.[7] These results led to the abandonment of minimally invasive fetoscopic surgery, in favor of open hysterotomy in the United States. Between 2003 and 2010, a randomized controlled trial, the Management of Myelomeningocele trial (MOMs trial), which compared open hysterotomy in-utero repair to postnatal closure was conducted. The MOMs trial results showed that in-utero repair decreased the risk of hydrocephalus and improved lower extremity motor function compared to patients who had a traditional postnatal closure. However, not all patients who underwent in-utero closure achieved these benefits and the trial showed significant risks to the mother and fetus, including thinning of the uterine wall or dehiscence at the repair site, prematurity, and fetal death. The MOMs trial established in-utero closure of MMC as a treatment option for pregnant mothers; however, it also documented the risk of significant maternal and fetal complications with fetal intervention.

Highly specialized centers across the world now offer in-utero MMC repair, most via the open hysterotomy technique, and some via minimally invasive fetoscopic closure. Now that the benefit of in-utero closure has been shown, most programs are working to improve outcomes by careful patient selection and minimization of postoperative complications.

Etiology

The etiology of MMC is complex, incompletely understood, and involves both genetic and environmental factors. Neural tube defects occur because of incomplete closure of the neural tube during the third to fourth week of embryonic development. Cerebrospinal fluid and neural tissue are exposed through the dorsal spinal canal defect. Known risk factors for MMC include trisomy 13 and 18, Waardenburg syndrome, Fraser syndrome, and a family history of spina bifida. Factors during pregnancy such as maternal obesity, diabetes, febrile illness early in the pregnancy, folate deficiency, and the use of anti-epileptic medications (especially valproate and carbamazepine) have all been shown to increase the risk of MMC. In the majority of cases, however, no risk factor can be identified.

Taking vitamin B and folic acid supplementation significantly reduces the risk of NTDs. In many countries, breads, grains, rice, and pastas are fortified with folic acid and this lowers the incidence of NTDs by ~46%.[8] Women considering pregnancy should take a dose of folic acid of 400 mcg/day, at least one month prior to conception, and continue this dose through the first trimester to reduce the risk of NTDs. For women with a history of NTDs in previous pregnancies, the recommended dose is 4,000 mcg/day during that same time period.

Diagnosis

Prenatal testing for open NTDs is highly sensitive. The diagnosis of MMC can be made accurately as early as 18 weeks of gestation, and almost always prior to 23 weeks of gestation. Testing involves a combination of maternal serum alpha-fetoprotein screening at 15–18 weeks, high-resolution obstetrical ultrasonography, amniocentesis, and in some cases fetal magnetic resonance imaging (MRI).

In the majority of fetal patients with MMC, high-resolution obstetrical ultrasonography through the cerebral ventricles will show ventriculomegaly and the frontal bone scalloping sign (Lemon sign), as shown in Figure 10.2a. Imaging through the cerebellum will show the Chiari II malformation (Banana sign); see Figure 10.2b. These changes in the brain are

(a)

(b)

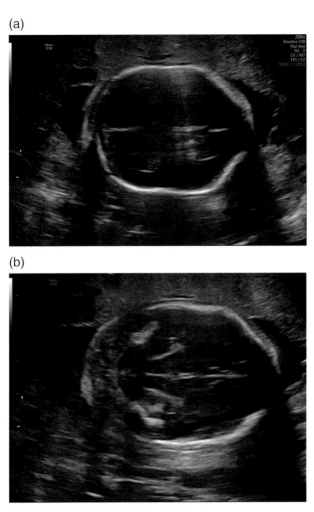

Figure 10.2 (a) Fetal head ultrasound depicting frontal bone scalloping sign (Lemon sign). (b) Ultrasound showing the Banana sign: compressed/elongated cerebellum resulting from downward pull of the spinal cord. Images courtesy of Texas Children's Fetal Center.

secondary to CSF leak at the site of the NTD and are highly reliable. It is more difficult to detect the actual lesion in the spine using ultrasound, especially when the lesion is not cystic but flat (myeloschisis); however, when the fetus is in a good position within the uterus, axial images through the spine can reveal the anatomic level of the lesion and associated spine deformities (e.g. scoliosis and/or gibbus deformity). Ultrasound can also be used to detect lower extremity movement and clubbing of the feet. This information is very useful in prenatal counseling as families consider treatment options.[9]

Fetal MRI complements ultrasound imaging but is not necessary to diagnose MMC. It can be useful to obtain when considering patients for fetal surgery. Primarily, it confirms the presence of hindbrain herniation, which needs to be present to consider a patient for fetal surgery (Figure 10.3). Fetal MRI can be useful in surgical planning and is helpful in

(a) (b)

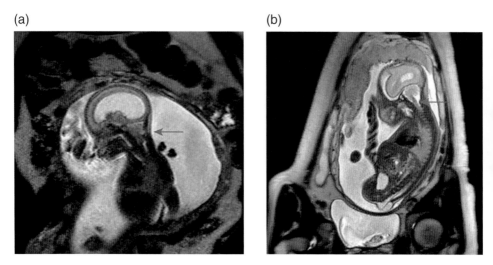

Figure 10.3 MRI of a fetus with significant hindbrain herniation. Image courtesy of Texas Children's Fetal Center.

screening patients for other congenital anomalies that may affect the decision to perform fetal surgery. Amniocentesis is seldom necessary to confirm the diagnosis of MMC but is typically obtained in patients considering fetal surgery to evaluate karyotype. In the MOMs trial, patients with an abnormal karyotype were excluded from the study.

Occasionally, it is difficult to distinguish between MMC, meningocele, and myelocystocele (a closed NTD). In general, the absence of hindbrain herniation, the presence of a thick-walled sac, and normal values of amniotic fluid alpha-feto protein and acetylcholinesterase strongly suggest a skin-covered dysraphism (closed NTD).[10] This differentiation is important because closed NTDs are not candidates for fetal intervention.

Pathophysiology

Failure of neural tube closure early in embryonic development is the underlying event for all open NTDs. The human neural tube forms and fuses dorsally between the first 18 and 27 days of human embryogenesis in a piecemeal fashion along the entire length of the neural tube. When the brain is affected at the rostral end of the neural tube, the outcomes are very poor (i.e. craniorachischisis or anencephaly), with most affected pregnancies ending in fetal death. Failure of closure over the spine results in a myelomeningocele. Patients with myelomeningoceles have a variable prognosis determined by a variety of factors including karyotype, degree of brainstem dysplasia and Chiari II malformation, and the level of the defect.[1]

A "two-hit" hypothesis has been proposed for MMC pathogenesis: (1) failure of neural tube formation; (2) spinal cord and nerve root injury from exposure to the potentially neurotoxic uterine environment and trauma.[2,11] At the site of the open NTD, the exposed spinal cord and nerve roots have variable function.

The nomenclature, Chiari II malformation is named for Hans Chiari, a pathologist who practiced at the German University in Prague. He first described this condition in a series of patients published in 1891.[12] The Chiari II malformation is seen most commonly in patients with MMC. The malformation has profound effects throughout the brain, skull, and spine; but the hallmark change is caudal displacement of the cerebellar vermis, fourth ventricle, and brainstem through an enlarged foramen magnum.[13] Other changes seen with Chiari II malformations include absence of the spinous processes and lamina, a decrease in the size of the vertebral bodies, a decrease in pedicle height, polymicrogyria, medullary kinking, a large massa intermedia, tectal beaking, gray matter heterotopias, callosal agenesis with a small posterior fossa, a low-lying confluence of the dural sinuses, an enlarged incisura, and an enlarged foramen magnum. The driving force behind these changes according to McLone and Knepper's unified theory of Chiari II malformation,[1] is the continuous leakage of CSF through the open NTD during formation of the central nervous system. As a result, CSF does not accumulate in the ventricles and both neural and calvarial development are affected by the lack of ventricular distension. The deflated ventricular system results in a small posterior fossa. The normal growth of the rhombencephalon, in this setting, results in the cerebellum growing both rostrally through the incisura and caudally into the spinal canal. Neuronal migration within the brainstem becomes disordered, leading to dysplasia. In some cases (3–8%), this leads to cranial nerve palsies and can result in the need for a tracheostomy and gastric tube. Similarly, supratentorial polymicrogyria, enlargement of the massa intermedia, and low-lying confluence of the sinuses are all produced secondary to the lack of ventricular distension in the telencephalon.[13]

Indications for Intervention (Surgical Management)

Several clinical criteria must be met by mother and fetus prior to fetal surgery. Careful patient selection decreases the risks of the procedure and increases the chances of a successful intervention. The MOMs trial criteria should be considered in every patient interested in fetal intervention. The inclusion criteria were that patients had to be greater than 18 years of age, between 19 weeks and 26 weeks of gestational age, of normal karyotype, and with MMC at level T1 through S1 with hindbrain herniation. Patients were excluded if they had a multifetal pregnancy, insulin-dependent pre-gestational diabetes, significant fetal anomaly not related to MMC (e.g. abnormal fetal ECHO), spinal column kyphosis in the fetus of 30 degrees or more, current or planned cerclage or documented history of incompetent cervix, placenta previa, placental abruption, short cervix (< 20 mm measured by cervical ultrasound), maternal obesity defined as a body mass index of 35 or greater, previous spontaneous singleton delivery prior to 37 weeks, maternal HIV or hepatitis-B positive or hepatitis-C positive, uterine anomaly such as large or multiple fibroids, and maternal hypertension that would increase the risk of preeclampsia or preterm delivery. Eligible mothers were also required to have a full-time support person to assist them after surgery so that no strenuous activity was undertaken during the period between fetal surgery and delivery.

Since publication of the MOMs trial, additional post-hoc analysis of data from the trial suggests that ventricular size prior to intervention predicts hydrocephalus outcomes (Table 10.1).[14] A fetus with ventricular size less than 10 mm across the atrium of the lateral ventricle at the time of prenatal counseling has the most significant reduction in risk of hydrocephalus; 20% incidence of hydrocephalus with fetal surgery versus ~80% with postnatal closure. Similarly, a fetus with ventricular size 10–15 mm has a less significant reduction in the risk of hydrocephalus, 45% incidence of hydrocephalus with fetal surgery versus 86% without. For fetuses with large ventricles (> 15 mm), no significant reduction in

Table 10.1 Fetal ventricular size at counseling and rate of hydrocephalus by type of surgical treatment

Ventricular size	Prenatal closure (%) (*n*=91)	Postnatal closure (%) (*n*=92)
<10 mm	20	79
10–15 mm	45	86
>15 mm	79	88

From Tulipan et al., 2015.[14]

the risk of hydrocephalus was observed following fetal surgery (78% versus 88%). These data are very useful in counseling prospective patients and help select patients with the greatest chance of achieving a benefit from fetal intervention. It makes little sense to choose fetal surgery in an attempt to avoid the diagnosis of hydrocephalus when the fetal ventricular size is greater than 15 mm.

Additionally, it is useful during the time of screening to assess lower extremity motor function using ultrasound. Fetal surgery has been shown to improve motor function in patients by protecting the neural elements from neurotoxic effects of amniotic fluid, which occur over the course of the pregnancy as well as in-utero traumatic injury as the fetus moves within the uterus. Therefore, patients whose fetuses have normal movement and muscle mass of the lower extremities at the time of screening are better candidates for fetal surgery because there is potential to preserve that function with surgery. However, patients who already have significant paraplegia and clubbing of the lower extremities are less likely to demonstrate a motor benefit because fetal surgery does not restore function.

Surgical Closure (Open and Fetoscopic)

The goals of a fetal MMC closure are the same as a postnatal closure: protect the functional neural elements and obtain a water-tight skin closure to prevent a CSF leak. The closure is similar to a postnatal closure but with some modifications because of the fragile nature of the fetus and fetal tissue.

Open NTDs of the spine can be divided into three anatomical types. The most common are the cystic myelomeningoceles, which have a dorsally displaced neural placode sitting on top of a large, cystic collection of CSF (Figure 10.4a). Myeloschisis is a second type (Figure 10.4b). This type of lesion is flat with the neural placode displaced ventrally and within the spinal canal. Overall, there is less tissue to close but the defect has the same associated central nervous system malformations as the cystic myelomeningoceles.[15] The third type, a hemi-myelomeningocele, is extremely rare. In these cases, there is a split-cord malformation with a myelomeningocele on one hemi-cord and the other hemi-cord is closed. This type of lesion requires a more extensive operation to untether and repair and therefore is not a candidate for fetal intervention. Although the lesions can be subdivided into three simple categories, there is significant variation from one lesion to another; "no two are alike."[15] The surgeon needs to be able to adapt the closure technique based on the size, shape, and complexity of the lesion to obtain the best closure and achieve the surgical goals. The closure is performed in layers and any of the following layers can be incorporated into the repair: pia, dura, fascia, and skin. However, it is not necessary nor is it usually possible to close them all.

(a)

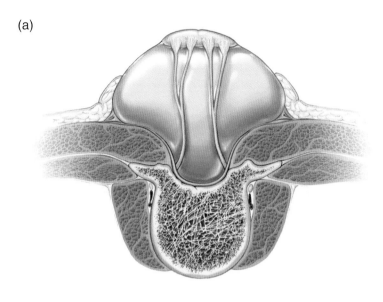

(b)

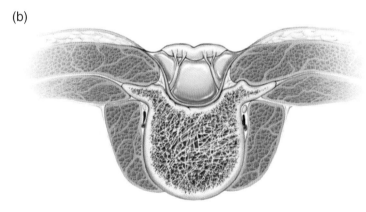

Figure 10.4 (a) Schematic diagram depicting cystic myelomeningocele. A cystic swelling of the dura and arachnoid, protrudes through the spina bifida defect in the vertebral arch. (b) Schematic diagram depicting myeloschisis. This defect is characterized by a cleft spinal cord resulting from the failure of the neural plate to fuse and form a complete neural tube.
Pictures courtesy of Katherine Relyea, MS, CMI.

Step one in the fetal surgical procedure is visualization of the back lesion, and identification of critical structures including the neural placode, and the junctional zone (Figure 10.5). Next, as in a postnatal repair, the neural placode is untethered from the surrounding skin. This is usually accomplished by cutting the arachnoid membrane between the placode edge and the junctional zone. Care is taken to visualize dorsal nerve roots, which can be adherent to the underside of the arachnoid membrane. When this adherence is observed, the nerves are bluntly dissected off the arachnoid membrane and allowed to hang down in the spinal canal so an incision can be made safely through the arachnoid membrane. This cut should be made at least 2 mm from the edge of the placode and the surgeon should

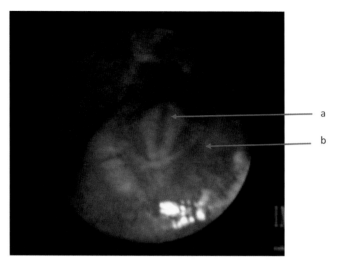

a

b

Figure 10.5 Intraoperative photo of fetal myelomeningocele showing the (a) placode and (b) junctional zone. Photo courtesy of Dr. William Whitehead.

exclude any epidermal remnants from the tissue attached to the placode to decrease the risk of an epidermoid inclusion cyst forming later in life. Alternatively, when the edge of the placode and the junctional zone are too difficult to discern, an initial incision can be made in the skin lateral to the junctional zone and the zona epitheliosa. This incision is extended through the dura and the fascia and completely encircles the defect. The arachnoid sac is then sharply mobilized medially and all remnants of epithelial tissue are trimmed off up to the placode edge (Figure 10.6).[16,17]

Closure of the neural placode is the next step, but this is not necessary to achieve the goals of surgery, and not all surgeons will perform this step. This is performed by placing a fine, monofilament suture through the pial edge on each side of the placode. Tying this suture brings the pial edges together and rounds out the neural placode. It is believed that this step reduces the amount of scarring between the spinal cord and dura, which would minimize the difficulty of untethering surgery if this should become necessary in the future. In some cases, the placode is quite large and wide, making this step difficult. "Tubularizing" the placode can cause the spinal cord to bulge dorsally making it difficult to close the dura. Additionally, placing sutures into the pial edges may cause trauma or bleeding within the spinal cord and diminish function.

The dura is closed next, when possible. A good dural closure over the placode can also minimize the challenge of future tethered cord release surgery because of the easily identified plane it creates over the spinal cord. As in traditional postnatal closure, the dura is incised laterally and mobilized medially for primary closure in the midline. When there is very minimal dural tissue, a patch can also be sewn to the dura. A variety of dural substitutes have been utilized, including collagen patches and bovine pericardium.[18] The dural layer in the fetus, however, is often quite fragile and usually tears during the dissection or the tying of sutures. For this reason, a primary water-tight closure, as described above performed for postnatal repairs, is usually very difficult to achieve. Often, other strategies are required to achieve dural closure.

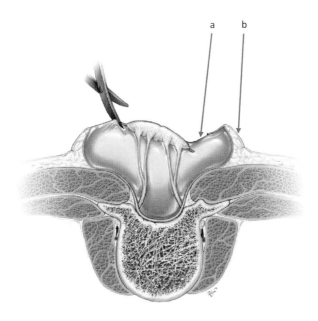

Figure 10.6 Separation of the placode from the skin. Incisions can be made at site 'a' or 'b'. If the skin is incised at 'b' the arachnoid is also trimmed and removed up to point 'a'.
Picture courtesy of Katherine Relyea, MS, CMI.

One alternative strategy for dural closure is to leave the dura attached to the underlying fascia and develop a paraspinal myofascial flap by cutting through dura, fascia and muscle laterally. This flap is then folded over toward the midline and the entire tissue layer is closed with a running or interrupted suture (Figure 10.7). Essentially, this strengthens the tissue layer of the dura by keeping it attached to the underlying fascia during dissection, mobilization, and suturing.[16]

A second alternative is to leave the dura intact all the way up to the junctional zone and place wide-based vertical mattress sutures through the skin and dura. This technique leaves the dura intact and everts the skin edges; the fascia and paraspinal muscles are also left intact, as in a postnatal closure (Figure 10.8).[19] Because the dura is quite thin and atrophic closer to the junctional zone, the first stitch should be ~6–9 mm from the skin edge (aka: junctional zone). It should also pierce the dura layer as laterally as possible. In addition, because this single layer of tissue can be thin, a dura-substitute patch should be placed on-lay over the placode. The patch should be slightly larger than the placode itself. This patch serves as a spacer to help keep the placode within the spinal canal and creates an additional layer between the placode and dura. The use of a patch at this stage covers the placode and protects it from trauma as the next layer is closed. Placing a patch over the placode may decrease adhesions and scarring; it may also serve as an additional layer or barrier in the closure which may reduce the rate of CSF leak. The effect of an on-lay patch over the placode on the rate of cord tethering and on reduction of CSF leaks remains unknown, however. This on-lay patch technique was one of a variety of techniques used in the MOMs trial.

The final layer is the skin, which can be closed with either a running or an interrupted stitch. Care is taken not to tear the skin as the stitch is being tightened. In the event that skin

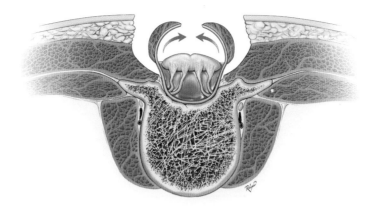

Figure 10.7 Schematic showing myofascial flap dissection.
Picture courtesy of Katherine Relyea, MS, CMI.

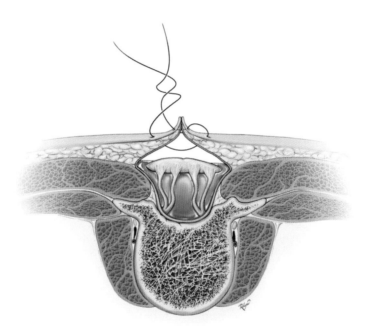

Figure 10.8 Single-layer closure with vertical mattress sutures.
Picture courtesy of Katherine Relyea, MS, CMI.

closure is under tension, several techniques to achieve closure have been described. One option is to aggressively undermine the skin in the plane just over the fascia to help mobilize the skin medially for primary closure. This technique is commonly used for a postnatal closure. A second option is to use a skin-substitute patch such as alloderm. A third option involves creation of lateral relaxing incisions 2–3 cm lateral to the skin edge, to help mobilize the skin medially (Figure 10.9).[20] The use of rotational flaps has also been

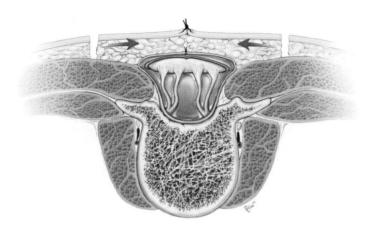

Figure 10.9 Lateral relaxing incisions to allow a midline, primary closure of skin. Picture courtesy of Katherine Relyea, MS, CMI.

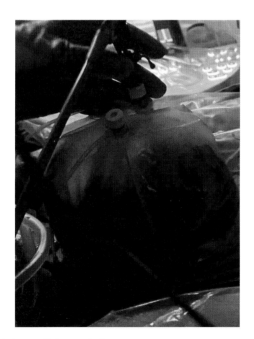

Figure 10.10 Exteriorized uterus with two port sites.

described.[21] Of all the layers, the skin layer is the most important and it is critical to achieve a water-tight closure.

The process of closure of the fetal defect is the same regardless of whether the approach is via an open approach or a fetoscopic approach. The fetoscopic approach is utilized routinely in some centers and performed under a research protocol in others. The fetoscopic approach is of two variants: one is repair of the fetal myelomeningocele entirely via fetoscopy, and the other is characterized by fetoscopic repair of the fetal myelomeningocele via maternal laparotomy. In the latter approach, the uterus is exteriorized and fetoscopes are used to repair the spine defect through either two or three ports (Figure 10.10). Regardless of the exact approach, fetoscopic repair of myelomeningocele has been associated with decreased uterine dehiscence. This may facilitate vaginal deliveries for subsequent pregnancies in contrast to the mandated cesarean delivery following open fetal surgery.[22,23]

Stopping the CSF leak with closure of the defect, allows re-expansion of the CSF spaces, and this drives growth and expansion of the posterior fossa, leading to reversal of the hindbrain herniation. It also provides a layer of protection over the neural elements preventing further damage from blunt trauma in-utero and exposure to the neurotoxic effects of amniotic fluid.

Anesthetic Considerations and Management

Myelomeningocele repair is the most common indication for prenatal surgery. The American College of Obstetrics & Gynecology recommends open fetal surgery for MMC because of the associated benefits after the baby is born.[24–27] Preoperatively, a multidisciplinary team, including perinatologists, fetal surgeons, neurosurgeons, anesthesiologists, social workers, nurse coordinators, neonatologists, radiologists, and cardiologists, meet individually and collectively with the patient to discuss the diagnosis and planned intervention. The anesthetic plan is developed, keeping in mind the maternal medical history, expected fetal stimulation, as well as surgeon and patient preferences.[24–27]

Surgery for MMC repair is typically offered between 20 and 25 weeks of gestation. A fetus begins to perceive noxious stimulus at about 18–20 weeks of gestation, therefore it is important to provide the fetus with adequate analgesia during surgery. During surgery, weight-based anesthetic medications are administered to the fetus by direct intramuscular injection to either the shoulders or buttocks. The estimated fetal weight for drug calculations and appropriate dosing of medications is obtained from fetal imaging studies.

For the surgery, the mothers typically receive general anesthesia along with epidural analgesia. To avoid intraoperative hemodynamic lability as a result of high volatile anesthetic requirements for uterine relaxation, local anesthetics are not administered through the epidural until after completion of the fetal intervention. The goals of anesthetic management during fetal surgery are to avoid hypotension, hypoxia, and acidosis, to ensure that adequate uteroplacental blood flow occurs throughout surgery. In addition to maintaining adequate uteroplacental blood flow, perioperative uterine relaxation is also essential. Nifedipine or indomethacin is administered preoperatively for tocolysis, while volatile anesthetics and magnesium sulfate are administered intra- and postoperatively, respectively, to maintain uterine relaxation. Volatile anesthetics are titrated during surgery to between 1 and 3 MAC (minimum alveolar concentration) based on surgeon feedback regarding the uterine tone. Uterine tone is assessed by manual palpation. In the rare event that inadequate uterine relaxation is obtained with the volatile anesthetic, supplemental medications such as intravenous nitroglycerin may be administered although this is rarely indicated. Postoperative tocolysis is achieved with any combination of the following: nifedipine (10 mg orally, every six hours), indomethacin (25 mg orally, every four hours for 48 hours), subcutaneous terbutaline (0.25 mg for two doses), and intravenous magnesium (4–6 g bolus followed by a 2 g/hour infusion), as indicated.[27–29]

Prior to surgery, the mother is typed and cross-matched for blood. While intra-uterine blood transfusion for the fetal repair is rare, irradiated, leukocyte-reduced, O-negative blood is prepared for the fetus. A few key physiologic considerations for surgery include left uterine displacement to avoid hypotension secondary to aortocaval compression, use of a higher oxygen concentration to compensate for the high oxygen consumption in pregnancy, and rapid desaturation during airway manipulation. The latter occurs because of lower functional residual capacity and can be further complicated by the higher incidence of difficulty in securing the airway in pregnancy.

At our institution, patients who present for open MMC repair have an epidural placed in the preoperative holding area with administration of only a test dose. A combined spinal epidural with intrathecal fentanyl allows the patient to easily tolerate the foley catheter placement in the operating room. Next, intra-arterial and peripheral venous catheters are obtained either in the preoperative holding area, or immediately upon arrival in the operating room. To decrease exposure to anesthesia, the urinary catheter is placed while awake, and the patient is positioned, prepped, and draped for surgery, prior to induction of general anesthesia. Based on the anesthesiologist's preference, the mother may receive intravenous analgesia and sedation during this stage or a combined spinal epidural may have been placed preoperatively, in which 15 mcg of intrathecal fentanyl only is administered; this will allow for placement of the urinary catheter with minimal discomfort. After surgical time-out has been performed, the patient then undergoes rapid-sequence induction and intubation. Intraoperative uterine relaxation is obtained using sevoflurane. Ephedrine and/or phenylephrine boluses and/or an infusion of phenylephrine may be required to keep the systolic blood pressure within 20% of awake baseline values, and maintain uteroplacental perfusion. Once access to the fetus is achieved, a medication cocktail is administered to the fetus via a direct intramuscular injection. The medication cocktail consists of an opioid, anti-cholinergic and muscle relaxant, namely: fentanyl 5–10 mcg/kg, atropine 20 mcg/kg, and vecuronium 0.4 mg/kg; this combination medication is re-dosed every 45–60 minutes until the end of surgery. These medications are all drawn up prior to the start of surgery and handed over to the scrub technician in a sterile fashion. Additionally, epinephrine (1 mcg/kg and 10 mcg/kg) and calcium gluconate (30 mg/kg) are also prepared in sterile fashion, in case intraoperative fetal resuscitation becomes necessary. Intermittent intraoperative monitoring of the fetus is conducted via echocardiography. Fetal heart rate (FHR) is used as an indicator of fetal well-being during intervention. Fetal bradycardia (< 100 bpm) is managed pharmacologically, and, when needed, chest compressions are performed. Intermittent measurement of FHR is conducted using Doppler ultrasound. The steps in fetal resuscitation are, first to improve uteroplacental blood flow by giving fluids and/or vasoactive agents; increase inspired maternal oxygenation; enhance tocolysis; and relief of any possible cord compression by repositioning the fetus and/or amnioinfusion. If these steps are unsuccessful, then epinephrine, atropine, fetal crystalloid infusion, or fetal packed red blood cells infusion should be utilized. The last step is to initiate fetal chest compressions. In a fetus that has reached viability, the fetus is delivered, and resuscitation is continued post delivery.

Once closure of the fetal defect has been completed, uterine closure begins. A loading dose of magnesium (4–6 g, based on surgeon preference) is started, and is followed by an infusion of 2 g/hour. Local anesthetics are administered via the epidural catheter, and the infusion is started. The patient is then extubated awake and transferred to the recovery room. The epidural infusion consists of local anesthetic (ropivacaine) and an opioid.

Postoperative epidural analgesia is continued for ~48 hours and the patient is transitioned to oral opioids. Patients that have undergone fetoscopic myelomeningocele repair have the epidural in place for one day postoperatively and patients that have undergone open fetal MMC repair have the epidural in place for 2–3 days as they have a larger uterine incision in contrast to port access points in fetoscopic surgery. To decrease postoperative opioid consumption, the patients receive a tranversus abdominis plane block at the time the epidural catheter infusion is discontinued. To prevent local anesthetic overdose, the infusion is typically stopped for ~2–4 hours prior to placement of the block.

Post surgery

After discharge, the patient returns every week for follow-up. Once 30–32 weeks of gestation is reached, the follow-up is spaced out to monthly intervals and includes a comprehensive ultrasound. When the pregnancy reaches 34 weeks of gestation, weekly biophysical profiles and Doppler studies are performed. For fetuses that have undergone the fetoscopic repair, a vaginal delivery is possible if all other obstetrical indications are met. Once the baby is delivered, the neonate is admitted to the NICU for a comprehensive evaluation by neonatology, neurosurgery, and urology.[29]

References

1. McLone DG, Knepper PA. The cause of Chiari II malformation: a unified theory. Pediatr Neurosc. 1989;15:1–12.

2. Heffez DS, Aryanpur J, Hutchins GM, Freeman JM. The paralysis associated with myelomeningocele: clinical and experimental data implicating a preventable spinal cord injury. Neurosurgery. 1990;26:987–992.

3. Meuli M, Meuli-Simmen C, Hutchins GM, et al. In utero surgery rescues neurological function at birth in sheep with spina bifida. Nat Med. 1995;1:342–347.

4. Meuli M, Meuli-Simmen C, Yingling CD, et al. Creation of myelomeningocele in utero: a model of functional damage from spinal cord exposure in fetal sheep. J Pediatr Surg. 1995;30:1028–32; discussion 32–3.

5. Michejda M. Intrauterine treatment of spina bifida: primate model. Z Kinderchir. 1984;39:259–261.

6. Bruner JP, Tulipan NE, Richards WO. Endoscopic coverage of fetal open myelomeningocele in utero. Am J Obstet Gynecol. 1997;176:256–257.

7. Farmer DL, von Koch CS, Peacock WJ, et al. In utero repair of myelomeningocele: experimental pathophysiology, initial clinical experience, and outcomes. Arch Surg. 2003;138:872–878.

8. Blencowe H, Cousens S, Modell B, Lawn J. Folic acid to reduce neonatal mortality from neural tube disorders. Int J Epidemiol. 2010;39 Suppl1: i110–121.

9. Maroto A, Illescas T, Melendez M, et al. Ultrasound functional evaluation of fetuses with myelomeningocele: study of the interpretation of results. J Matern Fetal Neonatal Med. 2017;30:2301–2305.

10. Midrio P, Silberstein HJ, Bilaniuk LT, Adzick NS, Sutton LN. Prenatal diagnosis of terminal myelocystocele in the fetal surgery era: case report. Neurosurgery. 2002;50:1152–1154; discussion 4–5.

11. Heffez DS, Aryanpur J, Rotellini NA, et al. Intrauterine repair of experimental surgically created dysraphism. Neurosurgery. 1993;32:1005–1010.

12. Ueber HC. Veränderungen des Kleinhirns infolge von Hydrocephalie des Grosshirns. Deutsche Medicinische Wochenschrift. 1891;17:1172–1175.

13. Stevenson KL. Chiari Type II malformation: past, present, and future. Neurosurg Focus. 2004;16:E5.

14. Tulipan N, Wellons JC, 3rd, Thom EA, et al. Prenatal surgery for myelomeningocele and the need for cerebrospinal fluid shunt placement. J Neurosurg Pediatr. 2015;16:613–620.

15. McComb JG, Mittler M. Myelomeningoceles and meningoceles. In: Albright AL, Pollack IF, Adelson PD, eds. *Operative Techniques in Pediatric Neurosurgery*. New York: Thieme; 2001:75–88.

16. Heuer GG, Adzick NS, Sutton LN. Fetal myelomeningocele closure: technical considerations. *Fetal Diagn Ther*. 2015;**37**:166–171.

17. Kohl T. Percutaneous minimally invasive fetoscopic surgery for spina bifida aperta. Part I: surgical technique and perioperative outcome. *Ultrasound Obstet Gynecol*. 2014;**44**:515–524.

18. Adzick NS, Thom EA, Spong CY, et al. A randomized trial of prenatal versus postnatal repair of myelomeningocele. *N Engl J Med*. 2011;**364**:993–1004.

19. Cheek WR, Laurent JP, Cech DA. Operative repair of lumbosacral myelomeningocele. Technical note. *J Neurosurg*. 1983;**59**:718–722.

20. Bennett KA, Carroll MA, Shannon CN, et al. Reducing perinatal complications and preterm delivery for patients undergoing in utero closure of fetal myelomeningocele: further modifications to the multidisciplinary surgical technique. *J Neurosurg Pediatr*. 2014;**14**:108–114.

21. Meuli M, Meuli-Simmen C, Mazzone L, et al. In utero plastic surgery in Zurich: successful use of distally pedicled random pattern transposition flaps for definitive skin closure during open fetal spina bifida repair. *Fetal Diagn Ther*. 2018;**44**:173–178.

22. Belfort MA, Whitehead WE, Shamshirsaz AA, et al. Fetoscopic repair of meningomyelocele. *Obstet Gynecol*. 2015;**126**:881–884.

23. Kabagambe SK, Jensen GW, Chen YJ, et al. Fetal surgery for myelomeningocele: a systematic review and meta-analysis of outcomes in fetoscopic versus open repair. *Fetal Diagn Ther*. 2018;**43**:161–174

24. Ferschl M, Ball R, Lee H, Rollins MD. Anesthesia for in utero repair of myelomeningocele. *Anesthesiology*. 2013;**118**:1211–1223.

25. Grivell R, Andersen C, Dodd J. Prenatal versus postnatal repair procedures for spina bifida for improving infant and maternal outcomes. *Cochrane Database Syst Rev*. 2014;**10**:CD008825.

26. Van de Velde M, De Buck F. Fetal and maternal analgesia/anesthesia for fetal procedures. *Fetal Diagn Ther*. 2012;**31**:201–209.

27. Committee Opinion No. 720: Maternal–Fetal Surgery for Myelomeningocele. *Obstet Gynecol*. 2017;**130**:e164–167.

28. Hoagland MA, Chatterjee D. Anesthesia for fetal surgery. *Pediatr Anesth*. 2017;**27**:346–357.

29. Belfort MA, Whitehead WE, Shamshirsaz AA, et al. Fetoscopic open neural tube defect repair: development and refinement of a two-port, carbon dioxide insufflation technique. *Obstet Gynecol*. 2017;**129**:734–743.

Chapter 11

Lung Masses

Candace C. Style, Mariatu Verla, Olutoyin A. Olutoye, and Oluyinka O. Olutoye

Introduction/Overview

Congenital lung masses comprise a variety of lesions resulting from developmental abnormalities of the bronchial tree, pulmonary vasculature, or the foregut. Pathologic variants include bronchopulmonary sequestrations, bronchogenic cysts, bronchial atresia, and congenital cystic adenomatoid malformations[1] (Figure 11.1). These space occupying lesions can vary in size from small to large, and can be detected in the prenatal period incidentally, or following evaluation for specific signs and symptoms. Very large lesions may cause compression and distortion of structures in the thoracic cavity resulting in shifting of the mediastinum, impairment of growth of adjacent normal lung tissue, compromised venous return and cardiac compression leading to decreased cardiac output, fetal distress, and ultimately fetal demise if left untreated. Severe symptoms in the fetal period are rare and the majority of these lesions will remain asymptomatic at birth to be observed or treated with elective surgical resection.[2]

Congenital lung malformations occur in about 1 in 3,500 live births with some variability based on the pathology of the lesion.[3] Prior to the widespread use of high-quality fetal ultrasonography, minor lesions were undiagnosed until adulthood, so the true incidence is unknown. There is little evidence of a genetic component being linked to any of the specific types although some will occur in the setting of other fetal anomalies.[4] There is no predilection for either gender except in the case of congenital lobar emphysema where there is a male to female predominance of 3:1. Mass location is typically evenly distributed

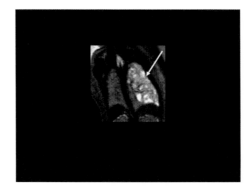

Figure 11.1 Fetal lung mass MRI. The arrow depicts a left upper lobe cystic lung lesion with the larger cysts more prominent as bright areas within the lesion, in contrast to the less intense lower lobe and contralateral lung.

between both sides of the thorax. Although this disease process has been extensively studied, the etiology remains unclear. Despite this, the prenatal management has advanced extensively improving outcomes.

Embryology of the Lung

Development of the lung begins at the fourth week of gestation and is divided into five histological stages: the embryonic stage at 4–7 weeks' gestation, the pseudoglandular stage at 5–17 weeks, the cannicular stage at 16–26 weeks, the saccular stage at 24–36 weeks, and the alveolar stage at 36 weeks to two years of age.[5,6] What results is a well-coordinated process facilitated by mesenchymal and epithelial interactions involving a multitude of transcription factors, growth factors, and adhesion molecules. In the embryonic stage, the foregut branches into the ventral trachea and the dorsal esophagus induced by paracrine signals from the surrounding mesenchyme of the notochord, heart, and septum transversum.[4] The tracheal rudiment is then proliferated by growth factors culminating in the formation of the primary lung buds. Vasculogenesis occurs simultaneously during this stage with the origination of the pulmonary arteries.[7–9] In the pseudoglandular stage, airway branching and blood vessel proliferation generate the bronchial tree, systematically shaping the secondary planar and tertiary three-dimensional branching design of the airway.[10] The cannalicular phase is defined by progressive thinning of the pulmonary tree and formation of a dense capillary network within the mesenchyme.[11] During the saccular stage, the terminal bronchioles widen to form air sacs and there is deposition of elastic fibers in preparation for the alveolar stage. In the final alveolar stage, the lung undergoes continuous maturation, restructuring, and microvascularization. This process continues well after birth and helps to modulate compensatory lung growth after resection.[12–14]

Although lung development is tightly regulated, congenital lung masses can result from disordered embryologic interactions at any stage during fetal lung development. While the actual molecular pathogenesis is not completely understood, several theories have been postulated. Many theorize that environmental factors cause decreased cellular apoptosis and persistent expression of early lung development markers, causing genetic defects that lead to interruption of lung morphogenesis.[15,16] Concurrently, vascular traction, insufficiency, or prolonged ischemia has been proposed as an alternate mechanism for the development of lung masses. Recent studies have also suggested that a genetic or epigenetic defect in the lung epithelium plays a central role in pathogenesis.[17] In one such animal study, cystic formation developed when lung branching was inactivated by knocking out *DICER*, an mRNA processing enzyme, in the lung epithelium of the mice model.[18,19] However, given the variety of lesion types, the malformation is likely multimodal with molecular pathogenetic specifications for each histologic subtype. Thus, additional studies are needed to fully illuminate the complex and likely multifaceted molecular mechanisms for each histologic variant.

Congenital Cystic Adenomatoid Malformation

Congenital cystic adenomatoid malformations or CCAMs, also referred to as congenital pulmonary airway malformations (CPAMs), are the most common form of lung masses. They develop as a result of decreased bronchial maturation with simultaneous mesenchymal overgrowth.[20] Albeit cystic in nature, CCAMs are often described as hamartous lesions because of the appearance of seemingly normal pulmonary tissue in a disorganized spatial arrangement. This tissue, however, does not participate in normal gas exchange, but there is some communication with the trachea-bronchial tree as evidenced by air trapping.[21]

The characteristics of CCAMs, including the tissue type, shape and size of cysts, and location, can vary from infant to infant. In 1977, Stocker et al. developed a classification scheme based on the sizing and spacing of the cysts and the histological appearance. The classification was originally subdivided into three stages.[22] Type I lesions are the most common, accounting for up to 50% of CCAMs and are described as large mucinous cysts characterized by one or more cysts of variable size up to 10 cm. Type II lesions are hyperechogenic, microcystic, and may occur with associated anomalies. Type III lesions, originally thought to confer the poorest prognosis of CCAM lesion type, are mostly solid and typically result in mediastinal shift. This classification scheme has since been updated to include both a type 0 and type IV.[23] Type 0, which represents acinar dysplasia, is a very rare malformation that is mainly lethal and incompatible with life if bilateral.[1] Type IV consists of nonmucinous cysts lined by alveolar cells.[1,23] The malformations can also coexist as hybrid lesions with pulmonary sequestrations. Although the Stocker classification is useful as a pathologic identification system, it has not been proven to be an accurate predictor of antenatal outcome given that many CCAMs do not fit succinctly into just one category. Thus for clinical management it has been most useful to classify the lesions as either macro (> 5 cm) or microcystic (< 5 cm) based on ultrasound diameters as proposed by Adzick et al.[4,24]

Bronchopulmonary Sequestration

Bronchopulmonary sequestrations (BPS) are the second most common type of lung malformations diagnosed. This results from the formation of a supernumerary lung bud, which can be either intralobar or extralobar.[25] The lesions are microscopic cystic masses of nonfunctioning pulmonary tissue, which do not communicate with the tracheobronchial tree and have a systemic vascular supply usually from the thoracic descending aorta or below the diaphragm. Additionally, BPS lesions can be present in the thoracic or abdominal cavity. Intralobar sequestrations (ILS) exist within the same pleural envelope as the normal surrounding lung tissue while extralobar sequestrations (ELS) are discrete from the normal lung and enveloped in a separate visceral pleura.[4,26] These can be also be distinguished from each other based on either pulmonary (ILS) or systemic (ELS) venous drainage. While there is no known genetic aberration associated with BPS, this lung mass is often associated with other fetal anomalies, such as congenital diaphragmatic hernia and ELS. As with other lung lesions, symptomatology varies. Fetuses may be asymptomatic or develop a pleural effusion, mediastinal shift, and/or polyhydramnios. In severe cases, nonimmune hydrops fetalis may develop.

Bronchogenic Cyst

Bronchogenic cysts (BC) are formed from aberrant budding of the foregut during the embryonic stage of development. These cysts may contain cartilage, muscle, and glands, and therefore have similar pathology to esophageal duplication cysts. Bronchogenic cysts are usually fluid-filled and rarely communicate with the airway. They are often located adjacent or adherent to the distal trachea in the anterior mediastinum and can cause mass effect on the trachea or bronchus.[4] However, despite their nomenclature, these cysts can be found in a variety of locations including the esophageal wall, below or within the diaphragm, in the head and neck region, and even the spine.[27] The cysts are unilocular and can grow as large as 10 cm in diameter. Histologically, the lesions are typically lined with respiratory epithelium and contain cartilage in the wall of the cyst. These lesions can, but rarely, cause symptoms in the fetal period. Yet, the risk of subsequent obstructive symptoms, malignancy, and infection necessitate the need for postnatal surgical intervention.

Bronchial Atresia

Bronchial atresia (BA) is defined as a focal airway obstruction resulting from interruption of a lobar, segmental, or mainstem bronchus and mucus impaction. This results in hyperinflation of the obstructed lung segment,[28–30] and will often coexist with other lung lesions, most commonly CCAMs. Lobar and segmental BA are largely benign and often discovered incidentally. For these subtypes, fetal symptoms are rare, but the condition can manifest as recurrent pulmonary infections after birth. Mainstem bronchial atresia (MBA), however, is a rare and lethal lesion that results in malformation of an entire lung which becomes overextended from hyperinflation. This leads to severe mediastinal compression and ultimately fetal demise.[31]

Congenital Lobar Emphysema

Congenital lobar emphysema (CLE) is often referenced as a differential diagnosis for lung masses. It occurs rarely and represents an overinflation of a lobe of the lung from trapped inspired air.[32] In the fetus, it may present as an echogenic lobe of the lung. The exact etiology is unclear. Unlike bronchial atresia, the bronchus appears to be normal but is thought to contain dysplastic bronchial cartilage.[33] It is rarely diagnosed in the prenatal period and is often diagnosed when neonates present with respiratory distress shortly after birth. Chest radiographs shortly after birth may reveal a portion of the lung which is more radio-opaque than the rest as the lung fluid within this portion of the lung is not completely expelled in the normal birthing process. As the lung lymphatics gradually clear the retained airway fluid, the alveoli fill with air and the affected lung becomes progressively more radiolucent as air trapping occurs. This process of air trapping is aggravated by positive pressure ventilation. The distended lobe may be so engorged as to cause a severe contralateral mediastinal shift and compression of adjacent normal lung tissue. Prompt treatment in this instance, will require a decompressive thoracotomy and lobectomy of the affected lobe of lung.

Congenital High Airway Obstruction Syndrome

Although extremely rare, congenital high airway obstruction syndrome, or CHAOS, should also be considered when evaluating for lung masses. This condition results from obstruction of the central airway, most commonly caused by laryngeal or tracheal atresia.[34] This obstruction results in bilateral lung hyperplasia. As a result of balanced bilateral overgrowth, the heart maintains a central position, but the diaphragm becomes flattened or everted as a result. The increased intrathoracic pressure is gradual, and fairly well tolerated in the fetus. Therefore, while signs of frank hydrops (ascites, body wall edema, placentomegaly) may be present, cardiac function is well-preserved suggesting that the fluid accumulation occurs as a result of elevated hydrostatic pressure and lymphatic obstruction and not from cardiac dysfunction. The central location of the obstruction results in bilateral echogenicity of the fetal lungs. In cases where bilateral CPAMs are suspected, CHAOS should be ruled out. The fetus is often able to tolerate a prolonged "hydropic" state if the cardiac function remains preserved. In-utero intervention to traverse a short (membranous) obstruction in the trachea can be attempted. Attempts at fetal tracheostomy to relieve the airway obstruction have also been considered. Most fetuses with CHAOS will be delivered preterm. An EXIT procedure is required to secure airway access while on placental support to avert birth asphyxia and death.[35] These newborns have an extremely high total body water content so tremendous fluid shifts and diuresis complicate the neonatal management. In the absence of prenatal diagnosis and plans for an EXIT procedure, almost all cases with CHAOS are fatal or associated with severe birth asphyxia.

Diagnosis of a Lung Mass

The widespread use of prenatal ultrasound has increased the diagnosis of fetal chest or lung malformations in the prenatal period. While the most common fetal chest mass detected prenatally is congenital diaphragmatic hernia, lung masses are also now commonly diagnosed between 18 and 20 weeks' gestation. Lung masses are distinguished on ultrasound by the appearance of increased echogenicity of the affected portion of the lung and/or the presence of cysts in the thoracic cavity and/or rarely in the abdominal cavity.[36] These general findings are similar for the major histologic diagnoses including pulmonary sequestrations, CCAMs, bronchial atresia, congenital lobar emphysema, or tracheal obstruction. Additional ultrasonographic features can be utilized to further distinguish the type of lesion. For instance, pulmonary sequestrations have Doppler evidence of a systemic arterial supply arising from the aorta or the celiac artery. The direction of pulmonary venous drainage can also help distinguish an ILS or ELS. The size and location of the entire lesion and the sizes of internal cysts can also be assessed by ultrasound.

Ultrasonography is a safe and effective method of detecting lung masses in the prenatal period; however, it can be difficult to predict the actual pathology and outcome solely by ultrasound.[37] For this reason, magnetic resonance imaging (MRI) is used as an imaging adjunct, enabling quantification of the congenital lesion size and the volume of the involved lung to allow for better prognostication. This can be advantageous when evaluating atypical tumors or large masses. Of importance in lung masses, compressed lung tissue can still be visualized on MRI allowing for better definition of the lobar anatomy. Additional imaging typically includes a fetal echocardiogram to assess for cardiac dysfunction and concomitant heart defects. The option for amniocentesis or umbilical cord sampling for fetal karyotyping is also offered to further assess the fetus, although these lesions are not typically associated with major chromosomal anomalies. Once a diagnosis is established, biweekly ultrasounds should be scheduled for continuous monitoring.

Prognosis

Regardless of pathologic variant, outcome of lung masses is mostly dependent on size of the lesion and the degree of fetal distress.[3] The natural history of lung masses is early rapid growth between 18 and 28 weeks' gestation. After this time period, many lesions shrink and often spontaneously resolve with no further sonographic detection.[38,39] The exact mechanism by which these masses regress or spontaneously resolve is unknown but this has been reported to occur in 10–40% of lesions identified prenatally.[40–42] Sonographic resolution does not always infer histologic resolution. As lung fluid production decreases in late gestation, there is less fluid within the lesions to permit discrimination by ultrasound.

Postnatal cross-sectional imaging has identified most of these lesions that were no longer apparent on late gestation ultrasound. A number of these lesions were no longer identifiable even on postnatal cross-sectional imaging. Lung masses may also continue to increase in size and cause symptoms. Large lesions present a significant risk of compression of surrounding thoracic structures and must be closely monitored. Compression of normal lung tissue may result in pulmonary hypoplasia. Esophageal compression interferes with fetal swallowing, and may result in polyhydramnios which increases the risk of preterm labor.[43] Larger lesions also cause a mediastinal shift which can ultimately lead to impaired venous return, cardiac compression, and impaired cardiac function or cardiac tamponade physiology. This, along with compression of the vena cavae, can result in accumulation of fluid manifesting as ascites, pleural effusion, pericardial effusion, skin/scalp edema, and/or placentomegaly. Nonimmune hydrops fetalis is diagnosed when there is fluid accumulation in two or more of these compartments in a fetus who does not have anemia from alloimmunization. The prognosis is markedly worse for the hydropic fetus, and if left untreated in-utero demise may occur. Lung mass symptoms are not only harmful to the fetus, but also the mother is at risk for severe preeclampsia and edema; these mimic the fetal condition and this is therefore referred to as "mirror syndrome," which can be fatal but may be reversed if the underlying cause is treated. With improvements in imaging, it has become apparent that not all hydropic fetuses are at imminent risk of in-utero demise. A careful assessment of the fetal cardiac function is an important differentiator.

Although symptomatic fetal lesions are rare, the consequences can be morbid thus it is imperative to risk stratify each fetus. The CCAM volume ratio, or CVR, is used to detect fetuses at risk for poor prognosis. First introduced by Crombleholme et al. in 2002, CVR is the estimated volume of lesion calculated by determining the volume of a prolate ellipse (length × height × width × 0.52) divided by the head circumference. On review of 43 cases with a diagnosis of CCAM, a CVR > 1.6 was predictive of hydrops.[44] Although CVR was developed with CCAMs, recent studies have further shown that CVR is predictive of the fetal outcome of most lung masses. A CVR of > 0.8 is predictive of polyhydramnios and a risk of respiratory distress. A higher CVR of > 2.0 is indicative of the need for fetal intervention.[3,45] Other parameters such as lung-to-head ratios, fetal lung volumes, and mass-to-thorax ratios have been studied as potential predictors of fetal outcome; however, CVR remains the most predictive and widely used.[46]

Following diagnosis of fetuses with large lesions, or those whose lesions are expected to continue to grow into a large lesion, mothers should be referred for evaluation at a tertiary treatment facility to undergo detailed evaluation and nondirective multidisciplinary counseling with pediatric surgery, maternal fetal medicine, neonatology, anesthesia, and cardiology. Evaluation will include a detailed high-resolution fetal ultrasound, ultrafast fetal MRI, fetal echocardiography, and possibly chromosomal analysis. Serial ultrasonography should be performed throughout the course of pregnancy to monitor for signs of ascites, skin/scalp edema, placentomegaly, and pleural effusions.[47] Based on the fetal and maternal symptoms, a delivery plan is developed. In the absence of any additional maternal or fetal complications, fetuses with asymptomatic masses and a persistently low CVR can be safely delivered at term at the parental treatment facility of choice. Symptomatic lesions should be closely monitored by a fetal center with continuous assessment for the need for fetal intervention, special delivery precautions, or fetal and maternal anesthetic concerns. Subsequent to delivery, the neonate should be closely monitored by a neonatologist for signs of respiratory distress.

Treatment

Maternal Steroids

Fetal lung mass characteristics and associated symptoms determine the option for fetal intervention.[48] For masses that are large and microcystic, high-dose maternal corticosteroid administration is a noninvasive treatment option utilized to reduce fetal symptoms by decreasing the growth of the mass. While the degree of improvement from maternal steroids is variable, particularly for non-CCAM congenital lung lesions, it has gradually become the first-line therapy for rapidly growing high-risk malformations considering the absence of major maternal side effects. Not all patients will respond to a steroid treatment;[49,50] however, a 2010 study by Curran and colleagues reported a negative CVR growth rate in 82% of the fetuses with CCAM after a single dose of betamethasone.[49] Yet, given the high rate of spontaneous regression without any intervention, the true efficacy of maternal steroids remains debatable.[51] Furthermore, some patients require multiple courses of steroids to respond. Whether the medication eventually takes effect, or the fetus gradually grows to a gestational age where relative decrease in mass size is part of the natural history, remains a topic of debate.

Minimally Invasive Fetal Intervention

For fetuses with macrocystic lesions (> 2 cm cysts), thoracocentesis and/or thoracoamniotic shunting is a technique that rapidly reduces the mass effect by draining the fluid in the large cysts. This is typically indicated for lung lesions in fetuses < 32 weeks' gestation who have a pleural effusion or a large macrocystic lesion in the setting of mediastinal shift with or without hydrops that is amenable to drainage. Multiple reports have shown this to be efficacious in fetuses with a CVR > 1.6;[52,53] drainage close to time of delivery allows for easier immediate postnatal ventilation.

An ultrasound scan is performed to define the appropriate site of entry into the maternal abdomen and this site is then infiltrated with local anesthesia to the level of the myometrium. Under continuous ultrasound guidance, a needle or cannula is inserted into the amniotic cavity, through the fetal chest and into the cyst. Thoracocentesis is a temporizing measure and fluid will gradually reaccumulate, therefore a shunt is often placed after initial fluid drainage. While the procedure can provide maternal and fetal relief, the role of thoracoamniotic (TA) shunting in fetuses without hydrops is also controversial. The risk vs. benefit profile must be carefully weighed as complications of TA shunts include bleeding, infection, shunt failure by occlusion or migration,[54,55] and premature rupture of membranes or premature delivery which could range from 0 to 16% for the procedure.[43,44,56] However, in a hydropic fetus with a large macrocyst, this procedure is gaining clinical momentum as an alternative to fetal surgery which is more invasive, as published experience has shown a fetal survival rate as high as 74% after TA shunt placement.[54] It has also been proposed that drainage can reduce the degree of pulmonary hypoplasia thereby minimizing the degree of neonatal distress at birth.

Other noteworthy fetal intervention strategies for lung masses include amnioreduction, laser therapy, or fetal sclerotherapy. Amnioreduction, or aspiration of excess amniotic fluid, reduces severe polyhydramnios, thereby lessening the risk of preterm labor[57] and alleviating maternal discomfort. This can be performed as a single procedure or multiple times throughout gestation. For sequestrations, interruption of the blood supply to the lung mass has been described using interstitial laser therapy or ultrasound-guided fetal sclerotherapy of either etanolamine or aethoxysclerol as described by Cavoretto et al.[40] There are very few cases of the use of laser ablation or sclerotherapy in the literature and outcomes are variable. Ablative techniques are associated with initial swelling prior to undergoing atrophy. The swelling may be a challenge in a fetus who already has significant mass effect from the lesion.

Anesthetic Considerations

Anesthesia for minimally invasive procedures such as thoracoamniotic shunt placement, amnioreduction, cyst aspiration, or laser ablation, entails maternal intravenous sedation in conjunction with local anesthetic infiltration. Preoperative medications commonly include intravenous antacids such as ranitidine, and oral citric acid and sodium citrate (Bicitra®) for acid aspiration prophylaxis; a necessity as any of these procedures could trigger labor which may not be adequately suppressed in a patient with a viable fetus. Following placement of standard American Society of Anesthesiologists (ASA) monitors (noninvasive blood pressure, electrocardiogram, pulse oximetry, and temperature), sedation is achieved with bolus administration of medications such as midazolam, opioids (fentanyl), and propofol. Most scenarios typically involve bolus administration of these medications in addition to an ongoing infusion of either remifentanil or dexmedetomidine. The latter medication is especially helpful in patients who have a high body mass index as it preserves spontaneous ventilation while providing patient sedation; an attractive feature in patients with diagnosed sleep apnea or those prone to airway obstruction while sleeping.[58] Often times, only light sedation of the patient is required. This allows the patient to respond to instructions such as a request to minimize deep breaths or holding breaths for brief periods of time, actions which might be necessary to aid surgeons in performing precise maneuvers.

Open Fetal Surgery

Direct fetal observation and surgical intervention dates back as far as the nineteenth century in animal models, but it was not until the 1960s and 1970s that surgeons ventured into human fetal surgery for treatment of immune hydrops fetalis. In the decades since, there have been several celebrated milestones in fetal surgery, including the first documented fetal resection of a CCAM at the University of California San Francisco in 1984 by Dr. Harrison and colleagues.[59–61] With advances in non- and minimally invasive treatment, open fetal surgery for lung masses is becoming less common and should be reserved as a last resort to prevent impending fetal demise after poor, or no response to conservative treatment measures. In recent times, open fetal surgery for lung masses has been limited to the hydropic fetus, less than 28 weeks' gestation, with a microcystic or solid lung mass, with CVR typically > 2.0, and evidence of impending heart failure on echocardiogram.[62]

All potential candidates for fetal surgery should be verified to have a normal karyotype and absence of any confounding anatomic abnormalities. Extensive counseling is undertaken during which the benefits of fetal intervention are weighed against the risks to both the fetus and the mother.

Anesthetic Considerations for In-Utero Fetal Thoracotomy

The pregnant woman is prepared for general anesthesia. Preoperative routine laboratory studies are evaluated. Blood products (packed red blood cells (PRBCs)) are cross-matched for the mother and O-negative irradiated PRBCs are made available for the fetus, An overnight fast is supplemented with clear liquids up to two hours before the planned procedure. Indomethacin is administered for tocolysis prior to induction of anesthesia. Intravenous and oral antacids are also administered. Prior to induction of anesthesia, fetal ultrasound evaluation is performed to confirm fetal well-being, placental location, planned uterine access, and estimated fetal weight (EFW). The EFW is used to calculate the dosage of fetal medications. Single-dose syringes (approximately three syringes each) of high- and low-dose epinephrine (10 mcg/kg and 1 mg/kg, respectively), calcium gluconate (15–30 mg/kg), sodium bicarbonate(0.5–1 mEq/kg), and a mixture of vecuronium (0.2–0.4 mg/kg), fentanyl (5–10 mcg/kg), and atropine (20 mcg/kg) are prepared and transferred to the scrub technician in a sterile fashion prior to the start of the case. Approximately three 10cc syringes of albumin should also be handed to the scrub technician in sterile fashion as administration of albumin to the fetus prior to exteriorization of the lung mass may be necessary during surgery. This serves to counteract the decrease in systemic vascular resistance that occurs once the lung mass is exteriorized. A baseline fetal echocardiogram is obtained prior to the induction of anesthesia. An epidural catheter is placed for post-operative pain management; this may be placed prior to patient arrival in the operating room or when the patient is in the operating room. In the operating room, the patient is positioned on the operating table with left lateral uterine displacement to prevent aortocaval compression, although during surgery, the position may be supine or lithotomy based on the surgeon's preference. Standard ASA monitors are placed plus an arterial line for close hemodynamic monitoring. To limit the duration of fetal exposure to anesthetic agents, the pregnant woman may be positioned, prepped, and draped prior to rapid sequence induction of anesthesia and endotracheal intubation. Choice of anesthetic gases for maintenance of anesthesia include sevoflurane and desflurane, with the latter having a greater effect on cardiac depression. Some centers have opted for total intravenous anesthesia (with remifentanil and propofol) to decrease the duration of anesthetic gas exposure. In this scenario, the depth of anesthesia is initially maintained with intravenous anesthetic agents to enable laparotomy and uterine exposure. Prior to uterine incision, the inhalational anesthetics are increased to decrease uterine tone and facilitate uteroplacental blood flow.[63] The use of magnesium sulfate as a tocolytic is an integral part of open fetal surgery. Historically, this was initiated towards the end of surgery to provide uterine relaxation in the postoperative phase; however, more recently, this infusion is being initiated after induction to help achieve uterine relaxation and decrease the high dose of inhalational anesthetics.[64] Some of the maternal inhalational agents pass across the placenta to anesthetize the fetus. This is supplemented by additional anesthesia and analgesia in the form of an intramuscular injection of a muscle relaxant, opioid for analgesia, and an anticholinergic (i.e. combination of vecuronium, fentanyl, and atropine, respectively). The anticholinergic, atropine helps to limit bradycardia resulting from fetal handling. Intravenous fluids are administered judiciously to prevent pulmonary edema that commonly occurs following open fetal surgery. This also depends on the duration of surgery with fluid administration ranging from 500mL to 2 L.[65]

Once the fetus is exposed, a pulse oximeter is placed on an extremity to monitor fetal heart rate and oxygen saturation. The available extremity for pulse oximeter monitoring depends on the fetal position for surgery, which is in turn dependent on the laterality of the lesion. Continuous fetal echocardiography by the fetal cardiologist on the operating field is invaluable in determining the cardiac function and fluid status of the fetus. It is also immensely helpful in tailoring the resuscitation as required while the chest is decompressed of the large mass.

Fetal Thoracotomy

The uterus is exposed via a Pfannenstiel incision and the adequacy of uterine relaxation is confirmed by the surgeon's manual assessment. Using ultrasound guidance, the fetus is maneuvered into adequate position for surgery, and the site of the hysterotomy identified to be devoid of placenta tissue at least 5 cm from the placental edge. The hysterotomy is performed using standard technique with hemostatic staplers. The fetus is partially delivered once exposed, the side of the lesion is verified by the operating team, and the ipsilateral arm brought out of the uterus. A pulse oximeter is placed, and a peripheral intravenous cannula is inserted into the ipsilateral hand. The remainder of the fetal head and torso remains in the intrauterine cavity. During partial exposure of the fetus, uterine volume is maintained by infusion of warm lactated Ringer's solution which also serves to keep the fetus warm and avoid umbilical cord compression. Responsibility for regulation of this warm lactated Ringer's solution should be assigned to a surgical team member as well as an operating room staff member who will follow the request of the surgery team member to regulate the fluid release from a Level 1® or Belmont® rapid infuser off the surgical field.[65]

With the fetal chest exposed, a fetal surgery timeout is performed to confirm correct surgical site, and a posterolateral incision is made centered over the fifth intercostal space. A generous incision is usually needed to eviscerate the large mass. Care is taken to deliver the mass without disruption and bleeding. Because of the anticipated drop in systemic vascular resistance once the mediastinal compression is relieved, the fetus is volume loaded with 5% albumin prior to exteriorizing the mass. We have also learnt that a gradual decompression of the chest with continuous echocardiographic monitoring allows the fetal heart to better tolerate the volume shifts. Once the mass is completely exteriorized, the extent of involvement of the other lobes of the lung is noted. Typically, the growth of the mass has resulted in the stretching of the hilum which allows the pedicle of the affected lobe to be easily stapled off, en-bloc, with a vascular stapler. Occasionally, additional dissection of the hilum is needed to preserve the bronchial and vascular anatomy to the adjacent lobes. Time is of the essence in these operations and unwarranted dissection should be avoided. With the mass removed, the heart and mediastinum can be directly observed. Transient cardiac resuscitation may be required during excision of the lung mass and if needed, direct cardiac massage can be performed or fluid, medications, and/or blood products administered directly into the existing peripheral venous catheter. Alternatively resuscitation fluids may be administered into the vena cava or atrium using a 23-gauge butterfly needle. Once resection has been completed, hemostasis is verified, and adequate cardiac function is confirmed. The thoracotomy incision is then closed in layers. No chest drain is placed. Any external items placed for monitoring or surgery (pulse oximeter and intravenous catheter) are removed and the exteriorized portion of the fetus is returned to the uterus. The amniotic fluid displaced by surgery is replaced with warm lactated Ringer's solution infused with antibiotics (cephazolin).[66] The uterus is then closed in a watertight fashion and the abdominal incision closed in layers. Following surgery, the mother is closely monitored and treated to maintain uterine quiescence to optimize for term delivery.[60,62]

Possible maternal complications include preterm labor, placental abruption, and an increased risk of intraoperative hemorrhage through the induced deep uterine relaxation.[67,68]

Despite the multilayer repair, the uterine scar remains at risk for rupture at delivery which persists with subsequent pregnancies. Therefore, women who have undergone open fetal surgery, should be delivered by cesarean section for the index pregnancy and for all subsequent pregnancies.[68]

If left untreated, true fetal hydrops, with cardiac compromise, will result in 100% mortality for patients with CCAMs. Survival is increased in hydropic fetuses that have undergone surgery. Adzick reported a 54% survival in 24 hydropic CCAM patients that underwent resection, including one pneumonectomy.[21] In all survivors, mediastinal shift and hydrops fetalis resolved in the setting of compensatory lung growth of the normal tissue. In the absence of cardiac compromise, even with a large chest mass, ascites, and skin edema, open fetal surgery may be deferred, and the fetus monitored closely. Progressive somatic growth of the fetus and treatment with steroids may help reduce the relative size and compressive effects of the mass. Nevertheless, those fetuses may still be left with a large thoracic mass that may impact ventilation at the time of delivery. Such fetuses should be evaluated for the need for resection of the lesion at the time of delivery via an EXIT-to-Resection procedure, as described below.

The Ex-Utero Intrapartum Treatment (EXIT)-To-Resection Procedure

The ex-utero intrapartum therapy (EXIT) procedure was originally designed for reversal of tracheal occlusion in fetuses with congenital diaphragmatic hernia (CDH) who underwent in-utero tracheal occlusion. The EXIT procedure is the process of partial delivery of the fetus with the maintenance of placental support for stabilization while transitioning from fetal to neonatal life.[69] The procedure has since evolved to be used for conditions where advanced fetal resuscitation is required, and a gradual transition needed from fetal to neonatal life. Such conditions include obstructing fetal neck masses to ensure an airway can be safely secured, and large congenital lung masses with mediastinal compression particularly when there is a concern for respiratory compromise. When this procedure includes resection of a mass during the period of transition from fetal to neonatal life, it is referred to as EXIT-to-resection.

Indications for an EXIT-to-resection for lung masses are persistent mediastinal shift and elevated CVR (> 2.0) after 32 weeks' gestation. The concern with the lung masses is that the lesion may increase in size with ventilation as it air-traps and will worsen the mass effect on the mediastinum. A decompressive thoracotomy at the time of the EXIT allows the lesion to be exteriorized from the confined thoracic cage. As with open fetal surgery, candidates must have a normal fetal karyotype, no additional congenital anomalies, or maternal medical concerns.[70] Similar to fetal surgery, during the EXIT procedure, high concentrations of inhalational anesthetics and additional tocolytics are used to maintain uterine relaxation and placental perfusion. Once complete uterine relaxation is obtained, a hysterotomy is performed under ultrasound guidance.

Location of the hysterotomy is determined by placental location. A low-segment uterine incision is preferred for the EXIT procedure. If there is a low-lying placenta, the benefit of the EXIT procedure must be weighed against the risk of a hysterotomy in the active uterine segment. The head, shoulders, and arms of the fetus are delivered followed by establishment of the airway and securing with an endotracheal tube. Depending on a predetermined plan, the infant will undergo one of two established clinical pathways: (i) a thoracotomy with immediate resection of the mass or (ii) mere exteriorization of the abnormal lung mass prior to separation of the fetus from placental support followed by initiation of ventilation and stabilization of the neonate. In cases of large lung masses, even after thoracotomy and resection of the mass, the residual compressed lung may be ill-prepared to immediately sustain the infant's ventilation. In such settings, extracorporeal membrane oxygenation (ECMO) may be utilized as a bridge for several days until the lung is well recruited and expanded. Fortunately, this is a rare situation.

The EXIT procedure survival rates are high, ranging from 80% to 95% as reported in the literature.[67,69-71] The EXIT-to-Resection procedure provides a smooth hemodynamic transition from placental support to ventilator support by removing the compressive effect of the large mass prior to initiating ventilation. Although operative times for the EXIT procedure are longer compared to traditional cesarean section, hospital length of stay for the mother and the infant have not been significantly different.

Postnatal Treatment

Symptoms in the fetal period are rare and asymptomatic fetal lung masses have favorable outcomes with survival rates > 90%. Babies with small lesions can be routinely observed in a mother-baby unit and are typically discharged home with the mother. With adequate prenatal imaging and follow-up, most babies with lung masses do not need any imaging in the newborn period as long as they remain asymptomatic. Some centers would obtain a chest radiograph but there is no indication for cross-sectional imaging in an asymptomatic neonate. However, all infants, including those whose lesions may have "disappeared" prenatally, should undergo cross-sectional imaging after at least six weeks of age. This allows time for retained fluid within the lungs to be absorbed. A computed tomography (CT) scan of the chest with intravenous contrast is best to identify the vascular anatomy of the lesions. The timeline for imaging and treatment is accelerated for symptomatic patients. The onset of symptoms in the neonatal period warrants resection. For babies that remain asymptomatic, there is still considerable debate about observation or preemptive surgical resection. For those who favor surgical resection, the optimal timing of the surgery is unclear, but many surgeons favor surgery earlier in childhood to take advantage of the compensatory lung growth. Most of these procedures are now being performed via thoracoscopy and are well tolerated. Recent studies suggest that, in experienced hands, lobectomies for lung masses performed in infants prior to three months of age are just as safe as later in infancy,[72] but with the theoretical advantage of avoiding any preoperative infection of the lesions. The outcomes for elective resection of asymptomatic lung lesions are very favorable. Survival is close to 100% in experienced hands.[73] To date, there have been no long-term studies to determine the natural history of the lesion if not removed, but many surmise that given the minimal risk of infection and < 1% risk of malignancy, it is reasonable to closely monitor these children throughout childhood.[74,75] Further studies are needed to validate this approach and the decision to resect or observe the asymptomatic lung lesion remains surgeon dependent.

References

1. Fowler DJ, Gould SJ. The pathology of congenital lung lesions. *Semin Pediatr Surg.* 2015;24(4):176–182.

2. Kim YT, Kim JS, Park JD, et al. Treatment of congenital cystic adenomatoid malformation–does resection in the early postnatal period increase surgical risk? *Eur J Cardiothorac Surg.* 2005;27(4):658–661.

3. Cass DL, Olutoye OO, Cassady CI, et al. Prenatal diagnosis and outcome of fetal lung masses. *J Pediatr Surg.* 2011;**46**(2):292–298.

4. Correia-Pinto J, Gonzaga S, Huang Y, Rottier R. Congenital lung lesions–underlying molecular mechanisms. *Semin Pediatr Surg.* 2010;**19**(3):171–179.

5. Mullassery D, Smith NP. Lung development. *Semin Pediatr Surg.* 2015;**24**(4):152–155.

6. Herriges M, Morrisey EE. Lung development: orchestrating the generation and regeneration of a complex organ. *Development.* 2014;**141**(3):502–513.

7. Chen F, Desai TJ, Qian J, et al. Inhibition of Tgf beta signaling by endogenous retinoic acid is essential for primary lung bud induction. *Development.* 2007;**134**(16):2969–2979.

8. Mendelsohn C, Mark M, Dolle P, et al. Retinoic acid receptor beta 2 (RAR beta 2) null mutant mice appear normal. *Dev Biol.* 1994;**166**(1):246–258.

9. Miura T. Modeling lung branching morphogenesis. *Curr Top Dev Biol.* 2008;**81**:291–310.

10. Metzger RJ, Klein OD, Martin GR, Krasnow MA. The branching programme of mouse lung development. *Nature.* 2008;**453**(7196):745–750.

11. Boucherat O, Jeannotte L, Hadchouel A, et al. Pathomechanisms of congenital cystic lung diseases: focus on congenital cystic adenomatoid malformation and pleuropulmonary blastoma. *Paediatr Respir Rev.* 2016;**19**:62–68.

12. Burri PH. Structural aspects of postnatal lung development – alveolar formation and growth. *Biol Neonate.* 2006;**89**(4):313–322.

13. Kitaoka H, Burri PH, Weibel ER. Development of the human fetal airway tree: analysis of the numerical density of airway endtips. *Anat Rec.* 1996;**244**(2):207–213.

14. Wilkinson GA, Schittny JC, Reinhardt DP, Klein R. Role for ephrinB2 in postnatal lung alveolar development and elastic matrix integrity. *Dev Dyn.* 2008;**237**(8):2220–2234.

15. Morotti RA, Cangiarella J, Gutierrez MC, et al. Congenital cystic adenomatoid malformation of the lung (CCAM): evaluation of the cellular components. *Hum Pathol.* 1999;**30**(6):618–625.

16. Cass DL, Quinn TM, Yang EY, et al. Increased cell proliferation and decreased apoptosis characterize congenital cystic adenomatoid malformation of the lung. *J Pediatr Surg.* 1998;**33**(7):1043–6; discussion 7.

17. Swarr DT, Peranteau WH, Pogoriler J, et al. Novel molecular and phenotypic insights into congenital lung malformations. *Am J Respir Crit Care Med.* 2018;**197**(10):1328–1339.

18. Harfe BD, Scherz PJ, Nissim S, et al. Evidence for an expansion-based temporal Shh gradient in specifying vertebrate digit identities. *Cell.* 2004;**118**(4):517–528.

19. Harris KS, Zhang Z, McManus MT, et al. Dicer function is essential for lung epithelium morphogenesis. *Proc Natl Acad Sci USA.* 2006;**103**(7):2208–2213.

20. Shanmugam G, MacArthur K, Pollock JC. Congenital lung malformations–antenatal and postnatal evaluation and management. *Eur J Cardiothorac Surg.* 2005;**27**(1):45–52.

21. Adzick NS. Management of fetal lung lesions. *Clin Perinatol.* 2009;**36**(2):363–76, x.

22. Stocker JT, Madewell JE, Drake RM. Congenital cystic adenomatoid malformation of the lung. Classification and morphologic spectrum. *Hum Pathol.* 1977;**8**(2):155–171.

23. Stocker JT. Congenital and developmental diseases. In: Dail DH Hammar SP, eds. *Pulmonary Pathology.* Springer; 2008, pp. 154–80.

24. Adzick NS, Harrison MR. Management of the fetus with a cystic adenomatoid malformation. *World J Surg.* 1993;**17**(3):342–349.

25. Azizkhan RG, Crombleholme TM. Congenital cystic lung disease: contemporary antenatal and postnatal

management. *Pediatr Surg Int.* 2008;**24**
(6):643–657.

26. Riley JS, Urwin JW, Oliver ER, et al.
Prenatal growth characteristics and pre/
postnatal management of
bronchopulmonary sequestrations. *J
Pediatr Surg.* 2018;**53**(2):265–269.

27. Mubang R, Brady JJ, Mao M, et al.
Intradiaphragmatic bronchogenic cysts:
case report and systematic review. *J
Cardiothorac Surg.* 2016;**11**(1):79.

28. Ramsay BH, Byron FX. Mucocele,
congenital bronchiectasis, and
bronchiogenic cyst. *J Thorac Surg.* 1953;**26**
(1):21–30.

29. Kinsella D, Sissons G, Williams MP. The
radiological imaging of bronchial atresia.
Br J Radiol. 1992;**65**(776):681–685.

30. Wang Y, Dai W, Sun Y, et al. Congenital
bronchial atresia: diagnosis and treatment.
Int J Med Sci. 2012;**9**(3):207–212.

31. Zamora IJ, Sheikh F, Olutoye OO, et al.
Mainstem bronchial atresia: a lethal
anomaly amenable to fetal surgical
treatment. *J Pediatr Surg.* 2014;**49**
(5):706–711.

32. Mourya M, Meena DS. Congenital lobar
emphysema: an approach of anesthetic
management. *J Clin Diagn Res.* 2016;**10**(8):
UD01–3.

33. Pariente G, Aviram M, Landau D,
Hershkovitz R. Prenatal diagnosis of
congenital lobar emphysema: case report
and review of the literature. *J Ultrasound
Med.* 2009;**28**(8):1081–1084.

34. Aslan H, Ekiz A, Acar DK, et al. Prenatal
diagnosis of congenital high airway
obstruction syndrome (CHAOS). Five case
report. *Med Ultrason.* 2015;**17**(1):115–118.

35. Vidaeff AC, Szmuk P, Mastrobattista JM, et
al. More or less CHAOS: case report and
literature review suggesting the existence of
a distinct subtype of congenital high airway
obstruction syndrome. *Ultrasound Obstet
Gynecol.* 2007;**30**(1):114–117.

36. Chowdhury MM, Chakraborty S. Imaging
of congenital lung malformations. *Semin
Pediatr Surg.* 2015;**24**(4):168–175.

37. Kane SC, Da Silva Costa F, Crameri JA, et
al. Antenatal assessment and postnatal
outcome of fetal echogenic lung lesions: a
decade's experience at a tertiary referral
hospital. *J Matern Fetal Neonatal Med.*
2019;**32**(5):703–709.

38. MacGillivray TE, Harrison MR, Goldstein
RB, Adzick NS. Disappearing fetal lung
lesions. *J Pediatr Surg.* 1993;**28**(10):1321–
1324; discussion 4–5.

39. Meagher SE, Fisk NM, Harvey JG, et al.
Disappearing lung echogenicity in fetal
bronchopulmonary malformations: a
reassuring sign? *Prenat Diagn.* 1993;**13**
(6):495–501.

40. Cavoretto P, Molina F, Poggi S, et al.
Prenatal diagnosis and outcome of
echogenic fetal lung lesions. *Ultrasound
Obstet Gynecol.* 2008;**32**(6):769–783.

41. Hadchouel A, Benachi A, Delacourt C.
Outcome of prenatally diagnosed
bronchial atresia. *Ultrasound Obstet
Gynecol.* 2011;**38**(1):119; author reply -20.

42. Kunisaki SM, Ehrenberg-Buchner S,
Dillman JR, et al. Vanishing fetal lung
malformations: Prenatal sonographic
characteristics and postnatal outcomes. *J
Pediatr Surg.* 2015;**50**(6):978–982.

43. Adzick NS, Harrison MR, Crombleholme
TM, et al. Fetal lung lesions: management
and outcome. *Am J Obstet Gynecol.*
1998;**179**(4):884–889.

44. Crombleholme TM, Coleman B, Hedrick
H, et al. Cystic adenomatoid malformation
volume ratio predicts outcome in
prenatally diagnosed cystic adenomatoid
malformation of the lung. *J Pediatr Surg.*
2002;**37**(3):331–338.

45. Ehrenberg-Buchner S, Stapf AM, Berman
DR, et al. Fetal lung lesions: can we start to
breathe easier? *Am J Obstet Gynecol.*
2013;**208**(2):151 e1-7.

46. Feghali M, Jean KM, Emery SP. Ultrasound
assessment of congenital fetal lung masses
and neonatal respiratory outcomes. *Prenat
Diagn.* 2015;**35**(12):1208–1212.

47. Mahle WT, Rychik J, Tian ZY, et al.
Echocardiographic evaluation of the fetus
with congenital cystic adenomatoid

malformation. *Ultrasound Obstet Gynecol.* 2000;**16**(7):620–624.

48. Peranteau WH, Boelig MM, Khalek N, et al. Effect of single and multiple courses of maternal betamethasone on prenatal congenital lung lesion growth and fetal survival. *J Pediatr Surg.* 2016;**51**(1):28–32.

49. Curran PF, Jelin EB, Rand L, et al. Prenatal steroids for microcystic congenital cystic adenomatoid malformations. *J Pediatr Surg.* 2010;**45**(1):145–150.

50. Morris LM, Lim FY, Livingston JC, et al. High-risk fetal congenital pulmonary airway malformations have a variable response to steroids. *J Pediatr Surg.* 2009;**44**(1):60–65.

51. Miller JA, Corteville JE, Langer JC. Congenital cystic adenomatoid malformation in the fetus: natural history and predictors of outcome. *J Pediatr Surg.* 1996;**31**(6):805–808.

52. Litwinska M, Litwinska E, Janiak K, et al. Thoracoamniotic shunts in macrocystic lung lesions: case series and review of the literature. *Fetal Diagn Ther.* 2017;**41**(3):179–183.

53. Schrey S, Kelly EN, Langer JC, et al. Fetal thoracoamniotic shunting for large macrocystic congenital cystic adenomatoid malformations of the lung. *Ultrasound Obstet Gynecol.* 2012;**39**(5):515–520.

54. Wilson RD, Johnson MP. Prenatal ultrasound guided percutaneous shunts for obstructive uropathy and thoracic disease. *Semin Pediatr Surg.* 2003;**12**(3):182–189.

55. Wittman BK, Martin KA, Wilson RD, Peacock D. Complications of long-term drainage of fetal pleural effusion: case report and review of the literature. *Am J Perinatol.* 1997;**14**(8):443–447.

56. Davenport M, Warne SA, Cacciaguerra S, et al. Current outcome of antenally diagnosed cystic lung disease. *J Pediatr Surg.* 2004;**39**(4):549–556.

57. Parikh DH, Rasiah SV. Congenital lung lesions: Postnatal management and outcome. *Semin Pediatr Surg.* 2015;**24**(4):160–167.

58. Shin H, Kim E, Hwang J, et al. Comparison of upper airway patency in patients with mild obstructive sleep apnea during dexmedetomidine or propofol sedation: a prospective, randomized, controlled trial. *BMC Anesthesiol.* 2018;**18**:120.

59. Harrison MR, Adzick NS, Jennings RW, et al. Antenatal intervention for congenital cystic adenomatoid malformation. *Lancet.* 1990;**336**(8721):965–967.

60. Adzick NS, Harrison MR, Flake AW, et al. Fetal surgery for cystic adenomatoid malformation of the lung. *J Pediatr Surg.* 1993;**28**(6):806–812.

61. Jancelewicz T, Harrison MR. A history of fetal surgery. *Clin Perinatol.* 2009;**36**(2):227–236, vii.

62. Cass DL, Olutoye OO, Ayres NA, et al. Defining hydrops and indications for open fetal surgery for fetuses with lung masses and vascular tumors. *J Pediatr Surg.* 2012;**47**(1):40–45.

63. Boat A, Mahmoud M, Michelfelder EC, et al. Supplementing desflurane with intravenous anesthesia reduces fetal cardiac dysfunction during open fetal surgery. *Paediatr Anaesth.* 2010;**20**(8):748–756.

64. Donepudi R, Huynh M, Moise KJ Jr., et al. Early administration of magnesium sulfate during open fetal myelomeningocele repair reduces the dose of inhalational anesthesia. *Fetal Diagn Ther.* 2019;**45**(3):192–196. doi: 10.1159/000487883.

65. Ferschl M, Ball R, Lee H, Rollins MD. Anesthesia for in utero repair of myelomeningocele. *Anesthesiology.* 2013;**118**(5):1211–1223. doi: 10.1097/ALN.0b013e31828ea597.

66. Adzick NS. Open fetal surgery for life-threatening fetal anomalies. *Semin Fetal Neonatal Med.* 2010;**15**(1):1–8.

67. Abraham RJ, Sau A, Maxwell D. A review of the EXIT (Ex utero Intrapartum Treatment) procedure. *J Obstet Gynaecol.* 2010;**30**(1):1–5.

68. Al-Refai A, Ryan G, Van Mieghem T. Maternal risks of fetal therapy. *Curr Opin Obstet Gynecol.* 2017;**29**(2):80–84.

69. Cass DL, Olutoye OO, Cassady CI, et al. EXIT-to-resection for fetuses with large

lung masses and persistent mediastinal compression near birth. *J Pediatr Surg.* 2013;**48**(1):138–144.

70. Hedrick HL, Flake AW, Crombleholme TM, et al. The ex utero intrapartum therapy procedure for high-risk fetal lung lesions. *J Pediatr Surg.* 2005;**40**(6):1038–1043; discussion 44.

71. Moldenhauer JS. Ex utero intrapartum therapy. *Semin Pediatr Surg.* 2013;**22**(1):44–49.

72. Style CC, Cass DL, Verla MA, et al. Early vs late resection of asymptomatic congenital lung malformations. *J Pediatr Surg.* 2019;**54**(1):70–74.

73. Tsai AY, Liechty KW, Hedrick HL, et al. Outcomes after postnatal resection of prenatally diagnosed asymptomatic cystic lung lesions. *J Pediatr Surg.* 2008;**43**(3):513–517.

74. Colon N, Schlegel C, Pietsch J, et al. Congenital lung anomalies: can we postpone resection? *J Pediatr Surg.* 2012;**47**(1):87–92.

75. Stanton M. The argument for a non-operative approach to asymptomatic lung lesions. *Semin Pediatr Surg.* 2015;**24**(4):183–186.

Chapter 12

Sacrococcygeal Teratoma

Kha Tran and Holly Hedrick

Introduction

Sacrococcygeal teratoma (SCT) is a common tumor of the newborn, with an incidence of approximately 1 in 40,000 births. The tumor is thought to arise from the totipotent stem cells in Hensen's node of the primitive streak in the developing gastrula.[1] These cells may have escaped normal inductive influence to differentiate into cell types that do not belong near the coccyx.[1-3] Small tumors may be managed in the postnatal period, but larger, prenatal tumors which are symptomatic are associated with increased maternal and fetal morbidity. These symptoms are secondary to mass effect, high output heart failure, or tumor rupture and hemorrhage. The management of a prenatally diagnosed large SCT is complex and often involves close prenatal assessment and multidisciplinary planning.

The SCT is classified anatomically before surgery and histologically after resection. Anatomical description has been based on the American Academy of Pediatrics Surgical Section (AAPSS) classification proposed by Altman et al. in 1974.[4] The tumors are described based on the amount of tumor that is either external to the body or internal (presacral/intrapelvic), and four types have been proposed. Type I tumor is all external, type II is primarily external with an internal component, type III is primarily internal with some small external component, and type IV is completely internal. This classification has implications on the time of diagnosis, relative ease of surgical resection, and potential for malignancy. Type I tumors tend to be diagnosed earlier, are more easily resected, and are less likely to be malignant, whereas type IV tumors lie on the other end of this spectrum. Histopathologic description will of course vary, as these cells are totipotent, but three broad groups have clinical implications.[5-8] The first group has tumor elements that are mature, with little or no mitotic activity, and good prognosis with a very little chance of malignant recurrence. In the second group with immature, embryonal cells present, there is a possibility of malignant recurrence after resection and metastatic potential. A third group demonstrates vitelline differentiation with the presence of yolk sac elements. This third group often experiences recurrences as a yolk sac carcinoma after resection, and prognosis is poor.[9]

Before the era of prenatal diagnosis, the management algorithms were more straightforward and included postnatal resection of the tumor when the child was deemed fit for surgery. Prenatal ultrasound has allowed for a much earlier detection of fetuses with SCT, which has dramatically expanded therapeutic options. Asymptomatic fetuses may be diagnosed by screening prenatal ultrasound, but the SCT may also cause symptoms of polyhydramnios in the mother which will prompt a focused diagnostic prenatal ultrasound. Screening maternal blood tests with elevations of alpha-fetoprotein will also prompt further investigation that may reveal SCT. Following a referral to a fetal treatment center, more detailed evaluation will include high level obstetric ultrasound, fetal echocardiography, magnetic resonance imaging (MRI), and other evaluations as needed. A team of surgeons, perinatologists, obstetricians, neonatologists, cardiologists, anesthesiologists, social workers, genetic counselors, and specialized nurses in all the disciplines should be involved in the care. The detailed diagnostic testing gives the team a sense of the anatomic classification of the tumor, as well as the degree of physiologic compromise of the fetus. Close surveillance is mandatory as the tumor size can change rapidly. Management options are tailored to the specific situation of the mother, fetus, and the family, taking into account such factors as psychosocial support, maternal health, degree of fetal compromise, anatomy, fetal lung maturity, speed of tumor growth, and clinical expertise of the treatment center.

Fetal and Maternal Complications

The SCT can have ill effects on both the fetus and the mother. The fetal problems can arise from simple mass effect of the tumor or from an undue metabolic burden caused by a "vascular steal" phenomenon that often results in high output heart failure.[10] The mother can suffer from polyhydramnios and maternal mirror syndrome, and is also at risk for preterm delivery.

The mass effects of the tumor are not immediately threatening to the fetus. Large tumors with internal components may compress and distort the genitourinary and gastrointestinal tracts.[11] Urinary obstruction may result in subsequent renal disease. Undiagnosed SCTs can cause problems during vaginal delivery, ranging from mild dystocia to complete arrest of descent.[12–14] A vaginal delivery may be converted emergently into a cesarean delivery and/or, the tumor may rupture and hemorrhage during delivery of the baby. Immediate and sometimes heroic efforts must be organized impromptu to deliver and resuscitate the child with an undiagnosed SCT. These efforts may include unplanned incisional drainage, hysterotomy with tumor drainage followed by vaginal delivery, and blind dissection of the tumor.

For a fetus with a prenatally diagnosed SCT, the increased cardiovascular burden of the tumor is more of a problem. This burden will vary with the size, rate of growth, and proportion of solid to cystic components of the tumor. Large, rapidly growing, and primarily solid tumors are the most metabolically demanding.[15] Increasing demand of the tumor places the fetus at risk for high output heart failure. The vascular architecture of some tumors may result in high flow arteriovenous fistulas and subsequent shunting of blood.[10,16] Hemorrhage into the tumor during fetal development will result in fetal anemia. All of these conditions place the fetus at risk for high output heart failure. Hydrops fetalis and fetal demise will often follow after a period of high output heart failure.

Fetal hydrops is defined as fluid collections or edema in at least two fetal compartments, which can include fetal skin, pleura, pericardium, or abdomen. Hydrops is associated with maternal polyhydramnios, which may result in premature delivery. The combination of immature lungs and heart failure complicates all aspects of care following delivery including resuscitation, surgical resection, and recovery. Maternal mirror syndrome is a rare, but potentially life-threatening condition in which fetal hydrops occurs in the presence of maternal edema.[17,18] The clinical picture may resemble preeclampsia, but the mother is usually hemodiluted, and not hemoconcentrated. The most worrisome aspect of maternal mirror syndrome is the development of pulmonary edema with potential respiratory failure. Mirror syndrome should not progress to eclampsia or HELLP syndrome (Hemolysis, Elevated Platelets, Low Platelets). Once mirror syndrome is present, the treatment for mother is delivery of the fetus.

Prenatal Assessment of the Fetus

Ultrasound, echocardiography, and MRI are the primary prenatal assessment tools used in diagnosis and formulation of management plans for fetal SCT.

Ultrasound

The initial diagnosis of SCT can be made during screening prenatal ultrasound of asymptomatic mothers or in mothers undergoing evaluation of polyhydramnios. If a sonographer discovers a caudal or intra-abdominal mass, SCT is suspected. However, other diagnoses must be excluded, such as myelomeningocele, meconium pseudocyst, chordoma, lipoma, and obstructive uropathy. If possible, a more detailed examination will further delineate intra-abdominal or intrapelvic extension. The base of the external component of the tumor may be characterized as pedunculated or broad-based. The characteristics of the tumor base will have implications for in-utero surgical intervention if this is the mode of therapy planned. Involvement of the fetal spine may be assessed, as well as the presence or absence of movement in the lower extremities. Compression of the bowel and urinary tract can also be assessed. The fetus should be examined for signs of hydrops, and the size of the placenta should be noted. A placenta thicker than 4 cm is considered to be larger than normal. While placentomegaly may be secondary to other causes, its presence in addition to signs of hydrops are dire findings. The diameter of the inferior vena cava (IVC) should be examined: Normal IVC diameter from 21 to 28 weeks' gestation ranges from 2.9 to 4.1 mm.[2] An IVC diameter > 6 mm is concerning as it may indicate a very vascular, rapidly growing tumor with high blood flow returning to the heart. Serial ultrasound exams are useful for the typical assessments of fetal well-being, such as biophysical profile, and blood flow in the umbilical vessel and middle cerebral artery. Serial ultrasounds are also needed to follow trends in SCT specific findings such as tumor size and growth, placental thickness, IVC diameter, and hydrops.[20–24] A higher ratio of tumor size to fetal weight is predictive of poor prognosis.[21,25] The frequency of ultrasound follow-up is dictated by the fetal condition. These patients must be evaluated early and frequently so intervention may occur at the appropriate time. While SCT is not characteristically associated with other syndromes or anomalies,[26] other anomalies have been noted in fetuses with SCT,[19,24] and the rest of the fetus' anatomy should be examined carefully. The presence or absence of other anomalies will inform the counseling of the family and management plans for the fetus.

Echocardiography

As high output heart failure is common in cases of large SCT, echocardiographic findings focusing on the effects of the tumor on the cardiovascular system are important. Fetal cardiac structure and function are measured. Left and right ventricular chamber measurements are recorded, along with shortening fraction. The combined cardiac output (CCO) is used to monitor the high output failure, and other scoring systems of cardiovascular compromise may also be used.[27,28] A normal CCO is about 425–550 mL/kg/min,[28] and flow in severely compromised fetuses can be in excess of 1,500 mL/kg/min.[2] A CCO > 750 mL/kg/min will often trigger intervention, such as debulking or delivery. Flow in the descending aorta can be assessed, and may be in excess of 1,000 mL/kg/min, with normal flow being 150–200 mL/kg/min. Umbilical venous flow may also be increased, with normal flow being about 110 mL/kg/min.[2] The increases in cardiac output, blood flow in the descending aorta, and umbilical vein, are all indicators of the increased cardiovascular and metabolic demand of the SCT. Serial echocardiography is the most important modality to measure trends and progression of disease.

MRI

A fetal MRI is performed on initial evaluation to closely delineate anatomic character-istics of the SCT. The MRI and ultrasound have some overlap, in that both modalities can be used to measure the size and extension of the tumor, as well as relative proportions of cystic or solid components. MRI provides more accurate assessment of the solid component of the tumor, and a larger proportion of solid mass is noted to be a predictor of adverse outcomes.[29] Additionally, MRI is able to more accurately deter-mine involvement of the spinal canal or neural tissue and intrapelvic or abdominal extension of the tumor with compression of the adjacent organs, such as the ureters and colon.[19,24,30]

Treatment Options

Once a fetus with prenatally diagnosed SCT develops high output cardiac failure, a fetal intervention or delivery is indicated. The treatment choice will depend on both tumor specific and fetal factors. Tumor specific factors, such as the type, growth rate, location, shape, and relative proportion of cystic or solid components, as well as fetal factors such as gestational age, comorbidities, presence of heart failure or hydrops, lung maturity, and additional congenital anomalies, will all impact the decision-making process. The majority of the options for fetal therapy occur in the second trimester. Options for SCT management include minimally invasive and open fetal surgery. Other options that are not specifically targeted to the fetus, but which involve the fetal care team are also discussed at the end of this section, such as planned delivery with immediate evaluation and surgery. Maternal medical and obstetric history, and expertise of the center performing the fetal therapy also contribute to the choice of therapy.

Minimally Invasive Fetal Therapy

Minimally invasive fetal therapy encompasses a wide range of options. While these options are novel and attractive in theory, their safety and outcomes require further study. The goal of minimally invasive procedures is typically to prevent and hopefully reverse the progres-sion of the high output heart failure to avoid further clinical deterioration and demise of the fetus. Treating the SCT may alleviate the fetal heart failure, prevent development of hydrops, and subsequently avert complications such as maternal mirror syndrome and premature delivery. Various therapies such as fetoscopic laser ablation of the tumor, ultrasound-guided vessel ablation, ultrasound-guided interstitial laser ablation, vascular coiling, alcohol embolization, and radiofrequency ablation (RFA) have all been described.[15,31–36] In practice, the collateral damage is difficult to control and unacceptable in some cases. Other minimally invasive therapy options are palliative in nature, such as cyst aspiration, or even amnioreduction.[19,24] In addition to the tumor and fetal factors men-tioned above, the choice of therapy is influenced by the preference and experience of the surgical team.

Minimally invasive ablation therapies can be divided into several categories, but there can be some overlap in the goals and techniques in individual cases. One category includes treatments where the goal is to destroy the actual tumor mass with energy from such devices as the radiofrequency probe or laser.[35,37] This technique has been described both for SCT and for lung lesions. Another category of ablative therapy targets the feeding vessels of the SCT, with techniques like laser, coiling, or alcohol embolization.[38–40] The terms "interstitial laser" and "laser ablation" can be confusing, and the studies should be read carefully to determine the actual technique used. Some authors use the term interstitial laser to describe direct laser ablation of the tumor,[32] whereas other authors use the term to describe placement of a laser fiber into the tumor to target a deep feeding vessel.[15] The term "laser ablation" may involve targeting of superficial vessels,[15,39] or targeting of deeper vessels.[39] Blood flow to the tumor is assessed with ultrasound after the intervention. Doppler ultrasound is also used to measure the peak systolic velocity of blood flow in the fetal middle cerebral artery, with higher velocities being indicative of anemia in nonhydropic fetuses. The rationale for targeting the vessels is to cause slow tumor regression. Some authors report a dual approach,[39] and other authors perform more palliative, symptomatic procedures, such as amnioreduction, cyst aspiration, or shunting.[19]

The literature evaluating these different techniques is sparse, given the relative rarity of the cases combined with the paucity of centers that perform the procedures. The case series are small, therefore data from other reports are consolidated to create more potentially generalizable knowledge. A series of five patients with a large SCT and evidence of heart failure were treated with minimally invasive interventions between 17 and 26 weeks' gestation.[39] One fetus at 26 weeks' gestation underwent laser ablation of a large superficial vessel of the SCT, developed fetal distress, was delivered by emergent cesarean section, underwent urgent tumor resection, and died at three days of age. A second fetus at 21 weeks underwent intrauterine transfusion and RFA of the tumor. The fetus developed bradycardia and asystole, was resuscitated, but died in-utero 24 hours later. Autopsy revealed tumor rupture as the likely cause of death. A third fetus at 26 weeks' gestation was treated with RFA. This child was delivered eight days after the procedure because of preterm labor. The tumor was debulked with a surgical stapling device at bedside at two days of age with complete resection at 10 days of age. This child had survived to three years of age at the writing of the study, which was published in 2014. The fourth case underwent coiling of a feeding vessel and interstitial laser ablation of a vessel at 17 weeks. Intrauterine fetal demise occurred one day after the procedure. The fifth patient in this series underwent attempted coiling and sequential interstitial laser ablation of two feeding vessels at 26 weeks' gestation in conjunction with intrauterine transfusion. This fetus was delivered at 28 weeks' gestation following rupture of membranes and subsequent labor. Emergency debulking occurred on the first day of life, and complete resection was performed at four months of age. This child had survived to nine months of age at the time of writing of the study. Neurodevelopmental data on the outcomes of the surviving premature infants are not available.

A more recent observational study describes minimally invasive intervention for five of 13 fetuses with large SCT and either hydrops or signs of heart failure.[32] The treatment plans offered to the families included termination, fetal intervention, delivery, or expectant management, and the treatment decisions were made after multidisciplinary team evaluation and counseling. The results of this nonrandomized study demonstrate improved survival in the cases of fetal intervention, but as this was a small, nonrandomized trial with differing approaches to fetal management, the results must be extrapolated with caution. A literature review included in this study consolidated the outcomes of 33 fetuses that underwent minimally invasive therapy. A vascular ablative approach was used in the management of 11 of these 33 cases, while the remaining 22 cases were interpreted as undergoing an interstitial tumor ablation. The survival rate of the vascular ablation group was 63.6% compared with 40.9% in the interstitial ablation group. These results should be interpreted cautiously.

Minimally invasive techniques for the management of SCT are risky, and our center does not advocate this approach. They can result in damage to adjacent tissue, and fetal demise may also occur during the course of the procedure.[32,34,39] The fetus is at risk for preterm delivery, and long-term neurodevelopmental data remain to be reported. A staged minimally invasive devascularization of the SCT may avoid abrupt changes in an already compromised fetal cardiovascular system and may also avoid widespread rapid tumor necrosis with subsequent bleeding and fetal demise. However a staged approach brings with it the risks of entering the amniotic space multiple times, that is membrane separation, rupture of membranes, infection, preterm labor, and prematurity. Much work remains to be done to adequately describe the safety and outcomes and also to define the optimal patients, techniques, and approaches to minimally invasive treatment of SCT.

Open Fetal Surgery

Mid-gestation open fetal surgery (OFS) for resection of SCT has been described.[24,25,41–44] This approach includes the standard techniques of OFS and a maternal laparotomy and hysterotomy. Open fetal surgery is offered only when there is increased CCO and early or impending hydrops. Once symptoms of maternal mirror syndrome are present, it is too late for fetal intervention and the fetus is delivered. The goal of OFS is to debulk the tumor and relieve the fetal cardiovascular system. This will hopefully reverse the progression of heart failure to hydrops and fetal demise. Maternal risks with OFS include bleeding, infection, membrane separation and rupture, preterm labor, preterm delivery, and required cesarean delivery for future pregnancies. The risks and benefits must be carefully weighed with the family. The anatomy of the fetal tumor must also be amenable to OFS. A pedunculated AAPSS type I or II tumor is much more favorable to OFS than a large type III or even a large type II tumor, which has a broad base of attachment to the fetus. The gestational age for OFS intervention is approximately 24 weeks. Ideally, OFS would be offered before 28 weeks' gestation.

Before the decision is made to proceed with OFS, a meeting is held where all members of the team openly discuss with the patient and family the clinical findings, indications for surgery, details of procedure and recovery, and risks to mother and fetus. On the morning of surgery, ultrasound is again performed to confirm placenta and fetal positioning, fetal well-being, and cervical length. After adequate general anesthesia is achieved, a Foley catheter is placed and the anterior abdomen is sterilely prepped and draped. The patient receives intravenous cefazolin or clindamycin. A transverse incision is made on the maternal abdomen at the level of the anterior iliac spines. Superior and inferior flaps are raised and a midline fascial incision extends from the umbilicus to the pubic bone. The uterus is exposed and the tone of the uterus (degree of uterine relaxation) is noted with frequent communication between the surgical and anesthetic teams. If version of the fetus is necessary to adequately position the fetus for surgery, then this is performed with frequent checks of the fetal heart rate and cardiac function. Version is performed prior to mobilizing the uterus or performing the hysterotomy. In some cases, if the placenta is anterior, then the uterus is mobilized from the abdominal cavity to expose the posterior wall. The placenta is mapped and an area for hysterotomy is chosen, ideally at least 6 cm from the placental edge. Stay sutures of 0-PDS are placed under ultrasound guidance. Electrocautery is used to divide the uterine muscle until the level of bulging membranes. The membranes are entered and uterine tone again reassessed by noting if the amniotic fluid remains in the uterus after opening or if the amniotic fluid rushes out under pressure. Bowel clamps are used to compress the uterine wall and then the uterine stapling device is deployed for at least two firings. Bleeding is addressed with 0-PDS. A Level I rapid infuser instills warmed lactated Ringer's fluid to replace lost amniotic fluid and maintain uterine volume. The fetal lower extremities are delivered into the wound and the SCT is exposed. A 24-gauge intravenous catheter and a pulse oximeter to monitor heart rate are placed in the lower extremity. Continuous echocardiography is performed once the hysterotomy is completed. Fluids, blood, and medications are administered to the fetus as indicated. A Rommel type tourniquet with umbilical tape and red rubber catheter segment are passed around the base of the tumor. An additional red rubber or Hegar dilator is placed in the rectum to avoid injury. A handheld harmonic scalpel is then used to debulk the tumor. The tourniquet is released and any areas of bleeding are oversewn with 4–0 PDS. The remaining skin edges are closed if feasible. The fetus is returned to the uterine cavity. Antibiotics are instilled into the amniotic fluid via the Level I catheter as it is withdrawn and the two-layer closure is completed. An omental flap is placed on the uterine closure and the maternal abdominal wall is closed. Indomethacin, magnesium sulfate, and nifedipine are administered for tocolysis.

The number of cases of open fetal surgery for SCT described in the literature is smaller than that of minimally invasive therapy. Case series have reported survival as high as three of four patients,[24] and as low as one of four patients.[43] Most published cases only represent the clinical course of a single patient. Van Mieghem[39] reviewed studies published from 1989 to 2011, and after accounting for overlapping studies reporting on the same patient, discerned a total of 12 cases of open fetal surgery. Overall survival was 50%, two intraoperative fetal deaths occurred, and the mean age of live born cases was approximately 30 weeks' gestation.[39] Between 2007 and 2015 our institution has performed five additional cases of open debulking of fetal SCT (unpublished). Of the nine total cases performed at our institution, six of the infants survived.

After completion of the fetal surgery, the fetus is at great risk for preterm delivery. In the series of patients with 75% survival after open fetal surgery, the mean duration of pregnancy after surgery was 5.1 weeks. The fetuses were born between 27 and 31 weeks' gestation. One of the four mothers required transfusion of packed red blood cells and one mother developed postoperative pulmonary edema requiring diuretic therapy. The neonates experienced complications such as patent ductus arteriosus, central apnea, pulmonary metastasis, rectal stenosis, sepsis, cholestasis, failure to thrive, and chronic lung disease.[24]

Early Delivery

Because the fetus with high-risk SCT can deteriorate precipitously, the managing team performs frequent assessment and follow-up (sometimes daily), and is on standby for emergent delivery. Some cases of hydrops may not manifest until after 28 weeks' gestation, which is later than the typically recommended gestational age to perform fetal surgery.

Delivery of the fetus before 32 weeks has previously not been recommended because of poor survival rates. Thus, the management of a rapidly decompensating fetus between 28 and 32 weeks' gestation presents a management quandary. The benefits of maintaining the pregnancy and improving lung maturity must be weighed against the costs of potential fetal demise because of a rapid evolution of heart failure or intrauterine tumor rupture. One report describes a higher than anticipated survival rate in these fetuses when managed with early delivery.[45] Between 1996 and 2009, nine fetuses with high-risk SCT were delivered before 32 weeks' gestation, and four of them survived. Of the four survivors, one was born at 27 weeks via ex-utero intrapartum therapy (EXIT procedure), two were delivered at 28 weeks via cesarean section, and one was delivered at 31 weeks via cesarean section. The five nonsurvivors were delivered via cesarean section between 26 and 31 weeks' gestation. Indications for delivery of the nine fetuses included preterm labor, rapid tumor growth, nonreassuring fetal heart rate, maternal mirror syndrome, evolving hydrops, and anhydramnios. While early delivery should not be undertaken without careful consideration, improvements in neonatal care, anesthetic and surgical care may allow better than expected survival.

Five of the eight infants that were delivered via cesarean section (two of the three survivors and three of the five nonsurvivors) were taken immediately to an adjacent operating room prepared for immediate neonatal resuscitation and tumor debulking. Three of the infants did not undergo immediate surgical debulking. The first infant had a large cystic SCT and was stable after delivery with Apgar scores of nine at both one and five minutes. Resection occurred on the second day of life. The second baby could not be resuscitated after delivery and received comfort care only. The third infant had significant abdominal ascites with respiratory insufficiency and died on the second day of life.

The fetus that survived and was delivered at 27 weeks via the EXIT procedure described in this series, deserves special mention. The EXIT procedure has typically been described for fetuses with airway obstruction or high-risk lung lesions.[46–48] This is the first known report of an EXIT for delivery of a fetus with SCT. The rationale for this course of action was informed by clinical experience with some of the other cases of early delivery of SCT. The EXIT approach can help scenarios that precipitate complications during delivery and resuscitation of the newborn with SCT, such as the need to warm and dry the baby, secure intravenous access and an airway, and transfer of the patient between operating rooms. These manipulations pose a significant risk of tumor rupture and hemorrhage. After debulking the tumor during the EXIT procedure the infant resuscitation occurred rapidly and relatively smoothly. Use of EXIT for SCT debulking is not an established standard of care, but this option certainly deserves some consideration in selected cases.

Anesthetic Management

Three goals of anesthesia care include patient safety, patient comfort, and facilitation of the procedure. In broad strokes, the factors that must be considered when devising a plan to achieve these goals include the physiology and disease state of the patient – the fetus, (or patients – mother and fetus), and the specific needs of the procedure. The physiology of the pregnant patient and the physiology of the fetus are discussed earlier in this book. General considerations for anesthetic management of fetal surgery have been described,[49] but specific details as they relate to fetuses with SCT will be elucidated below.

The pathophysiologic state of high output heart failure and hydrops fetalis is commonly present in fetuses with SCT. In addition to presenting a metabolic burden, the SCT functions as a large arteriovenous malformation, resulting in an increased preload and decreased afterload. In this scenario, the fetal CCO increases over time, as does the ventricular cavity wall stress. As the CCO increases, the heart compensates with a linear increase in size. Dilation of the heart chambers occurs and results in atrioventricular valve regurgitation. Normal CCO ranges from 425 to 550 mL/kg/min, but a fetus will typically not show signs of hydrops until the CCO reaches 700–800 mL/kg/min. During the 24 hours after open fetal surgery and even beyond this period, fetuses with SCT commonly display abnormal ventricular function, and a higher proportion of fetuses with SCT undergoing open fetal surgery have echocardiographic evidence of tricuspid regurgitation compared to fetuses undergoing fetal surgery for intrathoracic masses or myelomeningocele.[28,50]

While this knowledge is pertinent for the anesthesiologist, the treatment armamentarium of the anesthesiologist is small. The usual physiologic monitors on which the anesthesiologist relies are absent. Intermittent fetal heart rate and umbilical vessel Dopplers obtained by ultrasound are likely to be the only mechanisms for assessing fetal well-being in minimally invasive cases. Open fetal surgery affords more opportunity for monitoring, such as pulse oximetry and echocardiography. Blood gases may also be obtained in some circumstances. Traditionally, the anesthesiologist is accustomed to directly managing the cardiovascular system of the patient with the use of fluids, vasopressors, vasodilators, inotropes, chronotropes, and the like, but this is not the case in fetal surgery. The anesthesiologist is often far removed in proximity from the fetus. Depending on the nature of intervention, the anesthesiologist must effect change in the fetus via the maternal cardiovascular system, placenta, umbilical vessels, and the surgical team. Direct intravenous access to the fetus is typically only available during open fetal surgery. Close communication between the anesthesia, perinatal, cardiology, and surgical teams is crucial for successful anesthetic management of the fetus. Any surgical maneuvers that will affect the fetal cardiovascular system should be communicated clearly and performed gradually. Continuous echocardiography performed by the cardiologist during surgery, is often the best mode of monitoring for the anesthesiologist and assists in decision-making for all team members. Any anesthetic events that veer from the expected path should be communicated to the surgical team. All team members should understand the roles of the other team members, and everyone should be aware of the specific steps of each procedure.

Minimally Invasive

Preoperative evaluation of the mother should consist of a standard anesthetic history and physical examination. Further questioning and workup can be guided by the standard interview. The anesthesiologist should specifically seek a history of sleep apnea or airway obstruction. The ability of the patient to lie comfortably during a long prenatal ultrasound exam will give some insight into her ability to lie supine for a minimally invasive procedure. Complaints of back pain, light-headedness, nausea, dyspnea, or reflux symptoms during the ultrasound examinations, should alert the anesthesia team to proactively consider how these symptoms will be best managed during the procedure. Back pain will make positioning and sedation very challenging. Light-headedness or nausea may be indicative of supine hypotension. Dyspnea is often a result of the mechanical effect of the gravid uterus with polyhydramnios on the mother's breathing, but other causes such as pulmonary edema should be ruled out. The preoperative discussion and preparation of the patient are critical elements of these cases to establish trust and develop an adequate therapeutic plan. Preexisting maternal expectations about the degree of awareness during the minimally invasive procedures should be managed. Maternal anxiety and an expectation of being "completely asleep" make for a more challenging anesthetic. Therefore, setting expectations ahead of time will go a long way towards making the procedure easier to perform. Information about the fetus will typically not change the anesthetic management for these cases, but knowledge about the physiologic status of the fetus will help the anesthesiologist stay fully engaged in the procedure. The most recent estimated fetal weight, assessed by the maternal-fetal medicine specialists, allows the anesthesiologist to calculate weight-based drug dosages for the fetus if needed.

A wide range of anesthetic management options are available for the minimally invasive approach for SCT therapy. In any given institution, the anesthetic prescribed for minimally invasive treatment of SCT will likely be similar to the anesthetic that is provided for other conditions that are managed via a minimally invasive approach, such as laser ablation of placental vessels, RFA of the umbilical cord, or thoracoamniotic shunting. Standard fasting guidelines are given to the mothers for the day before surgery. Aspiration prophylaxis, standard monitors, and one intravenous catheter are often all that are required. The tocolytic regimen in the preoperative, intraoperative, and postoperative period is left to the discretion of the surgical team. Oral indomethacin may be all that is required.

The mother is typically positioned supine with left uterine displacement, but changes in positioning are sometimes required for adequate surgical access to the SCT. The specific needs of these cases include, first, a mother that is physiologically stable without respiratory distress in supine position, and second, a fetus that is in good position and immobile. Maternal sedation is not always needed, and local anesthetic infiltration may be all that is required. The fetus may receive an injection of opioid and muscle relaxant either intramuscularly or into umbilical vessels.[40] The needles and trocars or sheaths used to access the amniotic space and the fetus can be quite small, and maternal pain from insertion of these devices can often be attenuated simply with infiltration of local anesthetic.[37,51] In some institutions, maternal intravenous anxiolytics, sedatives, and analgesics are administered for minimally invasive cases. This practice has dual beneficial effects of increasing maternal comfort and possibly reducing fetal movement depending on the agents administered.[52] The particular combination of medicines administered to the mother will likely vary between institutions and also between anesthesiologists within institutions. The choice of medications per se is unlikely to have as much direct impact as the skill and vigilance of the anesthesiologist managing the patient. Medications commonly used for minimally invasive procedures at the authors' institution include midazolam and dexmedetomidine. Other combinations include midazolam and fentanyl with small boluses of propofol. Infusions of propofol may be used, but are not often required. Remifentanil, fentanyl, morphine, and diazepam use have all been described in pregnancy.[53–57] Previous concerns of teratogenic effects of benzodiazepines in pregnancy are unfounded.[58] A potential drawback to administering anesthetic medication to the mother is maternal partial airway obstruction. A moving fetus definitely makes the procedure technically more challenging, but maternal airway obstruction may lead to paradoxical motion of the abdomen, which also makes the procedure more technically challenging. The needs of a still fetus and maintenance of an adequate maternal airway tone can be very easily balanced in some cases, whereas in other cases, such balance cannot be achieved. Nonpharmacologic measures may be useful. Simple techniques such as hand holding and verbal reassurance can make a dramatic difference in the ability of the mother to tolerate the procedure. Music therapy may also be of some benefit.[59,60] While these procedures do not cause much maternal hemodynamic compromise and aggressive fluid administration is not necessary, phenylephrine or ephedrine should be readily available to treat maternal hypotension if it occurs. The anesthesiologist should also be prepared for conversion to a general anesthetic if needed. Backup plans should be in place, and discussions should be had about courses of action should fetal distress or demise occur. While pulmonary edema has been reported in a case of fetoscopic laser surgery,[61] the likelihood of pulmonary edema is quite low for most minimally invasive fetal procedures.

Open Fetal Surgery

In addition to the standard anesthetic history and physical examination, the preoperative evaluation should focus attention on symptoms of supine hypotension. At the typical gestational age for fetal surgery, 22–25 weeks, mothers are typically not excessively symptomatic in the supine position, but the polyhydramnios that likely comes with the diagnosis of SCT can exacerbate hypotension and breathing difficulties. Problems with previous general anesthetics, prior pregnancies, and experiences with neuraxial blockade are helpful to explore. The airway and spine exams are particularly important. The most recent estimated fetal weight is required to calculate doses of medications to be administered to the fetus. The anesthesiologist should have information regarding the type of SCT, the degree of fetal physiologic compromise, the planned surgical approach, location of the placenta, and contingency plans in case of fetal distress. These issues should be discussed in multidisciplinary team meetings before the day of surgery.

At our institution, mothers are encouraged to drink liberally in the days leading up to surgery to avoid problems with hypovolemia in the face of a very fluid-restrictive anesthetic. Standard fasting guidelines are advised for the night before surgery.

Complete blood count, serum electrolytes, chest x-ray, and baseline 12-lead electrocardiogram are obtained. Maternal blood is obtained for type and cross matching. Type O negative packed red blood cells for the fetus should be cross matched with the mother's sample as maternal antibodies can cross the placenta. Type AB positive fresh frozen plasma should also be obtained. Platelets and other blood products may be ordered as the team deems fit and the blood products should be as fresh as possible. Further laboratory or physiologic testing of the mother are dictated by findings in the history and physical examination. In general, a mother undergoing OFS should be very healthy with minimal comorbidities.

On the morning of surgery, intravenous access and an epidural catheter are secured while the patient is still awake. The epidural catheter is placed in the low thoracic or high lumbar intervertebral space so local anesthetic infused will cover a horizontal skin incision located a few centimeters inferior to the umbilicus. This incision is higher than a typical Pfannenstiel incision. While it is placed preoperatively, the epidural is used for postoperative analgesia, and is only tested preoperatively to rule out signs of intravascular or intrathecal placement. After administration of aspiration prophylaxis, the mother is positioned supine with left uterine displacement, and rapid sequence induction of general anesthesia and endotracheal intubation is performed. An orogastric tube is placed, together with a second large-bore intravenous catheter to allow for rapid administration of crystalloid and blood in the event that catastrophic maternal hemorrhage occurs. An arterial catheter is also placed for precise titration of vasopressor agents. Foley catheter placement is appropriate to monitor urine output, although low urine output rarely changes management intraoperatively. It is more helpful in the postoperative period to gauge response to small fluid boluses. Sequential compression devices should also be placed on the lower extremities to avoid venous stasis and deep venous thrombosis.

Profound uterine relaxation is a necessity and a hallmark of OFS. Decreased uterine tone allows for improved surgical exposure and better fetal perfusion.[62–64] Uterine relaxation can be accomplished in several ways. Nitroglycerin, terbutaline, nifedipine, indomethacin, magnesium, atosiban, and volatile anesthetics all decrease uterine tone. Indomethacin is usually administered prior to induction of anesthesia. Intraoperatively, the most commonly described tocolytic agents are volatile anesthetic agents and nitroglycerin. The rapid onset and offset of volatile anesthetic agents makes for easier titration and allows the anesthesia team to respond quickly in cases of increased uterine tone. High doses of volatile anesthetic, on the order of 1.5 to 2 times minimum alveolar concentration, are often utilized for open fetal surgery.[65] However, a disadvantage of these high doses of volatile anesthetic is an increased risk of fetal myocardial depression, which may lead to fetal bradycardia and cardiac arrest.[50,66] Some centers advocate decreasing the dose of volatile anesthetic and supplementing the anesthetic with propofol and remifentanil to decrease the risk of fetal adverse events.[66] In this series, the need for fetal resuscitative treatment decreased from 61% to 22%. This technique certainly deserves investigation,[67] and at the time of writing, anesthesiologists at the authors' institution are making efforts to minimize the doses of volatile anesthetic by supplementation with intermittent boluses of nitroglycerin. The baseline incidence of fetal adverse events at a given center[68] should be considered before making too many changes in an anesthetic that works well within expected parameters for a particular team. Postoperatively, magnesium sulfate and nifedipine are most commonly used for tocolysis, although intravenous magnesium is started intraoperatively once uterine closure begins. In Europe, atosiban is used in the place of magnesium. The use of volatile anesthetics comes with a risk-benefit consideration in addition to the concern for fetal myocardial depression. Maternal hypotension is common; given the risk of postoperative maternal pulmonary edema as a result of the required magnesium sulfate tocolysis postoperatively, the crystalloid administration for these cases is quite restrictive. Administration of 500–1,000 mL of crystalloid is common for open fetal procedures despite this surgery involving several hours of surgery and a maternal laparotomy. The preoperative oral hydration of these patients should therefore be taken seriously in light of the intraoperative fluid restrictions. Administration of either phenylephrine (boluses or infusion) or ephedrine boluses is common to maintain maternal blood pressure. The amount of maternal blood loss during OFS is rarely significant, for example, the maternal transfusion rates for fetal myelomeningocele repair are reported at 1%.[69]

After laparotomy, the uterus is exposed and the placenta is mapped. Uterine incision must be made carefully to avoid placental and fetal injury. After the fetus is exposed, an intramuscular injection of fentanyl (10–20 mcg/kg), atropine (20 mcg/kg), and vecuronium (0.2–0.4 mg/kg) is administered. A catheter is placed in the amniotic space and warmed crystalloid is administered to maintain warmth, amniotic fluid volume, and buoyancy of the fetus within the uterus. The fetus is monitored with continuous echocardiography and pulse oximetry. A peripheral intravenous catheter should be inserted into the fetus for administration of blood products and medications as a first step, prior to the occurrence of any problems. If an intravenous fluid line is utilized, it should be meticulously checked for air bubbles. Unit doses of emergency fetal medications are drawn up, handed over to the scrub technician in a sterile fashion and kept on the sterile field for intramuscular, intracardiac, or umbilical administration. The anesthesia team may also administer doses of emergency medications directly through the fetus' intravenous catheter after it has been placed. The estimated fetal weight and dosages of code medications can be documented on an operating room smart board to facilitate administration of the correct dose. Warmed blood is primed into the tubing in severe cases where intraoperative fetal blood transfusion is required. The "lining up" of the fetus and use of echocardiography has improved the success rate at our institution. Continuous echocardiography prompts continuous adjustments, and in the long run saves time.

All members of the team must remain in close communication to relay changes in maternal and fetal status and important events during the tumor debulking. Manipulation of the tumor can cause rapid shifts in preload and afterload. This is significant for a fetal heart that is already depressed from volatile anesthetics, and likely already dilated, hypertrophied, and in some degree of heart failure from the SCT. Tourniquets placed at the base of tumor and stapling of the feeding vessels and tumor mass will also cause changes in the fetal cardiovascular system. The presence of a cardiologist intraoperatively can guide the anesthesia and surgical team in its decision-making regarding fluid, blood, and medication administration. A preload bolus of crystalloid or blood (10–20 mL/kg) is often administered to the fetus prior to manipulation of the tumor while monitoring the effects by continuous echocardiography. In the event of fetal bradycardia or cardiac arrest, the anesthesia team should ensure and confirm adequate maternal oxygenation, ventilation, and hemodynamic stability. An empiric dose of a vasopressor may be warranted, but the cause of the bradycardia should be sought and directly addressed. Once maternal well-being is established, the integrity of the placental interface with the uterus must be confirmed, as well as the patency of the umbilical cord. Direct compression of the fetus may lead to bradycardia, and a lack of amniotic fluid may cause compression of the umbilical cord. Fetal hypovolemia is a clear danger in these cases and fetal hyperkalemia or hypocalcemia may occur, as well as fetal hypothermia, particularly if fetal blood transfusion occurs intraoperatively. As mentioned before, exposure of the fetus to volatile anesthetics may also cause fetal bradycardia. Robust data for OFS in the case of SCT is lacking. In the four cases of OFS reported from our institution, 50% of the fetuses had intraoperative bradycardia.[50] Inferences must be drawn from other sources. Fetuses delivered by the EXIT procedure for other indications also often have compromised cardiac function, similar to fetuses with SCT, but the fetuses in these cases tend to be much closer to term. A common reason for fetal bradycardia during EXIT procedures is umbilical cord compression.[68] In this series, 23% of fetuses delivered by EXIT procedure had a bradycardic event. Nine of the 15 events were determined to be secondary to umbilical cord issues. The incidence of bradycardia in open fetal surgery for myelomeningocele has been reported as 5% at our institution.[69] Since publication of this work, significant bradycardic events have been quite rare, and the clinical impression of the authors is that the rate of bradycardia is even lower than 5%. This rate must be placed in context, however, as fetuses with myelomeningocele do not have stressed cardiovascular systems such as those with SCT.

After the SCT has been debulked, and hemostasis is achieved, the venous catheter placed in the fetus is removed, and the surgical site and lower extremities of the fetus are replaced in the uterus. Intrauterine antibiotics are administered, the amniotic fluid volume is brought up to normal levels by replacing it with warmed crystalloid, and the uterus closed. After the uterus is closed, momentum is mobilized and sewn over the hysterotomy. The initial injection of fentanyl likely remains in the fetal circulation for much longer than it would in a neonate, so the fetal stress response should be attenuated for longer than a similar dose of fentanyl for a neonatal surgery.[70] Immaturity of the fetal liver and decreased pulmonary blood flow in the fetus contributes to the lasting effects of fentanyl. Either magnesium or atosiban is started with uterine closure, and the previously placed epidural catheter is bolused during the course of the abdominal closure. During the administration of the magnesium bolus, the volatile anesthetic is often able to be decreased, and as the volatile anesthetic is decreased, any vasoactive infusions are weaned. After abdominal closure, the mother is extubated awake. She is subsequently observed and managed by nurses and doctors in specially trained units that are familiar with postoperative management of open fetal procedures.

EXIT Procedure

The anesthetic considerations and techniques for an EXIT procedure for SCT management are largely similar to those of OFS. A similar process to OFS will take place, with preoperative evaluation, epidural placement, rapid sequence induction of general anesthesia with endotracheal intubation, and high-dose volatile anesthetic administration. There are some key differences, however, because the fetus will be delivered after completion of the EXIT procedure.

The staffing, resource utilization, and communication change considerably when EXIT is the planned procedure. A team of doctors and nurses from the neonatal intensive care unit are actively involved and prepared to receive the infant after the umbilical cord is clamped or emergently if the EXIT needs to be aborted for maternal issues. A second operating room staffed with a second team of operating room nurses and anesthesia staff is also ready to receive the infant, particularly if additional surgery may be required on the baby after the EXIT. These teams need to be prepared to assemble rapidly to care for the compromised baby during night-time and weekend emergencies. In a series of 65 EXITs from our institution, 32% of EXIT procedures happened earlier than expected, and 18% were deemed emergencies.[68] The second operating room is sometimes considered part of the backup plan in case the fetus does not tolerate the EXIT procedure, and it was utilized in 10 of the 65 cases. Reasons to use the second operating room could include placental abruption, refractory fetal bradycardia, or a need to complete the SCT debulking after the umbilical cord has been clamped. Extrapolation of these numbers from this series should be made cautiously, as most of these cases were not for SCT, but this is the largest series of EXIT procedures described in the literature. There should be redundancy of resuscitation equipment and medications, in the room dedicated to the mother's care as well as that dedicated to care of the newborn. The newborn may be managed by different care teams depending on the course of the surgery as well as the goals and needs of the surgical team. All team members need to be clear about the location of important resources, such as the blood products prepared for the fetus, surfactant, and emergency resuscitation medications.

As the fetus is going to be delivered via the EXIT, postoperative tocolysis is not required. Instead, the anesthesia team needs to be able to rapidly reverse profound uterine relaxation to avoid maternal postpartum hemorrhage after the umbilical cord is clamped and cut. Sometimes all that is required is discontinuation of the volatile anesthetics and administration of oxytocin, but postpartum hemorrhage is a real risk, and uterotonics such as methylergonovine and prostaglandin F2-alpha should be readily available. In a series of 65 EXIT procedures performed for a variety of fetal pathologies, 11 of 65 patients needed intramuscular injections of methylergonovine, and four of the 65 needed an intramuscular injection of prostaglandin F2-alpha. Two of the 65 also required rectal misoprostol. Estimated maternal blood loss during an EXIT procedure is reported to be 900±300 mL in 58 of the 65 mothers who did not require a transfusion of packed red blood cells. Seven of 65 of the mothers did require transfusion of packed red blood cells, and their estimated blood loss was 1,500±300 mL.[68] As magnesium tocolysis is not required, there is no concern for possible pulmonary edema after the EXIT procedure, and crystalloid administration can be liberalized as needed.

As with OFS, incremental boluses of local anesthetic through the epidural occur towards the end of the procedure, and the mother is extubated awake.

Delivery with Immediate Debulking/Resection

The planned delivery of a fetus with SCT, either early as mentioned previously,[45] or closer to term with plans for immediate tumor debulking, deserves mention in this chapter. While this situation is not truly a fetal surgical case, the team involved in a neonatal surgery immediately after birth is very likely the same team that would have been involved in a fetal surgical intervention. The literature regarding anesthetic management of SCT debulking or resection is sparse and largely limited to case reports or small case series.[71–76] Considerations for these types of cases include physiology, logistics, and communication. The first relatively large series of 32 cases focusing on the anesthetic management of SCT resection advocated hypothermia and controlled hypotension.[71] Deliberate hypothermia is not current practice at our institution.

The preoperative evaluation of the newborn with SCT is collated from three disparate sources. The first and most detailed source of information comes from weeks of prenatal evaluation of the mother and fetus. From ultrasound, echocardiography, and MRI, the team should have a wealth of detailed information about the size and type of tumor, tumor extension, heart structure and function, degree of heart failure, and associated anomalies. The second source of information will be from the parents' medical history. A vital piece of history to obtain is a maternal or paternal family history of malignant hyperthermia. While a primarily opioid-based anesthetic is recommended for these cases, a family history of malignant hyperthermia will mandate a nontriggering anesthetic for the neonate. The third source of information is gathered in the minutes between delivery and surgery.

Depending on practitioner preferences and institutional customs, the anesthesiologist may be an active participant in the neonatal resuscitation or simply a heavily invested observer. Both anesthesia and neonatology perspectives are important and need to be coordinated to optimize the outcome for the fragile neonate. Again, depending on institutional and provider preference, these activities can occur either in a neonatal resuscitation room or in the operating room where the debulking will take place. In many institutions, the location of the c-section and neonatal resuscitation rooms are not in proximity to the location of the operating room where the neonatal surgery will occur. The team members should carefully plan the physical path of the child after delivery. In high-risk cases, the room where the child is delivered and the room where the child will have surgery need to be immediately adjacent. If the neonatal resuscitation occurs in the operating room, every possible active measure must be taken to ensure that the neonate does not become hypothermic. The difficulty and importance of this task must be emphasized. The degree of surgical exposure required will make rewarming a hypothermic neonate a formidable task. After delivery, a rapid assessment of the degree of compromise of the infant must occur. A stable, crying infant with a broad-based tumor can be treated differently from one that is hemorrhaging. The usual priorities of airway, breathing, and circulation must be addressed. Handling and positioning of the baby and tumor must be discussed a priori, and it is often helpful to have one person specifically assigned to manage the tumor (Figure 12.1). If the child is stable, the resuscitation should consist of the usual warming, drying, and stimulation. Apgar scores should be assessed, standard monitors should be applied, and peripheral venous access should be obtained. Umbilical arterial and venous catheters should also be placed. Clinically, it seems that in some SCT patients, umbilical arterial lines rarely advance cephalad into the aorta, and they often end up in the iliac vessels. This may be a function of the greatly increased blood flow in the descending aorta, which may not allow the catheter tip to head "upstream." While this location is not ideal, it will suffice for drawing blood and for providing continuous invasive blood pressure measurement. Umbilical lines should be tied securely, as occult hemorrhage from these lines can occur intraoperatively and may not be recognized when the patient is prone. Intramuscular vitamin K should be administered, and erythromycin should be administered to the eyes. Blood samples should be obtained for type and cross matching, as well as measurement of glucose, hemoglobin, and blood gases.

Supine and lateral positioning of the infant each have their own merits. The supine position allows more space to work on the infant, and affords greater access to the airway and both upper extremities for placement of monitors and peripheral venous access. The supine position may allow pooling of blood into the tumor, however, with resulting impaired perfusion of the body. It is beneficial for the person managing the tumor position to consider the level of the tumor relative to the rest of the infant's body. Raising or lowering

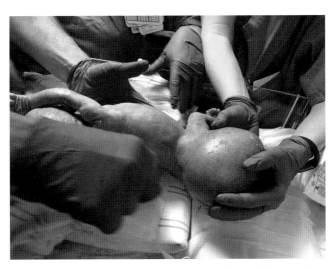

Figure 12.1 Neonate at the beginning of resuscitation. One team member is dedicated to keep control of the SCT. The team has several layered blankets and a chemical warming pad to keep the tumor positioned as neutrally as possible with respect to the body.
Courtesy of Holly Hedrick, MD.

the tumor with respect to the heart will likely impact the available preload for the heart. Kinking the tumor can have untoward effects. Appropriate pads, rolls, and other positioning devices must be available to allow the child to be supine without undue pressure on the tumor. Positioning the baby in the lateral position is another alternative. The lateral position may make management of the position of the tumor with respect to the body simpler, but access to the airway and endotracheal intubation more challenging as this is not a familiar position for anesthesiologists. Intubation in the lateral position is most easily accomplished with the left side down. In the lateral position, access to upper extremities and umbilical vessels is more limited. After resuscitation in the supine position, the child must be repositioned for surgery. In the lateral position, repositioning for surgery will be somewhat easier, and if the condition of the infant requires expeditious surgical control of bleeding, the debulking may be feasible in the lateral position. Prone positioning is more common, however, as it allows better access to the tumor (Figure 12.2). As with any critically ill neonate, great care must be taken to avoid mishaps with the endotracheal tube or vascular access. Extreme vigilance must take place with the positioning and handling of the child during these resuscitative measures, as well as during the intubation, as rupture of the tumor can be catastrophic.[45,72]

If the tumor has ruptured, in-utero, in the course of delivery, or during neonatal resuscitation, the greatest and immediate priority becomes control of the hemorrhage. The options and maneuvers to control the hemorrhage will vary depending on the tumor, the infant, and the team. In some cases, a tourniquet can be placed at the base of the tumor, in other cases manual pressure may be required (Figure 12.3). Many other scenarios can present, so the team must be vigilant, goal-directed, and sometimes creative in the strategies employed to stop the bleeding. Vascular access must be obtained immediately, and blood

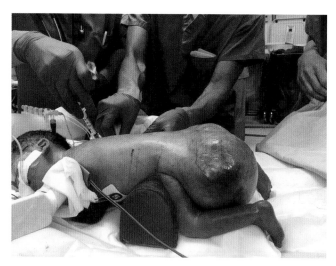

Figure 12.2 Neonate positioned prone for surgery. Note the gel rolls under the chest and pelvis. Chemical and forced air warmers are under the child, overhead warming lights are used, and the room temperature is set at 78–80° F. The head is turned to the side, peripheral intravenous lines are only in the upper extremities, and umbilical arterial and venous lines are secured tightly with umbilical tape and adhesive dressings. The upper extremities must also be used for pulse oximetry and noninvasive blood pressure.
Courtesy of Holly Hedrick, MD.

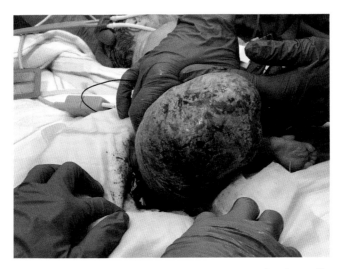

Figure 12.3 This neonate was delivered emergently after an ultrasound showed evidence of hemorrhage in-utero. Hemorrhage was confirmed at delivery, and the infant was rushed immediately into an adjacent operating room. Peripheral venous access was obtained and aggressive transfusion took place while team members held pressure on the base of the SCT to alleviate the bleeding. Concomitantly with administration of blood products, intubation and umbilical catheters were placed. Both the resuscitation and surgery were performed in the lateral position. Courtesy of Holly Hedrick, MD.

products should be administered to replace what has been lost. Just as for open fetal surgery and EXIT procedures, the team should have type O negative packed red cells cross matched against the mother's blood sample ready to give if bleeding occurs before the blood bank is able to process the infant's blood sample. Fresh frozen plasma and platelets should also be prepared. A retrospective review of a series of 112 patients with SCT operated on at our institution demonstrates highly variable transfusion requirements.[77] Infants at gestational age ≤ 30 weeks with AAPSS class I and II tumors were more likely to be transfused. If the tumor is predominantly solid, a greater transfusion volume is likely. Infants with cystic tumor morphology who were transfused received a mean volume of 63±69 mL/kg of all blood products combined. Infants with more solid tumor morphology required 148.9 ±177 mL/kg of all blood products combined.[77] An infant with a ruptured SCT will certainly lie on the higher end of the range of volume of blood transfused. A hemostatic transfusion strategy is recommended, at least with a 1:1 ratio of packed red cells and fresh frozen plasma. In some cases, an even more aggressive 1:1:1 ratio of packed red cells, plasma, and platelets may be required.

The operating room should be warmed as mentioned above, and the anesthesia team should be prepared with adequate intravenous lines, transducers for invasive hemodynamic monitoring, unit doses of emergency medications, infusions of vasopressors, an infusion of glucose-containing crystalloid, blood products, and equipment for point of care testing. If the team is planning on using component blood therapy, two blood warmers (one for packed red cells, one for plasma) will make for a much smoother transfusion workflow. Fresh whole blood would be a luxury, but the logistics of obtaining fresh whole blood for these cases are challenging. Acquiring recombinant factor VIIa ahead of time should also be considered as it is useful in cases of refractory medical bleeding.[74] If the infant is premature, the team may want to consider setting up a high-performance ventilator from the intensive care unit, or even a high-frequency oscillating ventilator. The drawback of these ventilators is the increased difficulty of measuring exhaled CO_2. Every effort should be made to minimize dead space in the breathing circuit. Inhaled nitric oxide may be useful in these cases, but it is typically more useful in cases of immediate resection of a lung tumor. Pre- and postductal oxygen saturations should be measured. Surfactant should be considered in those infants < 34 weeks' gestation. Ideally, peripheral venous access should be in the upper extremities, as the lower extremities may be prepped and included in the sterile field.

The intraoperative course can be tenuous for the debulking of SCT tumors. Oxygenation and ventilation can be challenging because of lung immaturity and also as a result of mechanical compression of the lungs by the tumor mass. Migration of the endotracheal tube may also occur. The cardiovascular system is already unstable from the SCT, and it is also subjected to abrupt changes of preload and afterload from tumor manipulation and tourniquet application. Hemorrhage may begin before surgery and continue well into the case. Intraoperative tumor manipulation is often associated with changes in oxygenation and ventilation. This may also occur because of the shifting of pooled blood from the tumor back into the infant's main circulating volume. Pressure on necrotic regions of tumor may release potassium into the circulation.[75] Transfusion of blood products will cause hypocalcemia and probably hyperkalemia. Neonatal acidosis may also occur secondary to respiratory and metabolic causes, and this acidosis will exacerbate hyperkalemia. Infants have an immature coagulation system, and SCT seems to predispose affected babies to disseminated intravascular coagulation.[78] Venous air embolism has also been reported.[76]

If the surgical and anesthetic teams are able to navigate this minefield, total resection of the SCT may be attempted, but signs of instability should prompt reevaluation of the surgical plan. Expeditious debulking of the tumor may be the most prudent course. This will allow the infant to transition from fetal to neonatal circulation faster. With the major mass of the tumor removed, the high output failure should resolve and the baby's heart may be able to remodel. A less dilated heart should decrease the severity of atrioventricular valve regurgitation. The subsequent completion of SCT resection several weeks later should be less problematic with smaller tumor mass, more mature lungs, a more compensated cardiovascular system, increased levels of coagulation factors, and more mature hepatic and renal function.

Future Directions

While SCT is the most common tumor of the neonatal period, it is still relatively rare, and the literature regarding prenatal evaluation and management is just now starting to develop. A Web of Science search for "sacrococcygeal teratoma" produces 943 publications from 1945 to 2016. More than a third of these publications (356) have been published since 2008. Avenues of future work include further refining of prenatal diagnosis and finding the most reliable predictors of prognosis. Prognostic indicators will help with counseling and patient selection for the most appropriate management, be it minimally invasive ablation, open fetal debulking, EXIT procedure, or early delivery. Minimally invasive techniques should be refined to avoid damage to adjacent fetal structures, adequately alleviate the high output heart failure, and avoid tumor necrosis and hemorrhage. Optimal anesthetic management of open fetal surgery remains to be determined. Minimizing fetal myocardial depression while providing adequate uterine relaxation should be an area of active research. With the increasing number of open fetal surgical procedures being performed around the world, contributions of anesthetic techniques to preterm labor and delivery may be determined, and anesthetic techniques can be adjusted.

References

1. Mintz B, Cronmiller C, Custer RP. Somatic cell origin of teratocarcinomas. *Proc Natl Acad Sci USA*. 1978;**75**(6):2834–2838.

2. Flake AW. Fetal sacrococcygeal teratoma. *Semin Pediatr Surg*. 1993;**2**(2):113–120.

3. Bale PM, Painter DM, Cohen D. Teratomas in childhood. *Pathology*. 1975;**7**(3):209–218.

4. Altman RP, Randolph JG, Lilly JR. Sacrococcygeal teratoma: American Academy of Pediatrics Surgical Section Survey–1973. *J Pediatr Surg*. 1974;**9**(3):389–398.

5. Bale PM. Sacrococcygeal developmental abnormalities and tumors in children. *Perspect Pediatr Pathol*. 1984;**8**(1):9–56.

6. Carney JA, Thompson DP, Johnson CL, Lynn HB. Teratomas in children: clinical and pathologic aspects. *J Pediatr Surg*. 1972;7(3):271–282.

7. Noseworthy J, Lack EE, Kozakewich HP, et al. Sacrococcygeal germ cell tumors in childhood: an updated experience with 118 patients. *J Pediatr Surg*. 1981;**16**(3):358–364.

8. Yao W, Li K, Zheng S, et al. Analysis of recurrence risks for sacrococcygeal teratoma in children. *J Pediatr Surg*. 2014;49(12):1839–1842.

9. Gonzalez-Crussi F, Winkler RF, Mirkin DL. Sacrococcygeal teratomas in infants and children: relationship of histology and prognosis in 40 cases. *Arch Pathol Lab Med*. 1978;**102**(8):420–425.

10. Bond SJ, Harrison MR, Schmidt KG, et al. Death due to high-output cardiac failure in fetal sacrococcygeal teratoma. *J Pediatr Surg*. 1990;**25**(12):1287–1291.

11. Partridge EA, Canning D, Long C, et al. Urologic and anorectal complications of sacrococcygeal teratomas: Prenatal and postnatal predictors. *J Pediatr Surg*. 2014;**49**(1):139–143.

12. Tanaree P. Delivery obstructed by sacrococcygeal teratoma. *Am J Obstet Gynecol*. 1982;**142**(2):239.

13. Weiss DB, Wajntraub G, Abulafia Y, Schiller M. Vaginal surgical intervention for a sacro-coccygeal teratoma obstructing labor. *Acta Obstet Gynecol Scand*. 1976;**55**(2):183–185.

14. Johnson JW, Porter J, Kellner KR, et al. Abdominal rescue after incomplete delivery secondary to large fetal sacrococcygeal teratoma. *Obstet Gynecol*. 1988;**71**(6 Pt 2):981–984.

15. Gucciardo L, Uyttebroek A, De Wever I, et al. Prenatal assessment and management of sacrococcygeal teratoma. *Prenat Diagn*. 2011;**31**(7):678–688.

16. Calenda E, Bachy B, et al. Sacrococcygeal teratoma and venous shunting through a tumor: biological evidence. *Anesth Analg*. 1992;**74**(1):165–166.

17. Braun T, Brauer M, Fuchs I, et al. Mirror syndrome: a systematic review of fetal associated conditions, maternal presentation and perinatal outcome. *Fetal Diagn Ther*. 2010;**27**(4):191–203.

18. van Selm M, Kanhai HH, Gravenhorst JB. Maternal hydrops syndrome: a review. *Obstet Gynecol Surv*. 1991;**46**(12):785–788.

19. Wilson RD, Hedrick H, Flake AW, et al. Sacrococcygeal teratomas: prenatal surveillance, growth and pregnancy outcome. *Fetal Diagn Ther*. 2009;**25**(1):15–20.

20. Ayed A, Tonks AM, Lander A, Kilby MD. A review of pregnancies complicated by congenital sacrococcygeal teratoma in the West Midlands region over an 18-year period: population-based, cohort study. *Prenat Diagn*. 2015;**35**(11):1037–1047.

21. Akinkuotu AC, Coleman A, Shue E, et al. Predictors of poor prognosis in prenatally diagnosed sacrococcygeal teratoma:

A multiinstitutional review. *J Pediatr Surg.* 2015;**50**(5):771–774.

22. Shue E, Bolouri M, Jelin EB, et al. Tumor metrics and morphology predict poor prognosis in prenatally diagnosed sacrococcygeal teratoma: a 25-year experience at a single institution. *J Pediatr Surg.* 2013;**48**(6):1225–1231.

23. Usui N, Kitano Y, Sago H, et al. Outcomes of prenatally diagnosed sacrococcygeal teratomas: the results of a Japanese nationwide survey. *J Pediatr Surg.* 2012;**47**(3):441–447.

24. Hedrick HL, Flake AW, Crombleholme TM, et al. Sacrococcygeal teratoma: prenatal assessment, fetal intervention, and outcome. *J Pediatr Surg.* 2004;**39**(3):430–438.

25. Rodriguez MA, Cass DL, Lazar DA, et al. Tumor volume to fetal weight ratio as an early prognostic classification for fetal sacrococcygeal teratoma. *J Pediatr Surg.* 2011;**46**(6):1182–1185.

26. Flake AW, Harrison MR, Adzick NS, et al. Fetal sacrococcygeal teratoma. *J Pediatr Surg.* 1986;**21**(7):563–566.

27. Statile CJ, Cnota JF, Gomien S, et al. Estimated cardiac output and cardiovascular profile score in fetuses with high cardiac output lesions. *Ultrasound Obstet Gynecol.* 2012;**41**(1):54–58.

28. Rychik J. Fetal cardiovascular physiology. *Pediatr Cardiol.* 2004;**25**(3):1–9.

29. Coleman A, Kline-Fath B, Keswani S, Lim F-Y. Prenatal solid tumor volume index: novel prenatal predictor of adverse outcome in sacrococcygeal teratoma. *J Surg Res.* 2013;**184**(1):330–336.

30. Danzer E, Hubbard AM, Hedrick HL, et al. Diagnosis and characterization of fetal sacrococcygeal teratoma with prenatal MRI. *AJR Am J Roentgenol.* 2006;**187**(4):W350–356.

31. Van Mieghem T, Al-Ibrahim A, Deprest J, et al. Minimally invasive therapy for fetal sacrococcygeal teratoma: case series and systematic review of the literature. *Ultrasound Obstet Gynecol.* 2014;**43**(6):611–619.

32. Sananes N, Javadian P, Schwach Werneck Britto I, et al. Technical aspects and effectiveness of percutaneous fetal therapies for large sacrococcygeal teratomas: cohort study and literature review. *Ultrasound Obstet Gynecol.* 2016;**47**(6):712–719.

33. Makin EC, Hyett J, Ade-Ajayi N, et al. Outcome of antenatally diagnosed sacrococcygeal teratomas: single-center experience (1993–2004). *J Pediatr Surg.* 2006;**41**(2):388–393.

34. Ibrahim D, Ho E, Scherl SA, Sullivan CM. Newborn with an open posterior hip dislocation and sciatic nerve injury after intrauterine radiofrequency ablation of a sacrococcygeal teratoma. *J Pediatr Surg.* 2003;**38**(2):248–250.

35. Paek BW, Jennings RW, Harrison MR, et al. Radiofrequency ablation of human fetal sacrococcygeal teratoma. *Am J Obstet Gynecol.* 2001;**184**(3):503–507.

36. Benachi A, Durin L, Vasseur Maurer S, et al. Prenatally diagnosed sacrococcygeal teratoma: a prognostic classification. *J Pediatr Surg.* 2006;**41**(9):1517–1521.

37. Ruano R, da Silva MM, Salustiano EMA, et al. Percutaneous laser ablation under ultrasound guidance for fetal hyperechogenic microcystic lung lesions with hydrops: a single center cohort and a literature review. *Prenat Diagn.* 2012;**32**(12):1127–1132.

38. Gucciardo L, Deprest J, Done E, et al. Prediction of outcome in isolated congenital diaphragmatic hernia and its consequences for fetal therapy. Best Pract Res Clin Obstet Gynaecol. 2008;**22**(1):123–138.

39. Van Mieghem T, Al-Ibrahim A, Deprest J, et al. Minimally invasive therapy for fetal sacrococcygeal teratoma: case series and systematic review of the literature. *Ultrasound Obstet Gynecol.* 2014;**43**(6):611–619.

40. Ruano R, Duarte S, Zugaib M. Percutaneous laser ablation of sacrococcygeal teratoma in a hydropic fetus with severe heart failure–too late for a surgical procedure? *Fetal Diagn Ther.* 2009;**25**(1):26–30.

41. Adzick NS, Crombleholme TM, Morgan MA, Quinn TM. A rapidly growing fetal teratoma. *Lancet*. 1997;**349**(9051):538–531.

42. Langer JC, Harrison MR, Schmidt KG, et al. Fetal hydrops and death from sacrococcygeal teratoma: rationale for fetal surgery. *Am J Obstet Gynecol*. 1989;**160**(5 Pt 1):1145–1150.

43. Graf JL, Albanese CT, Jennings RW, et al. Successful fetal sacrococcygeal teratoma resection in a hydropic fetus. *J Pediatr Surg*. 2000;**35**(10):1489–1491.

44. Grethel EJ, Wagner AJ, Clifton MS, et al. Fetal intervention for mass lesions and hydrops improves outcome: a 15-year experience. *J Pediatr Surg*. 2007;**42**(1):117–123.

45. Roybal JL, Moldenhauer JS, Khalek N, et al. Early delivery as an alternative management strategy for selected high-risk fetal sacrococcygeal teratomas. *J Pediatr Surg*. 2011;**46**(7):1325–1332.

46. Laje P, Peranteau WH, Hedrick HL, et al. Ex utero intrapartum treatment (EXIT) in the management of cervical lymphatic malformation. *J Pediatr Surg*. 2015;**50**(2):311–314.

47. Hedrick HL. Ex utero intrapartum therapy. *Semin Pediatr Surg*. 2003;**12**(3):190–195.

48. Hedrick HL, Flake AW, Crombleholme TM, et al. The ex utero intrapartum therapy procedure for high-risk fetal lung lesions. *J Pediatr Surg*. 2005;**40**(6):1038–1044.

49. Lin EE, Tran KM. Anesthesia for fetal surgery. *Semin Pediatr Surg*. 2013;**22**(1):50–55.

50. Rychik J. Acute cardiovascular effects of fetal surgery in the human. *Circulation*. 2004;**110**(12):1549–1556.

51. Klaritsch P, Albert K, Van Mieghem T, et al. Instrumental requirements for minimal invasive fetal surgery. *BJOG*. 2008;**116**(2):188–197.

52. Van de Velde M, Van Schoubroeck D, Lewi LE, et al. Remifentanil for fetal immobilization and maternal sedation during fetoscopic surgery: a randomized, double-blind comparison with diazepam. *Anesth Analg*. 2005;**101**(1):251–258.

53. Erkkola R, Kangas L, Pekkarinen A. The transfer of diazepam across the placenta during labour. *Acta Obstet Gynecol Scand*. 1973;**52**(2):167–170.

54. Kopecky EA, Simone C, Knie B, Koren G. Transfer of morphine across the human placenta and its interaction with naloxone. *Life Sci*. 1999;**65**(22):2359–2371.

55. Kan RE, Hughes SC, Rosen MA, et al. Intravenous remifentanil: placental transfer, maternal and neonatal effects. *Anesthesiology*. 1998;**88**(6):1467–1474.

56. Sia AT, Sng BL. Intravenous dexmedetomidine for obstetric anaesthesia and analgesia: converting a challenge into an opportunity? *Int J Obstet Anesth*. 2009;**18**(3):204–206.

57. Cooper J, Jauniaux E, Gulbis B, et al. Placental transfer of fentanyl in early human pregnancy and its detection in fetal brain. *Br J Anaesth*. 1999;**82**(6):929–931.

58. Koren G, Pastuszak A, Ito S. Drugs in pregnancy. *N Engl J Med*. 1998;**338**(16):1128–1137.

59. Wu P-Y, Huang M-L, Lee W-P, et al. Effects of music listening on anxiety and physiological responses in patients undergoing awake craniotomy. *Complement Ther Med*. 2017;32:56–60.

60. Vetter D, Barth J, Uyulmaz S, et al. Effects of art on surgical patients. *Ann Surg*. 2015;**262**(5):704–713.

61. Robinson MB, Crombleholme TM, Kurth CD. Maternal pulmonary edema during fetoscopic surgery. *Anesth Analg*. 2008;**107**(6):1978–1980.

62. Barrett JM. Fetal resuscitation with terbutaline during eclampsia-induced uterine hypertonus. *Am J Obstet Gynecol*. 1984;**150**(7):895.

63. Patriarco MS, Viechnicki BM, Hutchinson TA, et al. A study on intrauterine fetal resuscitation with terbutaline. *Am J Obstet Gynecol*. 1987;**157**(2):384–387.

64. Arias F. Intrauterine resuscitation with terbutaline: a method for the management

of acute intrapartum fetal distress. *Am J Obstet Gynecol.* 1978;**131**(1):39–43.

65. Tran KM. Anesthesia for fetal surgery. *Semin Fetal Neonatal Med.* 2010;**15** (1):40–45.

66. Boat A, Mahmoud M, Michelfelder EC, et al. Supplementing desflurane with intravenous anesthesia reduces fetal cardiac dysfunction during open fetal surgery. *Paediatr Anaesth.* 2010;**20** (8):748–756.

67. Ngamprasertwong P, Michelfelder EC, Arbabi S, et al. Anesthetic techniques for fetal surgery: effects of maternal anesthesia on intraoperative fetal outcomes in a sheep model. *Anesthesiology.* 2013;**118**(4):796–808.

68. Lin EE, Moldenhauer JS, Tran KM, et al. Anesthetic management of 65 cases of ex utero intrapartum therapy: a 13-year single-center experience. *Anesth Analg.* 2016;**123**(2):411–417.

69. Moldenhauer JS, Soni S, Rintoul NE, et al. Fetal myelomeningocele repair: the post-MOMS experience at the Children's Hospital of Philadelphia. *Fetal Diagn Ther.* 2015;**37**(3):235–240.

70. Tran KM, Maxwell LG, Cohen DE, et al. Quantification of serum fentanyl concentrations from umbilical cord blood during ex utero intrapartum therapy. *Anesth Analg.* 2012;**114**(6):1265–1267.

71. Robinson S, Laussen PC, Brown TC, Woodward AA. Anaesthesia for sacrococcygeal teratoma–a case report and a review of 32 cases. *Anaesth Intensive Care.* 1992;**20**(3):354–358.

72. Tran KM, Flake AW, Kalawadia NV, et al. Emergent excision of a prenatally diagnosed sacrococcygeal teratoma. *Pediatr Anesth.* 2008;**18**(5):431–434.

73. Kim J-W, Gwak M, Park J-Y, et al. Cardiac arrest during excision of a huge sacrococcygeal teratoma – A report of two cases. *Korean J Anesthesiol.* 2012;**63** (1):80–84.

74. Girisch M, Rauch R, Carbon R, et al. Refractory bleeding following major surgery of a giant sacrococcygeal teratoma in a premature infant: successful use of recombinant factor VIIa. *Eur J Pediatr.* 2004;**163**(2):118–119.

75. Reinoso-Barbero F, Sepulveda I, Pérez-Ferrer A, De Andres A. Cardiac arrest secondary to hyperkalemia during surgery for a neonatal giant sacrococcygeal teratoma. *Pediatr Anesth.* 2009;**19** (7):712–714.

76. Jafra A, Dwivedi D, Jain D, Bala I. Giant sacrococcygeal teratoma: Management concerns with reporting of a rare occurrence of venous air embolism. *Saudi J Anaesth.* 2017;**11** (1):124–125.

77. Isserman RS, Nelson O, Tran KM, et al. Risk factors for perioperative mortality and transfusion in sacrococcygeal teratoma resections. *Paediatr Anaesth.* 2017;**27** (7):726–732.

78. Murphy JJ, Blair GK, Fraser GC. Coagulopathy associated with large sacrococcygeal teratomas. *J Pediatr Surg.* 1992;**27**(10):1308–1310.

Chapter 13

Ex-Utero Intrapartum Therapy

James Fisher, Timothy C. Lee, and Mario Patino

Introduction

Ex-utero intrapartum therapy (EXIT) is a multidisciplinary approach utilized at the time of birth in select fetuses with congenital anomalies primarily affecting the upper airway. Commonly referred to as the EXIT procedure, it allows for life-saving measures such as establishment of a secure airway in the fetus/neonate while maintaining fetoplacental circulation and delivery of oxygenated blood to the fetus just prior to delivery. An EXIT procedure requires seamless coordination between anesthesiology, surgery, and neonatology teams. To facilitate such coordination, the steps of the EXIT procedure must be fully understood and well planned. To aid in the understanding of the EXIT procedure, this chapter will discuss the history, indications, and steps of an EXIT procedure as well as the outcomes following this procedure.

History

The acronym, EXIT, was first used in 1997;[1] however, multiple cases of similar procedures were published prior to the creation of the acronym. The concept of performing procedures on neonates prior to discontinuation of placental support was initially described in 1989.[2] The terminology "operation on placental support" or OOPS was used by Norris et al.[2] to describe the technique of maintaining fetoplacental or uteroplacental circulation during attempts at intubation in a preterm fetus with a large neck mass. Fetoplacental support was maintained for only 10 minutes in this initial case. One of the earlier accounts of maintaining fetoplacental circulation and providing uterine relaxation (a central tenet of the EXIT procedure) was published by Schwartz et al. in 1993.[3] In this report, a baby, just before 36 weeks' gestation, with a diagnosis of a large cervical vascular malformation causing polyhydramnios, was delivered via cesarean section and uterine relaxation was maintained using halothane. This case was associated with a prolonged period of fetoplacental circulation. During this delivery, the baby's airway was secured just prior to separation from placental support. The creation of the acronym, EXIT, occurred in conjunction with the description of the first series of neonates successfully treated on fetoplacental support prior to full delivery. In this series, Mychaliska et al. detailed the method of achieving uterine relaxation using high-dose isoflurane.[1] The authors stressed that maintenance of fetoplacental circulation, an absolutely essential component of the EXIT procedure, requires maximal uterine relaxation which is achieved by optimal anesthetic management. Consequently, the EXIT procedure has been adopted by centers worldwide to allow for successful management of fetal anomalies that may compromise the ability to oxygenate and ventilate the neonate following delivery.

Indications

The progression of fetal intervention, including the EXIT procedure, is mainly through the improvement of diagnostic tools such as imaging technology (ultrasound and magnetic resonance imaging). These have allowed for earlier, more precise prenatal diagnosis and subsequent targeted management. The approach of the EXIT procedure is also applied to other clinical scenarios apart from airway anomalies. These different scenarios in which the EXIT procedure is indicated, are generally described under different nomenclature namely "EXIT-to-airway" (for extrinsic neck masses which significantly compromise the airway, e.g. cervical teratoma, cystic hygroma, intrinsic airway obstruction caused by laryngeal atresia, laryngeal cysts, congenital high airway obstruction syndrome(CHAOS), as well as fetuses with previous endoscopic tracheal occlusion (FETO) which require balloon removal near term); "EXIT-to-resection" (for lung anomalies such as large congenital cystic adenomatoid malformation with significant pulmonary hypoplasia and tumors such as sacrococcygeal teratomas which can potentially lead to a high output heart failure with fetal hydrops); "EXIT-to-ECMO" (for significant cardiopulmonary disease requiring extracorporeal membranous oxygenation (ECMO)); and "EXIT-to-separation" (for conjoined twins). The fetal intervention in these different scenarios typically involves airway management such as endotracheal intubation by direct laryngoscopy, rigid bronchoscopy, retrograde wire intubation or tracheostomy; tumor resection, or the placement of ECMO cannulae prior to delivery.

EXIT-to-Airway

In the series establishing the EXIT acronym, the procedure was performed to provide fetoplacental circulation while the trachea was "unplugged" and the airway secured, in fetuses who had previously undergone tracheal plug placement for congenital diaphragmatic hernia (CDH).[1] These reports along with many others subsequently performed, have solidified the EXIT procedure as the standard approach for securing the airway in fetuses with an anticipated difficult airway (cervical teratomas, cervical lymphovascular malformations, or micrognathia). In each of these cases, polyhydramnios is used as a surrogate marker for the severity of tracheal and/or esophageal occlusion. Lazar et al.[4] have established a metric, the tracheoesophageal displacement index (TEDI) score, for determining the presence of a complicated airway in fetuses with neck masses. In this study, a TEDI score > 12 mm correlated with a complicated airway in 100% of cases. The TEDI score helps identify the potential need for an EXIT procedure. Another indication for the EXIT procedure is CHAOS. In these cases, the airway is obstructed by a congenital failure of canalization of the proximal trachea (intrinsic abnormalities) leading to characteristic findings during fetal ultrasound evaluation of enlarged, echogenic lungs with flattened diaphragms, dilated airways distal to the obstruction, and ascites/nonimmune hydrops.[5,6]

EXIT-to-Resection

The EXIT procedure is indicated in select cases of congenital pulmonary airway malformation (CPAM),[7,8] formerly referred to as congenital cystic adenomatoid malformation (CCAM). In these cases, the large size of the lung lesion causes significant mediastinal shift. When these lesions are filled with air, they compress the mediastinum further making oxygenation and ventilation difficult or even impossible despite intubation in some instances. When this occurs, immediate decompression by resection of the CPAM is necessary. To facilitate a controlled environment for the resection, an EXIT procedure is performed allowing for intubation of the neonate, thoracotomy, and exteriorization of the mass all on placental support, prior to initiation of ventilation. This prevents worsening of the mediastinal shift and cardiac compression if ventilation were to occur immediately after intubation. Some cervical lesions that preclude oral intubation or tracheostomy may also require EXIT-to-resection to permit intubation or tracheostomy. Indications for EXIT-to-resection can also be for certain tumors such as sacrococcygeal teratomas which are characterized by high output cardiac failure. In this situation, partial delivery of the tumor and immediate partial resection of the tumor with control of the feeding vessels responsible for the high output cardiac failure occur prior to full delivery of the neonate.

EXIT-to-ECMO

The EXIT procedures have been described to allow for ECMO cannulae insertion prior to cessation of fetoplacental circulation. Kunisaki et al.[9] described one of the initial experiences of EXIT-to-ECMO in neonates with severe CDH. However, subsequent studies have not shown a reduction in morbidity or mortality even with this approach to treatment.[10,11] It can also be considered for fetuses/neonates with airways that cannot be secured prior to the discontinuation of placental support.

EXIT-to-Separation

This is a uniquely described indication for the EXIT procedure which involves separation of conjoined twins. In the description of an EXIT-to-separation procedure by Mackenzie et al.,[12] fetoplacental circulation was maintained for a set of conjoined twins while the airway of both babies was secured, immediate vascular mapping of the shared cardiac circulation, and ultimate separation occurred, resulting in the survival of one of the twins. This application of the EXIT procedure allowed for the survival of at least one twin and prevented a double mortality which was almost certain had the separation been attempted off fetoplacental circulation.

Table 13.1 lists the different indications described for the EXIT procedure.

Anesthetic Considerations

The EXIT procedure involves performance of a hysterotomy followed by partial fetal exposure to proceed with therapeutic intervention while uteroplacental or fetoplacental flow (placental bypass) is preserved. Following the intervention, posterior clamping of the umbilical cord occurs with subsequent delivery of the newborn. It is important for the anesthesiologist to understand the implications of the fetal anomaly, the degree of severity, the necessary procedure required to treat the anomaly, possible alternative procedures, and the sequence of events that will occur. This information is essential to the formulation of an anesthetic plan.

Priority must be given to maternal safety under the principle of rendering beneficial fetal therapy, so an exhaustive discussion and understanding of the maternal risks is imperative.[13] Maternal selection is therefore, very important. The patient undergoing an EXIT procedure must not have serious comorbidities and must also have a complete understanding of the associated risks and benefits. During the preoperative evaluation,

Table 13.1 Indications for ex-utero intrapartum therapy

Type of EXIT	Specific indication
EXIT-to-airway	CHAOS (congenital high airway obstruction)
	Head or neck mass (teratoma, lymphatic malformation)
	Unilateral pulmonary agenesis
	Reversal of tracheal occlusion
EXIT-to-resection	CPAM (congenital pulmonary airway malformation)
	SCT (sacrococcygeal teratoma)
	Neck mass precluding intubation/tracheostomy
EXIT-to-ECMO	CDH (congenital diaphragmatic hernia) (recent outcomes have not shown benefit)
EXIT-to-separation	Bridge to separation of conjoined twins

comorbidities are evaluated to determine the degree of severity and also to decide if further optimization is necessary. Standard evaluation of previous anesthetic-related problems, as well as a physical examination with emphasis on the airway, cardiac, respiratory, and spine examination are crucial. A review of current medications including the preoperative administration of tocolytics such as indomethacin and calcium channel blockers is crucial as these medications may impact the patient's intraoperative hemodynamics. Evaluation of the preoperative imaging studies, such as fetal ultrasound and fetal MRI, is necessary to better define the disease process in the fetus, estimate the fetal weight for precise fetal drug administration, and also to identify the location of the placenta. The latter is necessary to determine if potential adjustments to either the patient position or surgical access will be required to facilitate access to the fetus. It is important to compare similar imaging studies performed at different gestational ages to evaluate the progress of the disease and the degree of severity. For instance, a CPAM can change in size and degree of severity during the prenatal period. Likewise, the degree of airway obstruction resulting from compression by a cervical tumor can also vary during this time. Finally, a thorough discussion of the informed consent and counselling must be part of the preoperative evaluation.[14]

Participation in the preprocedural multidisciplinary meetings provides an opportunity for the team members to listen in on the analysis of the outcomes to date of the different options for intervention, that is predelivery intervention on uteroplacental bypass versus postnatal intervention. Review of existing data facilitates the decision-making process by the multidisciplinary medical team. This decision algorithm may also be presented to the family when they meet with the team; however, some conditions have very limited evidence-based data. Including the patient in this preoperative meeting is extremely important so the patient can understand the plan, risks and benefits of the procedure. The multidisciplinary team involved in this meeting includes physicians from the following disciplines: maternal-fetal medicine, pediatric surgery, pediatric otolaryngology, pediatric anesthesiology, pediatric cardiology, pediatric neurosurgery, neonatology, and radiology. Genetic counsellors, neonatology and operating room nursing teams, as well as a social worker are also included in this multidisciplinary team. Important goals during the preoperative meeting are to discuss the case, potential challenges, and to understand the initial surgical approach, sequence of events, and the consideration of possible alternative plans. While this meeting may be held a few days before the actual procedure, a team huddle on the day of surgery is usually helpful so all participants remember their designated roles and the flow of events. Specific tasks must be assigned preoperatively to the different team members to facilitate the performance of sequential or simultaneous events in an effective and coordinated manner. Communication and teamwork are fundamental during the EXIT procedure to guarantee the best possible outcome.

Normal physiologic changes of pregnancy and its implications when providing general and regional anesthesia during cesarean section apply to the EXIT procedure. Important considerations include the need for prophylaxis against aspiration (usually with a nonparticulate antacid, H2 receptor antagonist, and/or metoclopramide) given that all pregnant women are considered to have a full stomach because of the increase in progesterone and estrogen levels (which decrease the lower esophageal tone), increased gastrin secretion by the placenta (increases gastric hydrogen secretion), and also as a result of the mechanical effects of the gravid uterus on the gastrointestinal tract.[15] Pregnancy is also associated with a lower minimal anesthetic concentration (MAC) even though electroencephalographic evaluation suggests similar responses to volatile agents in both pregnant and nonpregnant women.[16] This is important to note after endotrachaeal intubation and before uterine relaxation is required. Local anesthetic sensitivity is also increased during pregnancy.[17] The increased volume of soft tissues adjacent to the airway, airway edema, and capillary engorgement that are present in the pregnant patient require the consideration of the placement of smaller sized endotracheal tubes (6.0–6.5 mm).[18] Most of the coagulation factors are increased in concentration and this together with a decreased concentration of antithrombin III and tissue plasminogen activator (tPA) in pregnancy, result in a hypercoagulable state. Careful positioning of the patient on the operating room table is necessary to avoid aortocaval compression by the gravid uterus as this can lead to decreased venous return, cardiac output, and uteroplacental perfusion, with subsequent fetal acidosis.[19] It is important to realize that there is no autoregulation, and uteroplacental flow depends on uterine perfusion pressure. Engorgement of the epidural veins may also be present as a result of increased intra-abdominal pressure, and this may increase the incidence of intravascular epidural catheter placement.

Two operating rooms must be available in preparation for the EXIT procedure. One is dedicated to the mother, in which the fetal intervention will be performed on uteroplacental flow support. The equipment for fetal intubation in the mother's room, needs to be present on the surgical field and therefore must be sterile. Initial airway management may involve a direct laryngoscopy, rigid bronchoscopy, tracheostomy, retrograde airway intubation, or partial or complete surgical resection of a neck mass with further surgical airway manipulation.[20] A neonatology resuscitation team must be available in this first operating room to initiate the newborn care and resuscitation following delivery as deemed necessary. The maternal perioperative management usually includes placement of either an epidural catheter or spinal for neuraxial administration of opioids (morphine), which is considered the gold standard to provide postoperative analgesia. Equipotent doses of epidural and intrathecal opioids have a ratio of 20–30 to one.[21] An intrathecal dose of preservative-free morphine, 0.1–0.2 mg is commonly administered. Alternatively, the placement of an epidural catheter before induction of anesthesia with administration of 2–4 mg of epidural morphine at the end of the procedure has also been described. A meta-analysis examining the analgesic efficacy of intrathecal morphine versus epidural morphine found no difference with a similar duration of action of 12–24 hours.[21] The preoperative placement of an epidural catheter has the benefits of analgesic optimization during emergence from anesthesia as supplemental doses of local anesthetics can be administered through the epidural catheter. Administration of supplemental doses of epidural opioids, particularly long-acting opioids, is associated with risk of respiratory depression especially if unintentionally administered in the subdural or subarachnoid space in a catheter that is in a suboptimal location.

Cross-matched blood for the mother and Type O Rh negative blood for the fetus must be immediately available before proceeding with the induction of anesthesia. It is important to recognize that fetal blood transfusion may become necessary during placental support or after umbilical cord cross clamping. Therefore, blood for the fetus and appropriate blood transfusion equipment must be available not just in the operating room where the EXIT is performed, but the blood should also be transported to the adjacent operating room if the fetus has to be transferred to this room for further surgical care. The primary anesthetic is usually general anesthesia considering the goal of profound uterine relaxation and preservation of the uterine placental flow. During the induction of general anesthesia for an EXIT procedure, it is imperative to provide left uterine displacement and appropriate preoxygenation time to maintain adequate uteroplacental perfusion and adequate oxygenation. Given the decreased functional residual capacity and increase in oxygen consumption observed in pregnancy, rapid desaturation may occur after apnea in these patients. A three-minute preoxygenation prevents this rapid desaturation following induction. Rapid sequence induction and endotracheal intubation is performed as this is routine for term pregnant patients to protect against aspiration. Additionally, to optimize the patient's position for intubation, a shoulder ramp, or padding of pillows/blankets must be utilized to place the patient in a sniffing position in which the external auricular meatus lies in the same horizontal plane as the sternal notch. Alternative plans for intubation must be considered with all necessary equipment readily available in case a difficult intubation is encountered. Familiarity with the difficult airway algorithm in the obstetric patient is of extreme importance during the induction for an EXIT procedure.[22,23]

Large-bore venous access must be secured to facilitate administration of fluids and transfusion of blood products if necessary. Invasive monitoring of the patient's hemodynamic status with the use of an arterial line, is crucial for evaluation and optimization of the uteroplacental flow. Medications to facilitate the management of the fetus during the case are prepared and handed over to the surgical technician involved in the case, in a sterile fashion, preferably before the start of the procedure.

Sterile equipment available on the surgical field specifically for the management of the fetus includes angiocatheters for venous access in the fetus; short intravenous catheter tubing for administration of fluids to the fetus; a variety of endotracheal tube sizes appropriate for age; a sterile, disposable stethoscope; 10cc syringes with 5% albumin × 2; 10cc syringes with Ringer's lactate × 2; syringes with atropine, vecuronium, and fentanyl combination for intramuscular injection prior to laryngoscopy or incision; pulse oximeter probes; and an ambu bag to ventilate the fetus after umbilical cord clamping. A pulse oximeter cable is inserted in a sterile sleeve from the head of the operating table so it can be connected to the pulse oximeter applied to the fetus' finger once access to the fetus has been obtained. This allows for monitoring of fetal oxygen saturation.

The second room is prepared for the newborn to continue the fetal surgical intervention, continue further newborn resuscitation, or for establishment of a more definitive and secure airway. A separate anesthesia and nursing team must be designated for the baby's operating room to provide neonatal care. Ideally, the newborn is carried in warm blankets to the second operating room with some form of an airway, either an endotracheal tube or a tracheostomy. The airway may, however, need to be further secured, or, in instances where a partial resection of a neck mass occurred to establish the airway, closure of an open wound may be necessary. The anesthesiologist designated to take care of the newborn must be prepared to receive a neonate in a critical condition, with a partially secured airway or who will require further resuscitation. Therefore, blood products must be immediately available. Confirmation of a secure airway and establishment of adequate venous access are the initial tasks to perform on the baby following arrival to the baby's operating room. The pediatric surgical team continues care of the newborn in this second room while the maternal-fetal medicine team stays with the mother to close the abdominal incision and finalize the maternal procedure.

Maintenance of anesthesia during the EXIT includes maintenance of physiologic maternal partial pressure of carbon dioxide ($PaCO_2$) during mechanical ventilation, with a $PaCO_2$ of around 30 mm Hg.

The goals of anesthesia during the EXIT procedure are similar to that of mid-gestation interventions as uteroplacental flow must be preserved in conjunction with uterine relaxation. One important difference between this procedure and that of mid-gestation procedures is that delivery of the baby occurs immediately after the intervention and administration of tocolytics such as magnesium sulfate is avoided as uterine tone is quickly reestablished. During the EXIT procedure, fluid management is more liberal than during second trimester open fetal surgery as there is no similar concern regarding the potential for pulmonary edema with concurrent administration of magnesium sulfate. Knowledge of the pharmacokinetics of medications administered with emphasis on the fetal:maternal concentration ratios is crucial during the EXIT procedure. The placental transfer of medications depends on the maternal:fetal gradient, maternal protein binding, degree of liposolubility, the molecular weight and degree of ionization of the substance.[24] Table 13.2 shows different fetal:maternal ratios of medications following maternal administration.

The use of general anesthesia with volatile anesthetics provides optimal conditions for the EXIT procedure as appropriate uterine relaxation is maintained with the advantage of easy titration. There is a dose-dependent effect of volatile anesthetics on the degree of uterine relaxation. Volatile anesthetics at 0.75 MAC have been associated with uterine atony. The administration of high concentrations of volatile anesthetics (≥ 2 MAC) provides more potent uterine relaxation and is typically required during the EXIT procedure. However, significant maternal vasodilation usually results in subsequent hypotension and a decrease in the uteroplacental perfusion, which can compromise the fetal acid-base status. Vasopressors such as phenylephrine and ephedrine are therefore routinely administered intraoperatively to preserve uteroplacental perfusion. The hemodynamic goal is to maintain the blood pressure within a range of 10–20% of preoperative values with a mean arterial pressure ≥ 65 mm Hg. Phenylephrine, administered by either bolus or continuous infusion, has been shown to be the vasopressor of choice as it crosses the placenta less and is associated with less fetal acidosis compared to ephedrine.[25,26] While volatile anesthetics are used in some centers as the sole agents during the EXIT procedure, some centers utilize

Table 13.2 Fetal:maternal ratios of medications commonly used during EXIT procedures

Medications	Fetal:maternal ratio
Halothane	0.7–0.9
Isoflurane	0.7
Nitrous oxide	0.83
Thiopental	0.4–1.1
Etomidate	0.5
Propofol	0.5–0.85
Ketamine	1.2
Diazepam	1–2
Midazolam	0.76
Morphine	0.61
Fentanyl	0.16–1.2
Remifentanil	0.29–0.88
Sufentanil	0.81
Ephedrine	0.7
Phenylephrine	0.17
Nitroglycerin	0.18
Vecuronium	0.06–0.11
Rocuronium	0.16
Glycopyrrolate	0.2
Atropine	0.93
Dexmedetomidine	0.12

Note that the high molecular weight and poor lipid solubility of nondepolarizing muscle relaxants limit the transfer to the fetus.[24]

a combination of volatile agents and intravenous anesthesia. A retrospective study examining the effects of 2.5 MAC of desflurane in comparison to total intravenous anesthesia with remifentanil and propofol and addition of 1.5 MAC desflurane at the time uterine relaxation is required (SIVA, supplemented intravenous anesthesia), found moderate to severe left ventricular systolic dysfunction with a higher incidence of fetal bradycardia in the group of patients that had prolonged exposure and increased MAC of desflurane with an incidence of 61% versus 26% in the SIVA group. Uterine relaxation was determined to be appropriate by manual palpation of the uterus by surgeons, at 1.5 MAC of desflurane, and less hemodynamic consequences to the fetus were observed, thereby decreasing the need for fetal intervention or resuscitation.[27] A further study in sheep by the same group showed better maternal hemodynamics and fetal acid-base status in the SIVA group compared to the high-dose volatile anesthetic group, with no difference in fetal myocardial function examined by echocardiography.[28] Alternative options to provide uterine relaxation during the EXIT procedure which have been described, include administration of nitroglycerin, a vasodilator, at a bolus dose of 50–100 mcg and continuous infusion at 0.5–1 mcg/kg/min up to 20 mcg/kg/min in patients receiving a combined spinal epidural technique.[29,30] Beta 2 agonists such as terbutaline can be used as coadjuvants to provide uterine relaxation. The challenge with the use of nitroglycerin is the inability to titrate it to effect, and the side effect of persistent hypotension and pulmonary edema.[31]

To provide fetal analgesia, preserve fetal hemodynamics, and obtain fetal muscle relaxation, a combination of medications including atropine (20 mcg/kg), fentanyl (5–20 mcg/kg), and vecuronium (0.2–0.4 mg/kg) is administered to the fetus via an intramuscular injection and is usually repeated every 45 minutes for the duration of the fetal intervention. The fetus also receives volatile anesthetics from the mother via the placenta; the fetus is sensitive to the effects of these volatile agents with a lower MAC requirement.[32] To prevent hypothermia, the fetal exposure to the environment must be limited as much as possible, and the room temperature must be maintained at high temperatures. Temperatures of approximately 80 degrees Farenheit are not uncommon for this procedure; infusion of warmed fluids into the uterus during the procedure also helps to preserve fetal temperature. Despite these measures, the baby will still be relatively hypothermic after delivery and extra measures should be taken to warm the baby either when handed off to the neonatology team after the airway has been secured (EXIT-to-airway), or on arrival to the baby's operating room in the scenario where additional surgery is required. Keeping the baby's operating room also at a high temperature, use of radiant heat lamps at initial arrival in baby's room, taking time to wipe off some of the vernix with warmed wet cloths, wrapping the extremities with padding, covering the baby's head with a cap or wrapping in a warm blanket, placing the baby on a Bair Hugger, and utilization of a heat exchange moisturizer, are ways to minimize heat loss in the baby. Even if the airway has been secured in the scenario of an EXIT-to-airway procedure, ventilation of the baby's lungs while on uteroplacental bypass is still avoided, as ventilation can potentially induce changes from the fetal circulation to that of a neonate and compromise the benefit of uteroplacental bypass.

Fetal monitoring during the EXIT procedure includes the use of fetal pulse oximetry and echocardiography to evaluate fetal heart rate, contractility, and volume status. Normal values of fetal pulse oximetry range from 50% to 70%, with a normal fetal PaO_2 of 40 mm Hg. Fetal heart rate monitoring with the use of a fetal scalp monitor has also been described during EXIT procedures,[33] although this is not routinely used. Another parameter for evaluation of the fetus in conjunction with echocardiography, is the umbilical cord flow. The absence or reversal of diastolic flow in the umbilical arteries is associated with fetal distress and worse outcomes.[34] If fetal distress is detected during an EXIT procedure as evidenced by fetal bradycardia or fetal desaturation, a sequence of interventions must be rapidly implemented and the cause quickly determined. Fetal resuscitation must be initiated and this includes preservation of uterine placental flow by increasing the maternal blood pressure to 15–25% of baseline, appropriate maternal positioning to avoid aortocaval compression, confirmation of adequate uterine relaxation by the surgeons, detection and management of umbilical cord compression and/or maternal hemorrhage. An abrupted placenta must be ruled out. Correction of existing maternal hypothermia if present, administration of intramuscular or intravenous epinephrine to the fetus at doses of 1–

10 mcg/kg, and the need for administration of intravenous fluid boluses or O negative irradiated packed red blood cells (PRBCs) cross matched to mother, should all be considered. The necessity of fluid or blood administration can easily be determined by a quick assessment of the volume status of the fetal heart by the cardiologist performing the fetal echocardiography during the procedure. Emergent delivery with subsequent neonatal resuscitation must occur for persistent fetal distress. If fetal blood transfusion is required, careful consideration must be given to the volume of PRBCs administered to the fetus. The estimated blood volume of a baby is 110 mL/kg, 100 mL/kg, and 90 mL/kg in a mid-gestation fetus, preterm, and full term baby, respectively. For a more precise calculation of the fetal blood volume, the following formula based on gestational age has been developed:[35]

$$\text{Estimated fetal blood volume} = 11.2 \times \text{gestational age} - 209.4$$

After the umbilical cord is clamped at the end of the EXIT procedure, there is a risk of uterine atony because of the prolonged period of uterine relaxation required during the case. Uterine atony is a leading cause of maternal mortality. Given that approximately 10% of the maternal cardiac output supports uteroplacental perfusion, the blood loss during uterine atony can be considerable. Therefore, the concentration of inhaled anesthetics should be rapidly decreased once the fetal procedure has been completed and immediately before the umbilical cord is clamped. Uterotonic medications such as oxytocin must also be administered promptly. The administration of intramuscular prostaglandin F2 alpha (hemabate) 0.25 mg, methergine 0.2 mg, as well as PRBCs must be considered if persistent atony occurs despite the administration of oxytocin. In cases of massive obstetric hemorrhage, additional help must be called for immediately, large-bore venous access must be secured to facilitate the resuscitation, and the use of a rapid infuser for the transfusion of blood products must be established. The activation of a massive transfusion protocol must occur with an expected ratio of transfusion of 1:1 of PRBCs to fresh frozen plasma (FFP) with the administration of one unit of platelets for each 4–6 units of PRBCs. Cryoprecipitate must be administered if fibrinogen is < 100 mg/dL and factor VIIa must be given if bleeding persists in this scenario.

Complete reversal of neuromuscular blockade and awake extubation should be considered with confirmation of adequate analgesia upon extubation.

Surgical Steps of the EXIT Procedure

With effective uterine relaxation allowing for a prolonged period of fetoplacental support, a safe EXIT procedure can occur. Prior to administration of anesthesia, the patient is appropriately padded and placed in a supine position with a leftward displacement of the uterus. Sequential compression devices are also placed on both lower legs. The room is warmed appropriately to maintain adequate temperatures for the fetus during the potential prolonged exposure of the EXIT procedure. General anesthesia is commenced as detailed above, and prophylactic antibiotics are provided.

A low transverse (Pfannenstiel) incision is made large enough to allow for adequate control of the uterus during hysterotomy. Dissection is performed down to the fascia, which is then opened in a transverse fashion. The fascia is then dissected free from the underlying rectus abdominus muscle up to the level of the umbilicus superiorly and down to the level of the pyramidalis muscles inferiorly. The rectus abdominus muscle is split in the midline and the peritoneal cavity is accessed. If necessary, a bladder flap is created, giving more access to the lower uterine segment. At this time, the uterine tone is assessed via palpation. If the tone is adequately relaxed, then the placenta is mapped using intraoperative ultrasound to select a site for the hysterotomy which should be at least 5 cm away from the placental edge. If the site for hysterotomy is too close to the placenta, it can potentially lead to an abruption, increase the risk of significant maternal hemorrhage and greatly decrease the length of time that fetoplacental circulation can be maintained. A hysterotomy in the lower uterine segment is preferred; however, given the location of the placenta and that of the head of the fetus, a lower uterine segment hysterotomy may not be possible. In this situation, a fundal or posterior hysterotomy must be utilized. Once the hysterotomy site has been selected, the fetus is positioned away from this site. Under ultrasound guidance, a series of full-thickness, interrupted 2–0 PDS sutures are placed and tied down in a box formation. The amniotic cavity is then entered within the box allowing for enough room for a stapler. A vicryl stapler (US Surgical Corporation, Norwalk, CT, USA) or a GIA stapler (Medtronic, Minneapolis, MN, USA) is then inserted into the amniotic cavity, the position of the umbilical cord and fetus are confirmed clear of the stapler, and the hysterotomy is created (Figure 13.1). Additional firings of the stapler are necessary to allow for a hysterotomy large enough to allow for delivery of the fetal head, neck, upper torso (keeping the umbilical cord inside the uterine environment), and right arm. This hysterotomy should also be large enough to allow for delivery of a sacrococcygeal teratoma if resection is indicated, or for delivery of the portion of the conjoined twins that will serve as the site of separation. Prior to the partial delivery of the fetus, anchoring stitches using 2–0 PDS are placed at both staple line vertices to secure the staple line. The whole fetus is not delivered to allow for continued infusion of warmed Ringer's lactate solution via a rapid infusion device (Sims Level 1, Inc, Rockland, MA, USA) into the uterus; this provides an environment that protects the umbilical cord from compression and also prevents a premature separation of the placenta from the uterine wall.

At this time of partial delivery of the fetus, additional anesthesia is administered to the fetus in the form of an intramuscular injection of fentanyl, vecuronium, and atropine (as detailed above). A pulse oximeter is then placed on the right hand to allow for continuous monitoring of fetal oxygen saturation and heart rate, and fetal echocardiography is

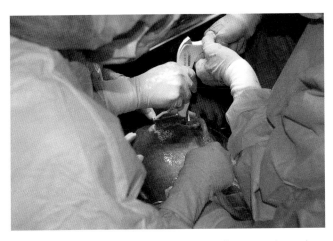

Figure 13.1 Making the hysterotomy during an EXIT procedure. This image shows the second firing of an absorbable stapler device for creation of the hysterotomy. This technique allows for appropriate hemostasis and securing the intrauterine membranes.
Photo courtesy of James Fisher, MD.

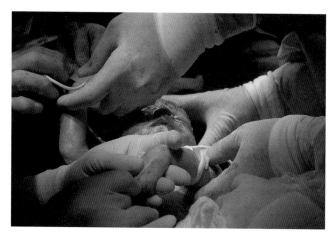

Figure 13.2 Fetal monitoring and intravenous access. The process of applying a pulse oximeter for fetal monitoring and securing peripheral intravenous access during an EXIT procedure are demonstrated in this image. Photo courtesy of James Fisher, MD.

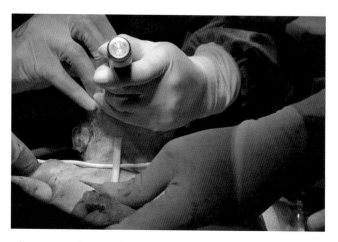

Figure 13.3 Direct laryngoscopy for intubation and securing the fetal airway. A first attempt to secure the fetal airway proceeds with direct laryngoscopy and endotracheal tube placement. Photo courtesy of James Fisher, MD.

performed. The pulse oximeter may need to be covered with a piece of foil together with a sterile towel to prevent light interference with the reading. A fetal peripheral intravenous cannula is also inserted (Figure 13.2). Once these measures for the fetus have been completed, the next steps allow for the airway of the fetus to be secured (Figure 13.3). This may be achieved by either direct laryngoscopy followed by intubation, rigid bronchoscopy with a preloaded endotracheal tube for intubation over the bronchoscope, retrograde intubation via cervical trachea access with a guide wire directed proximally through the vocal cords and mouth allowing for passage of an endotracheal tube along the wire, or tracheostomy if the aforementioned three methods are unsuccessful. Once intubation has occurred, endotracheal tube placement is confirmed by observation of chest rise, auscultation, and positive detection of end-tidal carbon dioxide. The endotracheal tube is then secured to the neonate's gums with sutures. If the fetal airway cannot be secured, then resection or partial resection of the extrinsic neck mass (in the case of EXIT-to-airway for airway obstruction), is performed to facilitate intubation or tracheostomy. If the airway cannot be secured in spite of this, then cannulation of the fetus for ECMO will likely be necessary. In the setting of CHAOS caused by a laryngeal or tracheal membrane, attempts will be made to perforate the membrane (if possible) to allow for insertion of the endotracheal tube into the trachea or a tracheostomy will be performed.

If an EXIT-to-resection is being performed, then the resection can proceed after the airway is secured. For example, a large CPAM can be resected via thoracotomy after intubation. The resection does not need to be completed while the baby is on fetoplacental support. The thoracotomy is made immediately after intubation to allow for decompression while on fetoplacental support, and this is followed by resection of the mass in the second operating room which has been prepared in advance for the baby's operation.

Regardless of the indication of the EXIT procedure, umbilical artery and venous catheters are placed prior to clamping and division of the umbilical cord. During the placement of these catheters, detailed communication is necessary between the surgery and anesthesia teams to allow for reduction of the inhalational anesthetic and prompt administration of maternal intravenous oxytocin. This will prevent uterine atony and subsequent maternal hemorrhage upon clamping and dividing the umbilical cord and delivery of the neonate. Following delivery, the neonate is wrapped in sterile towels and quickly transported to the adjacent operating room, for additional resuscitation or further operative procedures, as indicated. The neonate is then transported to the neonatal intensive care unit once those additional measures are completed. While the neonate is being attended to in the other room, the uterus is allowed to contract with spontaneous expulsion of the placenta. If prolonged uterine atony occurs, then medications such as hemabate and methergine are administered. If significant blood loss has occurred, transfusion of blood products should be considered. Depending on the severity of blood loss, the massive transfusion protocol may be indicated. If hemorrhage persists despite administration of uterotonic medications and correction of platelet and coagulation factor derangements, then balloon tamponade may become necessary. If bleeding cannot be controlled, then hysterectomy is indicated.

Once uterine tone is appropriate and adequate hemostasis has been achieved, the staple lines are excised and the hysterotomy is closed in layers. The peritoneum is approximated together along with the rectus abdominus muscles. The fascia is closed in a running fashion, the dermal space is approximated, and the skin is closed in a running subcuticular fashion.[36]

Outcomes

Outcomes of neonatal morbidity and mortality for EXIT procedures are not well established in the literature. However, there are multiple case series reported for cervical lesions (teratomas and lymphovascular malformations) detailing the success rates for securing the neonatal airway. In these series of identified high-risk fetuses, the success rates for intubation or tracheostomy are greater than 90%.[36–38] Additionally, the outcomes following EXIT-to-ECMO for CDH have been studied and these indicate that the neonates that underwent EXIT-to-ECMO had no improvement in morbidity or mortality compared to historical controls that did not utilize fetoplacental circulation while being cannulated.[10,11]

Despite the paucity of data for neonatal outcomes after an EXIT procedure, the utility of the EXIT procedure is still preserved because the lack of such an operation for these patients would almost certainly lead to their demise at birth.

Maternal outcomes following the EXIT procedure have also not been well established. There is a report from Noah et al.[39] describing the early experience at the University of California, San Francisco (UCSF) detailing early morbidity following an EXIT procedure. This report found a higher rate of maternal wound complications (15% vs 2%) and higher blood loss (1,104 mL vs 883 mL) in patients that underwent the EXIT procedure compared to those who underwent a standard cesarean section. This report did not detail any long-term complications such as uterine dehiscence, uterine rupture, or changes in fecundity. Zamora et al.[40] attempted to answer some of the questions regarding long-term maternal morbidity following an EXIT procedure. A questionnaire was sent out to women who underwent fetal surgery or an EXIT procedure with an 82% response rate. Of those responding, 21 had undergone an EXIT procedure. All women who attempted to become pregnant afterwards, were able to do so (13/13). The mean time to pregnancy after the EXIT procedure was 2.5 years with 11/13 conceiving spontaneously. Uterine dehiscence occurred in 1/13 of these pregnancies. Overall, the maternal morbidity, both short-term and long-term, appears to be acceptable based upon this study.

Conclusion

The identification of fetuses that will benefit from an EXIT procedure is continually improving. To provide the best outcomes for these patients, the EXIT procedure must be well coordinated by an experienced multidisciplinary team. Excellent communication and extreme attention to detail are of necessity during the surgical portion of the EXIT procedure. However, the maximum benefit and success of an EXIT procedure relies heavily on the appropriate level of uterine relaxation and maintenance of this state of relaxation until the umbilical cord is clamped. Although outcome data are limited, the EXIT procedure is viewed as a mandatory tool for neonatal survival in select cases, and will likely continue to be utilized as such in these specific cases.

References

1. Mychaliska GB, Bealer JF, Graf JL, et al. Operating on placental support: the ex utero intrapartum treatment procedure. *J Pediatr Surg.* 1997;32(2):227–230.

2. Norris MC, Joseph J, Leighton BL. Anesthesia for perinatal surgery. *Am J Perinatol.* 1989;6(1):39–40.

3. Schwartz MZ, Silver H, Schulman S. Maintenance of the placental circulation to evaluate and treat an infant with massive head and neck hemangioma. *J Pediatr Surg.* 1993;28(4):520–522.

4. Lazar DA, Cassady CI, Olutoye OO, et al. Tracheoesophageal displacement index and predictors of airway obstruction for fetuses with neck masses. *J Pediatr Surg.* 2012;47(1):46–50.

5. Mong A, Johnson AM, Kramer SS, et al. Congenital high airway obstruction syndrome: MR/US findings, effect on management, and outcome. *Pediatr Radiol.* 2008;38(11):1171–1179.

6. Saadai P, Jelin EB, Nijagal A, et al. Long-term outcomes after fetal therapy for congenital high airway obstructive syndrome. *J Pediatr Surg.* 2012;47(6):1095–1100.

7. Hedrick HL, Flake AW, Crombleholme TM, et al. The ex utero intrapartum therapy procedure for high-risk fetal lung lesions. *J Pediatr Surg.* 2005;40(6):1038–1043.

8. Cass DL, Olutoye OO, Cassady CI, et al. EXIT-to-resection for foetuses with large lung masses and persistent mediastinal compression near birth. *J Pediatr Surg.* 2013;**48**(1):138–144.

9. Kunisaki SM, Barnewolt CE, Estroff JA, et al. Ex utero intrapartum treatment with extracorporeal membrane oxygenation for severe congenital diaphragmatic hernia. *J Pediatr Surg.* 2007;**42**(1):98–104.

10. Stoffan AP, Wilson JM, Jennings RW, et al. Does the ex utero intrapartum treatment to extracorporeal membrane oxygenation procedure change outcomes for high-risk patients with congenital diaphragmatic hernia? *J Pediatr Surg.* 2012;**47**(6):1053–1057.

11. Shieh HF, Wilson JM, Sheils CA, et al. Does the ex utero intrapartum treatment to extracorporeal membrane oxygenation procedure change morbidity outcomes for high-risk congenital diaphragmatic hernia survivors? *J Pediatr Surg.* 2017;**52**(1):22–25.

12. Mackenzie TC, Crombleholme TM, Johnson MP, et al. The natural history of prenatally diagnosed conjoined twins. *J Pediatr Surg.* 2002;**37**(3):303–309.

13. Golombeck K, Ball RH, Lee H, et al. Maternal morbidity after maternal-fetal surgery. *Am J Obstet Gynecol.* 2006;**194**(3):834–839.

14. American College of Obstetricians and Gynecologists, Committee on Ethics; American Academy of Pediatrics, Committee on Bioethics. Maternal-fetal intervention and fetal care centers. *Pediatrics.* 2011;**128**(2):e473–478.

15. Gaiser R. Physiologic changes of pregnancy. In: Chestnut DH, ed. *Chestnut's Obstetric Anesthesia: Principles and Practice.* Elsevier Saunders, 2014;15–38.

16. Ueyama H, Hagihira S, Takashina M, et al. Pregnancy does not enhance volatile anesthetic sensitivity on the brain: an electroencephalographic analysis study. *Anesthesiology.* 2010;**113**(3):577–584.

17. Flood P, Rollins MD. Anesthesia for obstetrics. In: Miller RD, ed. *Miller's Anesthesia.* Saunders, 2015; 2328–2358.

18. Munnur U, de Boisblanc B, Suresh MS. Airway problems in pregnancy. *Crit Care Med.* 2005;**33**(10 Suppl):S259–268.

19. Kinsella SM, Lohmann G. Supine hypotensive syndrome. *Obstet Gynecol.* 1994;**83**(5 Pt 1):774–788.

20. Marwan A, Crombleholme TM. The EXIT procedure: principles, pitfalls, and progress. *Semin Pediatr Surg.* 2006;**15**(2):107–115.

21. Ng K, Parsons J, Cyna AM, et al. Spinal versus epidural anaesthesia for caesarean section. *Cochrane Database Syst Rev.* 2004;(**2**):CD003765.

22. Apfelbaum JL, Hagberg CA, Caplan RA, et al. Practice guidelines for management of the difficult airway: an updated report by the American Society of Anesthesiologists Task Force on Management of the Difficult Airway. *Anesthesiology.* 2013;**118**(2):251–270.

23. Balki M, Cooke ME, Dunington S, et al. Unanticipated difficult airway in obstetric patients: development of a new algorithm for formative assessment in high-fidelity simulation. *Anesthesiology.* 2012;**117**(4):883–897.

24. Zakowski MI, Geller A. The placenta: anatomy, physiology and transfer of drugs. In: Chestnut DH, ed. *Chestnut's Obstetric Anesthesia: Principles and Practice.* Elsevier Saunders, 2014;55–74.

25. Ngan Kee WD, Khaw KS, Ng FF. Comparison of phenylephrine infusion regimens for maintaining maternal blood pressure during spinal anaesthesia for Caesarean section. *Br J Anaesth.* 2004;**92**(4):469–474.

26. Ngan Kee WD, Lee A, Khaw KS, et al. A randomized double-blinded comparison of phenylephrine and ephedrine infusion combinations to maintain blood pressure during spinal anesthesia for cesarean delivery: the effects on fetal acid-base status and hemodynamic control. *Anesth Analg.* 2008;**107**(4):1295–1302.

27. Boat A, Mahmoud M, Michelfelder EC, et al. Supplementing desflurane with intravenous anesthesia reduces fetal cardiac dysfunction during open fetal surgery. *Paediatr Anaesth.* 2010;**20**(8):748–756.

28. Ngamprasertwong P, Michelfelder EC, Arbabi S, et al. Anesthetic techniques for fetal surgery: effects of maternal anesthesia on intraoperative fetal outcomes in a sheep model. *Anesthesiology.* 2013;**118**(4):796–808.

29. George RB, Melnick AH, Rose EC, et al. Case series: Combined spinal epidural anesthesia for Cesarean delivery and ex utero intrapartum treatment procedure. *Can J Anaesth.* 2007;**54**(3):218–222.

30. Clark KD, Viscomi CM, Lowell J, et al. Nitroglycerin for relaxation to establish a fetal airway (EXIT procedure). *Obstet Gynecol.* 2004;**103**(5 Pt 2):1113–1115.

31. El-Sayed Y, Riley E, Holbrook H, Cohen S, et al. Randomized comparison of intravenous nitroglycerin and magnesium sulfate for treatment of preterm labor. *Obstet Gynecol.* 1999;**93**(1):79–83.

32. Brusseau R, Mizrahi-Arnaud A. Fetal anesthesia and pain management for intrauterine therapy. *Clin Perinatol.* 2013;**40**(3):429–442.

33. Kaneko M, Tokunaga S, Mukai M, et al. Application of a fetal scalp electrode for continuous fetal heart rate monitoring during an ex utero intrapartum treatment. *J Pediatr Surg.* 2011;**46**(2):e37–40.

34. Müller T, Nanan R, Rehn M, et. al. Arterial and ductus venosus Doppler in fetuses with absent or reverse end-diastolic flow in the umbilical artery: longitudinal analysis. *Fetal Diagn Ther.* 2003;**18**(3):163–169.

35. Smith GC, Cameron AD. Estimating human fetal blood volume on the basis of gestational age and fetal abdominal circumference. *BJOG.* 2002;**109**(6):721–722.

36. Lazar DA, Olutoye OO, Moise KJ, et al. Ex-utero intrapartum treatment procedure for giant neck masses – fetal and maternal outcomes. *J Pediatr Surg.* 2011;**46**(5):817–822.

37. Laje P, Johnson MP, Howell LJ, et al. Ex utero intrapartum treatment in the management of giant cervical teratomas. *J Pediatr Surg.* 2012;**47**(6):1208–1216.

38. Laje P, Howell LJ, Johnson MP, et al. Perinatal management of congenital oropharyngeal tumors: the ex utero intrapartum treatment (EXIT) approach. *J Pediatr Surg.* 2013;**48**(10):2005–2010.

39. Noah MM, Norton ME, Sandberg P, et al. Short-term maternal outcomes that are associated with the EXIT procedure, as compared with caesarean delivery. *Am J Obstet Gynecol.* 2002;**186**(4):773–777.

40. Zamora IJ, Ethun CG, Evans LM, et al. Maternal morbidity and reproductive outcomes related to fetal surgery. *J Pediatr Surg.* 2013;**48**(5):951–955.

Index

alloimmunization, 64, 65
amniotic fluid, 26
anesthesia
  EXIT procedure, 181–182,
    193–200
  and fetal brain development,
    29–30
  fetal cardiac intervention,
    111–113
  fetal endoscopic tracheal
    occlusion (FETO)
    procedure, 97–98
  for fetal intrauterine
    transfusion, 72
  lung masses, congenital, 159
  for maternal intrauterine
    transfusion, 70–71
  multidisciplinary approach
    to maternal-fetal surgery,
    48–49
  myelomeningocele (MMC)
    surgical management,
    147–150
  open fetal surgery, 159–161,
    178–181
  selective fetoscopic laser
    photocoagulation (SFLP),
    91, 92
anesthesia, sacrococcygeal
    teratoma (SCT)
  background, 175–176
  early delivery with
    immediate debulking/
    resection, 182–186
  EXIT procedure, 181–182
  minimally invasive fetal
    therapy, 176–178
  open fetal surgery, 178–181
antenatal fetal
    surveillance (AFS)
  biophysical profile (BPP),
    127–128
  contraction stress test (CST),
    126–127
  Doppler evaluation of
    umbilical artery, 129–130
  and fetal blood sampling
    (FBS), 119
  during fetal surgery, 130–132

indications for, 119–120
  maternal-fetal movement
    assessment, 120
  modified biophysical profile
    (BPP), 128–129
  nonstress test (NST), 126
  objective of, 119

biophysical profile (BPP)
  for fetal surveillance,
    127–128
  modified, 128–129
blood pressure during
    pregnancy, 3
blood volume during
    pregnancy, 7
bronchial atresia (BA), 155
bronchogenic cysts (BC),
    154–155
bronchopulmonary
    sequestration (BPS), 154

cardiac output during
    pregnancy, 2
cardiovascular system during
    pregnancy
  anatomic changes, 1
  blood pressure, 3
  cardiac output, 2
  heart rate, 2
  hemodynamic changes, 2
  hemodynamic changes
    during labor, 3–4
  pulmonary vascular
    resistance, 3
  stroke volume, 2–3
  systemic vascular resistance
    (SVR), 3
cardiovascular system, fetal,
    22–26
central nervous system during
    pregnancy, 7
cesarean section, 58–60
Cincinnati staging system, 85
circulation system, fetal, 24
coagulation during pregnancy
    (blood), 8
communication in maternal-
    fetal surgery, 60

congenital cystic adenomatoid
    malformation (CCAM),
    153–154
congenital diaphragmatic
    hernia (CDH), 95–97
congenital high airway
    obstruction syndrome
    (CHAOS), 155–156
congenital lobar emphysema
    (CLE), 155
consent in maternal-fetal
    ethics, 39
contraction stress test (CST),
    126–127
critical titer, 67

endocrine system during
    pregnancy, 10–11
ethics in maternal-fetal surgery
  1982 conference on, 37
  consent, 39
  examples, 41–44
  fetal status paradigms, 39–40
  fetal therapy board, 37–39
  institutional review board
    standards, 60
  twins, 41
  work-up, 40–41
ethnicity and prevalence
    of Rh (D)negative blood
    type, 65
ex-utero intrapartum
    treatment. see EXIT
    procedure
EXIT procedure
  anesthesia for, 22, 193–200
  congenital lung masses,
    162, 193
  defined, 191
  history of, 191
  indications for, 192
  outcomes, 200–203
  procedure, 55–57
  sacrococcygeal teratoma
    (SCT) anesthesia, 181–182
  surgical steps, 200–203

fetal access sites
  free loop of cord, 72–73

fetal access sites (cont.)
intracardiac transfusion, 73
intraperitoneal transfusion
(IPT), 73
placental cord insertion, 72
fetal cardiac disease
extracardiac anomalies,
105–106
genetic conditions, 106
prevalence of, 103
fetal cardiac intervention
anesthesia for, 111–113
complications, 111
fetal echocardiography,
103–105
popularity of, 103
fetal cardiac intervention
categories
aortic valvuloplasty, 107–108
catheter-based fetal cardiac
intervention, 106–107
generalities, 106
fetal cardiac intervention
surgical approaches
catheter-based, 108–109
pulmonary atresia with
intact intraventricular
septum (PA/IVS), 111
pulmonary
valvuloplasty, 111
restrictive septum, 108–110
stent placement, 110
fetal endoscopic tracheal
occlusion (FETO)
complications, 100
history of, 97
fetal endoscopic tracheal
occlusion (FETO)
indications
congenital diaphragmatic
hernia (CDH), 95–96
severe pulmonary hypoplasia
from ePPROM, 96
fetal endoscopic tracheal
occlusion (FETO)
procedure
maternal and fetal
anesthesia, 97–98
mother remaining close
distance for, 60
postoperative
considerations, 98–99
preoperative
considerations, 97
tracheal occlusion balloon
insertion, 98

tracheal occlusion reversal,
99–100
fetal growth retardation (FGR),
129–130
fetal intervention phases
prenatal assessment, 53
preoperative preparation,
53–54
surgical intervention, 54–60
fetal intervention types, 59
fetal operating room nurse, 51
fetal pain, 27–30
fetal physiology
effects of drugs on, 21–22
environment, 17
placenta, 17–20
uteroplacental blood flow,
20–21
fetal physiology by system
amniotic fluid, 26
blood pressure, 24
blood volume, 24
cardiac development, 22–24
cardiovascular system, 22–26
circulation, 24
pulmonary, 24–26
renal system, 26
fetal therapy center, 45–46
fetal therapy nurse
coordinator, 50
fetal therapy review
board
composition of, 38–39
examples, 41–44
necessity of, 37–38
fetal thoracotomy, 161–162
fetoscopic surgery, 60
follow-up, maternal-fetal
surgery, 61

gallbladder changes during
pregnancy, 10
gastrointestinal system during
pregnancy
changes, 8–10
gallbladder, 10
liver, 10
genetics, 48

heart rate during pregnancy, 2
hematologic system
blood volume, 7
coagulation, 8
platelets, 8
red blood cells, 7
white blood cells, 8

hemodynamic changes during
labor, 3–4
hemodynamic changes during
pregnancy, 2
hemolytic disease of the fetus
and newborn (HDFN)
epidemiology, 64
etiology, 64
history of, 64
hypothyroidism, 10–11

intraperitoneal transfusion
(IPT), 73
intrauterine transfusion in
maternal-fetal surgery
epidemiology, 64
etiology, 64, 65
history of, 64
outcomes, 77
patient selection criteria,
65–66
intrauterine transfusion in
maternal-fetal surgery
anesthesia
fetal, 72
maternal, 70–71
intrauterine transfusion in
maternal-fetal surgery
complications
long-term, 76–77
procedural, 76
intrauterine transfusion in
maternal-fetal surgery
pre-procedure
blood preparation, 70
maternal preparation, 70
setting and staff, 69–70
timing, 69
intrauterine transfusion in
maternal-fetal surgery
procedure
fetal access site, 72–73
subsequent procedure
timing, 75–76
technique, 74–75
volume to transfuse,
73–74

liver changes during
pregnancy, 10
lung embryology, 153
lung masses, congenital
anesthesia for, 159
bronchial atresia (BA), 155
bronchogenic cysts (BC),
154–155

bronchopulmonary sequestration (BPS), 154
congenital cystic adenomatoid malformation (CCAM), 153–154
congenital high airway obstruction syndrome (CHAOS), 155–156
congenital lobar emphysema (CLE), 155
defined, 152
diagnosis, 156
EXIT procedure, 162–163
fetal thoracotomy, 161–162
incidence of, 152–153
open fetal surgery, 159–161
postnatal treatment, 163
prognosis, 156–157
treatment, 158–159
lung mechanics during pregnancy, 4–5

maternal-fetal medicine specialists (MFM), 48
maternal-fetal surgery
antenatal fetal surveillance (AFS), 119–132
congenital lung masses, 152–163
ethical considerations, 37–44
EXIT procedure, 191–204
fetal cardiac intervention, 103–113
fetal endoscopic tracheal occlusion (FETO) procedure, 95–100
intrauterine transfusion, 64–77
multidisciplinary approach to, 45–54
myelomeningocele (MMC), 137–150
phases of fetal intervention, 52–60
sacrococcygeal teratoma (SCT), 168–187
twin anemia polycythemia sequence (TAPS), 89–90
twin-twin transfusion syndrome (TTTS), 83–89
maternal-fetal surgery, day of
communication, 60
ethical oversight, 60
follow-up, 61
operating room, 61

preparation for, 54–60
simulation, 60–61
minimally invasive fetal therapy, 171–173, 176–178
multidisciplinary approach to maternal-fetal surgery
anesthesia, 48–49
cardiology, 49–50
clinical team, 46–47
fetal therapy center, 45–46
genetics, 48
imaging, 47
maternal fetal medicine specialists (MFM), 48
neonatology, 50
nursing, 50–52
obstetrics, 48
psychosocial services, 52
surgeons, 47
musculoskeletal system during pregnancy, 11
myelomeningocele (MMC)
defined, 137
diagnosis, 138–140
etiology, 138
incidence of, 137
pathophysiology of, 140–141
in-utero repair of, 137–138
myelomeningocele (MMC) surgical management
anesthesia for, 147–150
indications for, 141
post-surgery, 150
procedure, 142–147
ultrasound to assess motor function, 142

neonatal ICU nurse, 52
neonatal surgical advance practice nurse, 51–52
neurologic system during pregnancy
anatomic changes, 6
central nervous system, 7
nonstress test (NST)
accelerations, 122–123
baseline, 121, 122
categories, 121
contraction stress test (CST), 126–127
decelerations, 123–124
intrapartum fetal monitoring, 124–126
prevalence of, 121
sinusoidal pattern, 124–125

vibroacoustic stimulation, 121
nursing for maternal-fetal surgery
fetal operating room nurse, 51
fetal therapy nurse coordinator, 50
neonatal ICU nurse, 52
neonatal surgical advance practice nurse, 51–52
obstetric nurse, 51
perinatal advance practice nurse, 50–51

obstetric nurse, 51
open fetal surgery
anesthesia for, 159–161, 178–181
background, 159–161
post-surgery, 58
for sacrococcygeal teratoma (SCT), 173–174
operating room, maternal-fetal surgery, 61

pain, fetal, 27–30
perinatal advance practice nurse, 50–51
pharmacology, effect on fetus, 21–22
placenta
anatomy of, 18
at delivery, 19–20
functions of, 17–18
pathophysiology of during pregnancy, 18–19
placenta accreta spectrum, 19–20
platelets during pregnancy, 8
pregnancy
cardiovascular system, 1–4
endocrine system, 10–11
gastrointestinal system, 8–10
hematologic system, 7
musculoskeletal system, 11
neurologic system, 6–7
renal system, 10
respiratory system, 4
preterm premature rupture of membranes (ePPROM), 96
psychosocial services, 52
pulmonary system, fetal, 24–26
pulmonary vascular resistance during pregnancy, 3

Quintero staging system, 84–85

red blood cells during
   pregnancy, 7
renal system during
   pregnancy, 10
renal system, fetal, 26
respiratory system during
   pregnancy
   anatomic changes, 4
   factors affecting obstetric
      airway, 4
   gas exchange, 6
   lung mechanics, 4–5

sacrococcygeal teratoma (SCT)
   classification, 168
   defined, 168
   fetal and maternal
      complications, 169
   management options,
      168–169
sacrococcygeal teratoma (SCT)
   anesthesia
   background, 175–176
   early delivery with
      immediate debulking/
      resection, 182–186
   EXIT procedure, 181–182
   minimally invasive fetal
      therapy, 176–178
   open fetal surgery, 178–181
sacrococcygeal teratoma (SCT)
   prenatal assessment
   echocardiography, 170–171

magnetic resonance imaging
   (MRI), 171
ultrasound, 170
sacrococcygeal teratoma (SCT)
   treatment options
   early delivery, 174–175
   minimally invasive fetal
      therapy, 171–173
   open fetal surgery, 173–174
selective fetoscopic laser
   photocoagulation (SFLP)
   anesthesia for, 91
   complications, 93
   local anesthesia versus
      sedation, 92
   most popular approach, 88
   selective coagulation, 88–89
   ultrasound guidance of, 88
simulation, maternal-fetal
   surgery, 60–61
stroke volume during
   pregnancy, 2–3
surgical intervention steps
   cesarean section to
      immediate neonatal
      resection, 58–60
   clinical team
      requirements, 56
   day of, 54
   fetoscopic and ultrasound
      procedures, 58
   fetoscopic surgery, 60
   intraoperative phase, 55
   open and EXIT procedures,
      55–57

open fetal surgery, 58
postoperative, 58–60
preoperative preparation,
   54–55
systemic vascular resistance
   (SVR) during pregnancy, 3

thrombocytopenia, 8
tracheal occlusion balloon
   insertion, 98
   reversal, 99–100
twin anemia polycythemia
   sequence (TAPS), 89–90.
   see also twin-twin
   transfusion syndrome
twin-twin transfusion
   syndrome (TTTS). see also
   twin anemia polycythemia
   sequence
   etiology of, 83–84
   management, 87–89
   pathophysiology
      of, 83–84
   screening for, 84
   staging systems for, 84–87
twin-twin transfusion
   syndrome (TTTS)
   anesthesia
   intraoperative
      management, 92
   preoperative considerations,
      90–92

white blood cells during
   pregnancy, 8

Endorsed by:

N. Scott Adzick, MD
Surgeon-in-Chief, Children's Hospital of Philadelphia
C. Everett Koop Professor of Pediatric Surgery,
Perelman School of Medicine at the University of Pennsylvania
Founder and Director of the Richard D. Wood Jr. Center for Fetal Diagnosis
and Treatment